Full View of Yangtze River Pharmaceuticals Group (Taizhou, Jiangsu, China)

扬子江药业集团全景（中国·江苏·泰州）

A Newly Compiled
Practical English-Chinese Library
of Traditional Chinese Medicine
（英汉对照）新编实用中医文库

General Compiler-in-Chief Zuo Yanfu
总主编　左言富

Translators-in-Chief
Zhu Zhongbao Huang Yuezhong Tao Jinwen Li Zhaoguo
总编译　朱忠宝　黄月中　陶锦文　李照国（执行）

Compiled by Nanjing University of
Traditional Chinese Medicine
Translated by Shanghai University
of Traditional Chinese Medicine
南京中医药大学　主编
上海中医药大学　主译

GYNECOLOGY OF TRADITIONAL CHINESE MEDICINE

中医妇科学

Compiler-in-Chief	Tan Yong
Vice-compilers-in-Chief	He Guixiang
Translators-in-Chief	Li Zhaoguo
	Cheng Peili
Vice-Translators-in-Chief	Lan Fengli
	Qu Yusheng

主　编　谈　勇
副主编　何贵翔
主　译　李照国
　　　　成培莉
副主译　兰凤利
　　　　屈榆生

PUBLISHING HOUSE OF SHANGHAI UNIVERSITY
OF TRADITIONAL CHINESE MEDICINE
上海中医药大学出版社

Publishing House of Shanghai University of Traditional Chinese Medicine
530 Lingling Road，Shanghai，200032，China

Diagnostics of Traditional Chinese Medicine
Compiler-in-Chief Wang Lufen   Translator-in-Chief Li Zhaoguo   Bao Bai
(A Newly Compiled Practical English-Chinese Library of TCM General Compiler-in-Chief
Zuo Yanfu)

ISBN 7 - 81010 - 657 - 0/R • 623   paperback
ISBN 7 - 81010 - 682 - 1/R • 647   hardback

Printed in Shanghai Xinhua Printing Works

图书在版编目(CIP)数据

中医妇科学 / 谈勇主编；李照国，成培莉主译. —上海：上海中医药大学出版社，2002
(英汉对照新编实用中医文库/左言富总主编)
ISBN 7 - 81010 - 657 - 0

Ⅰ.中... Ⅱ.①谈...②李...③成... Ⅲ.中医妇科学-英、汉 Ⅳ.R271.1

中国版本图书馆 CIP 数据核字(2002)第 047655 号

中医妇科学   主编 谈 勇   主译 李照国 成培莉

上海中医药大学出版社出版发行   (零陵路 530 号 邮政编码 200032)
新华书店上海发行所经销   上海新华印刷厂印刷
开本 787mm×1092mm 1/18   印张 15.333   字数 366 千字   印数 1—3 600
版次 2002 年 10 月第 1 版   印次 2002 年 10 月第 1 次印刷

ISBN 7 - 81010 - 657 - 0/R • 623   定价 36.70 元

Compilation Board of the Library

《(英汉对照)新编实用中医文库》编纂委员会

Approval Committee of the Library

《（英汉对照）新编实用中医文库》审定委员会

Foreword Ⅰ

As we are walking into the 21st century, "health for all" is still an important task for the World Health Organization (WHO) to accomplish in the new century. The realization of "health for all" requires mutual cooperation and concerted efforts of various medical sciences, including traditional medicine. WHO has increasingly emphasized the development of traditional medicine and has made fruitful efforts to promote its development. Currently the spectrum of diseases is changing and an increasing number of diseases are difficult to cure. The side effects of chemical drugs have become more and more evident. Furthermore, both the governments and peoples in all countries are faced with the problem of high cost of medical treatment. Traditional Chinese medicine (TCM), the complete system of traditional medicine in the world with unique theory and excellent clinical curative effects, basically meets the need to solve such problems. Therefore, bringing TCM into full play in medical treatment and healthcare will certainly become one of the hot points in the world medical business in the 21st century.

Various aspects of work need to be done to promote the course of the internationalization of TCM, especially the compilation of works and textbooks suitable for international readers. The impending new century has witnessed the compilation of such a

序 一

人类即将迈入 21 世纪,"人人享有卫生保健"仍然是新世纪世界卫生工作面临的重要任务。实现"人人享有卫生保健"的宏伟目标,需要包括传统医药学在内的多种医学学科的相互协作与共同努力。世界卫生组织越来越重视传统医药学的发展,并为推动其发展做出了卓有成效的工作。目前,疾病谱正在发生变化,难治疾病不断增多,化学药品的毒副作用日益显现,日趋沉重的医疗费用困扰着各国政府和民众。中医药学是世界传统医学体系中最完整的传统医学,其独到的学科理论和突出的临床疗效,较符合当代社会和人们解决上述难题的需要。因此,科学有效地发挥中医药学的医疗保健作用,必将成为 21 世纪世界卫生工作的特点之一。

加快中医药走向世界的步伐,还有很多的工作要做,特别是适合国外读者学习的中医药著作、教材的编写是极其重要的方面。在新千年来临之际,由南京中医药大学

series of books known as *A Newly Compiled Practical English-Chinese Library of Traditional Chinese Medicine* published by the Publishing House of Shanghai University of TCM, compiled by Nanjing University of TCM and translated by Shanghai University of TCM. Professor Zuo Yanfu, the general compiler-in-chief of this Library, is a person who sets his mind on the international dissemination of TCM. He has compiled *General Survey on TCM Abroad*, a monograph on the development and state of TCM abroad. This Library is another important works written by the experts organized by him with the support of Nanjing University of TCM and Shanghai University of TCM. The compilation of this Library is done with consummate ingenuity and according to the development of TCM abroad. The compilers, based on the premise of preserving the genuineness and gist of TCM, have tried to make the contents concise, practical and easy to understand, making great efforts to introduce the abstruse ideas of TCM in a scientific and simple way as well as expounding the prevention and treatment of diseases which are commonly encountered abroad and can be effectively treated by TCM.

This Library encompasses a systematic summarization of the teaching experience accumulated in Nanjing University of TCM and Shanghai University of TCM that run the collaborating centers of traditional medicine and the international training centers on acupuncture and moxibustion set by WHO. I am sure that the publication of this Library will further promote the development of traditional Chinese med-

主编、上海中医药大学主译、上海中医药大学出版社出版的《(英汉对照)新编实用中医文库》的即将问世,正是新世纪中医药国际传播更快发展的预示。本套文库总主编左言富教授是中医药学国际传播事业的有心人,曾主编研究国外中医药发展状况的专著《国外中医药概览》。本套文库的编撰,是他在南京中医药大学和上海中医药大学支持下,组织许多著名专家共同完成的又一重要专著。本套文库的作者们深谙国外的中医药发展现状,编写颇具匠心,在注重真实,不失精华的前提下,突出内容的简明、实用,易于掌握,力求科学而又通俗地介绍中医药学的深奥内容,重点阐述国外常见而中医药颇具疗效的疾病的防治。

本套文库蕴含了南京中医药大学和上海中医药大学作为 WHO 传统医学合作中心、国际针灸培训中心多年留学生教学的实践经验和系统总结,更为全面、系统、准确地向世界传播中医药学。相信本书的出版将对中医更好地走向世界,让世界更好地了解中医产生更

icine abroad and enable the whole world to have a better understanding of traditional Chinese medicine.

为积极的影响。

Professor Zhu Qingsheng

Vice-Minister of Health Ministry of the People's Republic of China

Director of the State Administrative Bureau of TCM

December 14, 2000 Beijing

朱庆生教授

中华人民共和国卫生部副部长

国家中医药管理局局长

2000 年 12 月 14 日于北京

Foreword II

Before the existence of the modern medicine, human beings depended solely on herbal medicines and other therapeutic methods to treat diseases and preserve health. Such a practice gave rise to the establishment of various kinds of traditional medicine with unique theory and practice, such as traditional Chinese medicine, Indian medicine and Arabian medicine, etc. Among these traditional systems of medicine, traditional Chinese medicine is a most extraordinary one based on which traditional Korean medicine and Japanese medicine have evolved.

Even in the 21st century, traditional medicine is still of great vitality. In spite of the fast development of modern medicine, traditional medicine is still disseminated far and wide. In many developing countries, most of the people in the rural areas still depend on traditional medicine and traditional medical practitioners to meet the need for primary healthcare. Even in the countries with advanced modern medicine, more and more people have begun to accept traditional medicine and other therapeutic methods, such as homeopathy, osteopathy and naturopathy, etc.

With the change of the economy, culture and living style in various regions as well as the aging in the world population, the disease spectrum has changed. And such a change has paved the way for the new application of traditional medicine. Besides,

序 二

在现代医学形成之前,人类一直依赖草药和其他一些疗法治病强身,从而发展出许多有理论、有实践的传统医学,例如中医学、印度医学、阿拉伯医学等。中医学是世界林林总总的传统医学中的一支奇葩,在它的基础上还衍生出朝鲜传统医学和日本汉方医学。在跨入21世纪的今天,古老的传统医学依然焕发着活力,非但没有因现代医学的发展而式微,其影响还有增无减,人们对传统医学的价值也有了更深刻的体会和认识。在许多贫穷国家,大多数农村人口仍然依赖传统医学疗法和传统医务工作者来满足他们对初级卫生保健的需求。在现代医学占主导地位的许多国家,传统医学及其他一些"另类疗法",诸如顺势疗法、整骨疗法、自然疗法等,也越来越被人们所接受。

伴随着世界各地经济、文化和生活的变革以及世界人口的老龄化,世界疾病谱也发生了变化。传统医学有了新的应用,而新疾病所引起的新需求以及现代医学的成

the new requirements initiated by the new diseases and the achievements and limitations of modern medicine have also created challenges for traditional medicine.

WHO sensed the importance of traditional medicine to human health early in the 1970s and have made great efforts to develop traditional medicine. At the 29th world health congress held in 1976, the item of traditional medicine was adopted in the working plan of WHO. In the following world health congresses, a series of resolutions were passed to demand the member countries to develop, utilize and study traditional medicine according to their specific conditions so as to reduce medical expenses for the realization of "health for all".

WHO has laid great stress on the scientific content, safe and effective application of traditional medicine. It has published and distributed a series of booklets on the scientific, safe and effective use of herbs and acupuncture and moxibustion. It has also made great contributions to the international standardization of traditional medical terms. The safe and effective application of traditional medicine has much to do with the skills of traditional medical practitioners. That is why WHO has made great efforts to train them. WHO has run 27 collaborating centers in the world which have made great contributions to the training of acupuncturists and traditional medical practitioners. Nanjing University of TCM and Shanghai University of TCM run the collaborating centers with WHO. In recent years it has, with the cooperation of WHO and other countries, trained about ten thousand international students from over

就与局限又向传统医学提出了挑战,推动它进一步发展。世界卫生组织早在 20 世纪 70 年代就意识到传统医学对人类健康的重要性,并为推动传统医学的发展做了努力。1976 年举行的第二十九届世界卫生大会将传统医学项目纳入世界卫生组织的工作计划。其后的各届世界卫生大会又通过了一系列决议,要求各成员国根据本国的条件发展、使用和研究传统医学,以降低医疗费用,促进"人人享有初级卫生保健"这一目标的实现。

世界卫生组织历来重视传统医学的科学、安全和有效使用。它出版和发行了一系列有关科学、安全、有效使用草药和针灸的技术指南,并在专用术语的标准化方面做了许多工作。传统医学的使用是否做到安全和有效,是与使用传统疗法的医务工作者的水平密不可分的。因此,世界卫生组织也十分重视传统医学培训工作。它在全世界有 27 个传统医学合作中心,这些中心对培训合格的针灸师及使用传统疗法的其他医务工作者做出了积极的贡献。南京中医药大学、上海中医药大学是世界卫生组织传统医学合作中心之一,近年来与世界卫生组织和其他国家合作,培训了近万名来自 90 多个国

90 countries.

In order to further promote the dissemination of traditional Chinese medicine in the world, *A Newly Compiled Practical English-Chinese Library of Traditional Chinese Medicine*, compiled by Nanjing University of TCM with Professor Zuo Yanfu as the general compiler-in-chief and published by the Publishing House of Shanghai University of TCM, aims at systematic, accurate and concise expounding of traditional Chinese medical theory and introducing clinical therapeutic methods of traditional medicine according to modern medical nomenclature of diseases. Undoubtedly, this series of books will be the practical textbooks for the beginners with certain English level and the international enthusiasts with certain level of Chinese to study traditional Chinese medicine. Besides, this series of books can also serve as reference books for WHO to internationally standardize the nomenclature of acupuncture and moxibustion.

The scientific, safe and effective use of traditional medicine will certainly further promote the development of traditional medicine and traditional medicine will undoubtedly make more and more contributions to human health in the 21st century.

Zhang Xiaorui
WHO Coordination Officer
December, 2000

家和地区的留学生。

在南京中医药大学左言富教授主持下编纂的、由上海中医药大学出版社出版的《（英汉对照）新编实用中医文库》，旨在全面、系统、准确、简要地阐述中医基础理论，并结合西医病名介绍中医临床治疗方法。因此，这套文库可望成为具有一定英语水平的初学中医者和具有一定中文水平的外国中医爱好者学习基础中医学的系列教材。这套文库也可供世界卫生组织在编写国际针灸标准术语时参考。

传统医学的科学、安全、有效使用必将进一步推动传统医学的发展。传统医学一定会在 21 世纪为人类健康做出更大的贡献。

张小瑞
世界卫生组织传统医学协调官员
2000 年12 月

Preface

The Publishing House of Shanghai University of TCM published *A Practical English-Chinese Library of Traditional Chinese Medicine* in 1990. The Library has been well-known in the world ever since and has made great contributions to the dissemination of traditional Chinese medicine in the world. In view of the fact that 10 years has passed since its publication and that there are certain errors in the explanation of traditional Chinese medicine in the Library, the Publishing House has invited Nanjing University of TCM and Shanghai University of TCM to organize experts to recompile and translate the Library.

Nanjing University of TCM and Shanghai University of TCM are well-known for their advantages in higher education of traditional Chinese medicine and compilation of traditional Chinese medical textbooks. The compilation of *A Newly Compiled Practical English-Chinese Library of Traditional Chinese Medicine* has absorbed the rich experience accumulated by Nanjing University of Traditional Chinese Medicine in training international students of traditional Chinese medicine. Compared with the previous Library, the Newly Compiled Library has made great improvements in many aspects, fully demonstrating the academic system of traditional Chinese medicine. The whole series of books has systematically introduced the basic theory and thera-

前　言

上海中医药大学出版社于 1990 年出版了一套《(英汉对照)实用中医文库》,发行 10 年来,在海内外产生了较大影响,对推动中医学走向世界起了积极作用。考虑到该套丛书发行已久,对中医学术体系的介绍还有一些欠妥之处,因此,上海中医药大学出版社特邀南京中医药大学主编、上海中医药大学主译,组织全国有关专家编译出版《(英汉对照)新编实用中医文库》。

《(英汉对照)新编实用中医文库》的编纂,充分发挥了南京中医药大学和上海中医药大学在高等中医药教育教学和教材编写方面的优势,吸收了作为 WHO 传统医学合作中心之一的两校,多年来从事中医药学国际培训和留学生学历教育的经验,对原《(英汉对照)实用中医文库》整体结构作了大幅度调整,以突出中医学术主体内容。全套丛书系统介绍了中医基础理论和中医辨证论治方法,讲解了中药学和方剂学的基本理论,详细介绍了 236 味中药、152 首常用方剂和 100 种常用中成药;详述

peutic methods based on syndrome differentiation, expounding traditional Chinese pharmacy and prescriptions; explaining 236 herbs, 152 prescriptions and 100 commonly-used patent drugs; elucidating 264 methods for differentiating syndromes and treating commonly-encountered and frequently-encountered diseases in internal medicine, surgery, gynecology, pediatrics, traumatology and orthopedics, ophthalmology and otorhinolaryngology; introducing the basic methods and theory of acupuncture and moxibustion, massage (tuina), life cultivation and rehabilitation, including 70 kinds of diseases suitable for acupuncture and moxibustion, 38 kinds of diseases for massage, examples of life cultivation and over 20 kinds of commonly encountered diseases treated by rehabilitation therapies in traditional Chinese medicine. For better understanding of traditional Chinese medicine, the books are neatly illustrated. There are 296 line graphs and 30 colored pictures in the Library with necessary indexes, making it more comprehensive, accurate and systematic in disseminating traditional Chinese medicine in the countries and regions where English is the official language.

This Library is characterized by following features:

1. Scientific　Based on the development of TCM in education and research in the past 10 years, efforts have been made in the compilation to highlight the gist of TCM through accurate theoretical exposition and clinical practice, aiming at introducing authentic theory and practice to the world.

2. Systematic　This Library contains 14 separa-

264 种临床内、外、妇、儿、骨伤、眼、耳鼻喉各科常见病与多发病的中医辨证论治方法；系统论述针灸、推拿、中医养生康复的基本理论和基本技能，介绍针灸治疗病种 70 种、推拿治疗病种 38 种、各类养生实例及 20 余种常见病证的中医康复实例。为了更加直观地介绍中医药学术，全书选用线图 296 幅、彩图 30 幅，并附有必要的索引，从而更加全面、系统、准确地向使用英语的国家和地区传播中医学术，推进中医学走向世界，造福全人类。

本丛书主要具有以下特色：(1) 科学性：在充分吸收近 10 余年来中医教学和科学研究最新进展的基础上，坚持突出中医学术精华，理论阐述准确，临床切合实用，向世界各国介绍"原汁原味"的中医药学术；(2) 系统性：本套丛书包括《中医基础理论》、《中医诊断学》、《中药学》、《方剂学》、《中医内

rate fascicles, i. e. *Basic Theory of Traditional Chinese Medicine*, *Diagnostics of Traditional Chinese Medicine*, *Science of Chinese Materia Medica*, *Science of Prescriptions*, *Internal Medicine of Traditional Chinese Medicine*, *Surgery of Traditional Chinese Medicine*, *Gynecology of Traditional Chinese Medicine*, *Pediatrics of Traditional Chinese Medicine*, *Traumatology and Orthopedics of Traditional Chinese Medicine*, *Ophthalmology of Traditional Chinese Medicine*, *Otorhinolaryngology of Traditional Chinese Medicine*, *Chinese Acupuncture and Moxibustion*, *Chinese Tuina (Massage)*, *and Life Cultivation and Rehabilitation of Traditional Chinese Medicine*.

3. Practical   Compared with the previous Library, the Newly Compiled Library has made great improvements and supplements, systematically introducing therapeutic methods for treating over 200 kinds of commonly and frequently encountered diseases, focusing on training basic clinical skills in acupuncture and moxibustion, tuina therapy, life cultivation and rehabilitation with clinical case reports.

4. Standard   This Library is reasonable in structure, distinct in categorization, standard in terminology and accurate in translation with full consideration of habitual expressions used in countries and regions with English language as the mother tongue.

This series of books is not only practical for the beginners with certain competence of English to study TCM, but also can serve as authentic textbooks for international students in universities and colleges of TCM in China to study and practice TCM. For those from TCM field who are going to go

科学》、《中医外科学》、《中医妇科学》、《中医儿科学》、《中医骨伤科学》、《中医眼科学》、《中医耳鼻喉科学》、《中国针灸》、《中国推拿》、《中医养生康复学》14 个分册,系统反映了中医各学科建设与发展的最新成果;(3) 实用性:临床各科由原来的上下两册,根据学科的发展进行大幅度的调整和增补,比较详细地介绍了 200 多种各科常见病、多发病的中医治疗方法,重点突出了针灸、推拿、养生康复等临床基本技能训练,并附有部分临证实例;(4) 规范性:全书结构合理,层次清晰,对中医各学科名词术语表述规范,对中医英语翻译执行了更为严格的标准化方案,同时又充分考虑到使用英语国家和地区人们的语言习惯和表达方式。

本丛书不仅能满足具有一定英语水平的初学中医者系统学习中医之用,而且也为中医院校外国留学生教育及国内外开展中医双语教学提供了目前最具权威的系列教材,同时也是中医出国人员进

abroad to do academic exchange, this series of books will provide them with unexpected convenience.

Professor Xiang Ping, President of Nanjing University of TCM, is the director of the Compilation Board. Professor Zuo Yanfu from Nanjing University of TCM, General Compiler-in-Chief, is in charge of the compilation. Zhang Wenkang, Minister of Health Ministry, is invited to be the honorary director of the Editorial Board. Li Zhenji, Vice-Director of the State Administrative Bureau of TCM, is invited to be the director of the Approval Committee. Chen Keji, academician of China Academy, is invited to be the General Advisor. International advisors invited are Mr. M. S. Khan, Chairman of Ireland Acupuncture and Moxibustion Fund; Miss Alessandra Gulí, Chairman of "Nanjing Association" in Rome, Italy; Doctor Secondo Scarsella, Chief Editor of YI DAO ZA ZHI; President Raymond K. Carroll from Australian Oriental Touching Therapy College; Ms. Shulan Tang, Academic Executive of ATCM in Britain; Mr. Glovanni Maciocia from Britain; Mr. David, Chairman of American Association of TCM; Mr. Tzu Kuo Shih, director of Chinese Medical Technique Center in Connecticut, America; Mr. Helmut Ziegler, director of TCM Center in Germany; and Mr. Isigami Hiroshi from Japan. Chen Ken, official of WHO responsible for the Western Pacific Region, has greatly encouraged the compilers in compiling this series of books. After the accomplishment of the compilation, Professor Zhu Qingsheng, Vice-Minister of Health Ministry and Director of the State Administrative Bureau of TCM, has set a high value on the books in his fore-

行中医药国际交流的重要工具书。

全书由南京中医药大学校长项平教授担任编委会主任、左言富教授任总主编,主持全书的编写。中华人民共和国卫生部张文康部长担任本丛书编委会名誉主任,国家中医药管理局李振吉副局长担任审定委员会主任,陈可冀院士欣然担任本丛书总顾问指导全书的编纂。爱尔兰针灸基金会主席萨利姆先生、意大利罗马"南京协会"主席亚历山大·古丽女士、意大利《医道》杂志主编卡塞拉·塞肯多博士、澳大利亚东方触觉疗法学院雷蒙特·凯·卡罗院长、英国中医药学会学术部长汤淑兰女士、英国马万里先生、美国中医师公会主席大卫先生、美国康州中华医疗技术中心主任施祖谷先生、德国中医中心主任赫尔木特先生、日本石上博先生担任本丛书特邀外籍顾问。世界卫生组织西太平洋地区官员陈恳先生对本丛书的编写给予了热情鼓励。全书完成后,卫生部副部长兼国家中医药管理局局长朱庆生教授给予了高度评价,并欣然为本书作序;WHO 传统医学协调官员张小瑞对于本丛书的编写给予高度关注,百忙中也专为本书作序。我国驻外教育机构,特别是中国驻英国曼彻斯特领事张益群先生、中国驻美国休斯敦领事严美华

word for the Library. Zhang Xiaorui, an official from WHO's Traditional Medicine Program, has paid great attention to the compilation and written a foreword for the Library. The officials from the educational organizations of China in other countries have provided us with some useful materials in our compilation. They are Mr. Zhang Yiqun, China Consul to Manchester in Britain; Miss Yan Meihua, Consul to Houston in America; Mr. Wang Jiping, First Secretary in the Educational Department in the Embassy of China to France; and Mr. Gu Shengying, the Second Secretary in the Educational Department in the Embassy of China to Germany. We are grateful to them all.

The Compilers
December, 2000

女士、中国驻法国使馆教育处一秘王季平先生、中国驻德国使馆教育处二秘郭胜英先生在与我们工作联系中,间接提供了不少有益资料。在此一并致以衷心感谢!

编 者
2000 年 12 月

Note for compilation   编写说明

Gynecology, one of the main clinical specialties in traditional Chinese medicine(TCM), is unique in theory, rich in therapeutic methods and significant in clinical curative effect. For the purpose of promoting the development of the theory and treatment of gynecology in TCM in the whole world for the benefit of mankind, we have compiled this book based on our clinical experience and other medical literature.

This book is composed of two major parts. The general introduction includes three chapters, concentrating on introducing the physiological features and pathological changes, the diagnosis based on the four diagnostic methods and syndrome differentiation as well as the therapeutic principles and treatment. Specific discussions is composed of 8 chapters and 31 kinds of diseases. The diseases are described, with the names of modern medicine, in terms of their definition, causes and pathogenesis as well as clinical characteristics. The part of key points for syndrome differentiation focuses on describing the history, symptoms and signs as well as differential diagnosis of the disease in question. The part of treatment based on syndrome differentiation mainly includes main symptoms, therapeutic methods, prescription and medicinal herbs as well as herbal modification. Other therapeutic methods include patent medicine of TCM, empirical and folk recipes, application, fumigation and lotion.

This book is easy to read, concise in description

中医妇科学是中医学中的主要临床学科之一,具有较为独特的理论和丰富的治疗方法,临床疗效卓著。为促进中医妇科学的学术理论、诊疗技术走向世界,造福于全人类,我们在总结多年临床实践经验和参阅大量文献资料的基础上,编成此书。

全书分总论、各论两大部分。总论共有三章,主要介绍中医对女性的生理、病理特点的认识;以四诊为纲,辨证为要,介绍妇科疾病的诊察要点,突出介绍妇科的特色;并提纲挈领地介绍妇科疾病的治法概要。各论部分共有八章,介绍常见病 31 种,临床各节以西医病名为纲,概述部分介绍该疾病的定义、病因病机、临床特征;诊断要点部分用简练明快的语言阐述本病病史、症状、体征以及鉴别诊断;辨证论治部分包括主要证候、治法、方药和加减;其他疗法部分包括了中成药、单验方、外敷薰洗等有确凿疗效的特色疗法、诊法及治疗内容。

全书内容深入浅出,简明扼

and practical in application. The content ranges from the ancient literature to the modern practice covering the concerned records in both the ancient and modern medical literature as well as the clinical experience of the doctors in the previous dynasties. The terms used in describing symptoms and treatment are selected in light of the Clinical Diagnostic and Therapeutic Terminology of TCM issued by the People's Republic of China and Gynecology of TCM in Medical Encyclopedia.

要,实用具体,编写内容及素材的取舍均来自于古今中医药文献记载与历代医家的临床实践,疾病的证候、治法等术语参照中华人民共和国国家标准《中医临床诊疗术语》、《医学百科全书·中医妇科学》。

Contents

目　录

1 General Introduction

1.1 Physiological and pathological characteristics of women

Gynecology of TCM is a clinical specialty and concentrates on studying the physiological and pathological characteristics, diagnostic and therapeutic principles and specific diseases related to women. Through a long history of two thousand years of practice and improvement, gynecology of TCM has developed a unique theory based on the physiological and pathological characteristics of women which are quite different from those of men. Women are characterized by uterus, uterine collaterals and uterine vessels in anatomy; menstruation, pregnancy, delivery and child-feeding in physiology; and disorders of menstruation, leukorrhea, pregnancy and delivery in pathology. It is just based on the cognition of uterus, menstruation, pregnancy, delivery and child-feeding as well as their relation with the viscera, meridians, qi and blood that gynecology of TCM studies the pathological characteristics of woman disease and the principles for prevention and clinical treatment.

总 论

第一章 女性的生理、病理特点

中医妇科学是根据中医学理论,研究女性的解剖、生理、病理特点,诊疗规律及其特有疾病的一门临床学科。在两千多年漫长的历史发展过程中中医药学经妇科临床的实践,形成了一个较为完整、系统的理论体系,这一体系的基础就在于女性的生理、病理特点,与男性有着根本不同之处。由于其有子宫、胞络和胞脉等解剖学方面的特征,就有了月经、胎孕、产育、哺乳等方面的生理变化特点,并可导致经、带、胎、产等的异常而产生妇科疾病。中医妇科学就是通过对子宫、月经、胎孕、产育、哺乳等与脏腑、经络、气血的关系的认识,来研究女性的病理特征,从而探索妇科疾病的特点及其防治的规律。

1.1.1　Physiological characteristics

1.1.1.1　Uterus

The uterus is located in the pelvis, like an upside down pear, posterior to the bladder and anterior to the rectum. The uterus is responsible for menstruation and conceiving fetus. Under physiological conditions, the uterus is to store essence and blood for menstruation or conception of fetus, demonstrating the "storage" function of the zang organs; and discharge menstruation or deliver baby, manifesting the "excretion" function of the fu organs. That is why it is called "extraordinary fu organ" in Neijing or Canon of Medicine. Such physiological functions of the uterus are closely related to meridians, viscera, qi and blood. The uterus is connected with the heart and kidney through meridians. The heart governs blood and the kidney stores essence. Only when the heart blood is sufficient and kidney essence is abundant can blood and essence flow into the uterus for the preparation of menstruation and pregnancy. Besides, the uterus is also closely related to thoroughfare vessel, conception vessel, governor vessel and belt vessel through meridians. Such an extensive relation with the meridians and vessels enables the uterus to connect with the viscera and well accomplish its function in managing menstruation and pregnancy.

第一节　生理特点

一、子宫

子宫亦称女子胞、子处、子脏、子肠、胞宫、子户等。其位置在下腹部盆腔之中,呈倒置的梨形,是个腔状器官,居于膀胱之后,直肠之前,是女性特有的生殖器官。它的作用是主行月经和孕育胎儿。在生理状态下,子宫的功能活动,平时蓄积精血,为月经的来潮或为胚胎的孕育奠定应有的物质基础,表现了脏的"藏"的功能;而在行经期排出月经,或在分娩时娩出胎儿,又表现了腑的"泻"的功能;由于有这种双重的功能,故《内经》称之为"奇恒之府"。子宫的这些生理功能与脏腑、经络、气血密切相关。首先,因为子宫在经络上与心肾相通,而心主血、肾藏精,心血畅旺,肾精充沛,通过经脉注入胞中,才具备了产生月经、胎孕的条件。其次,子宫还与奇经中的冲、任、督、带等经脉有密切联系,并通过这些经脉与十二经及脏腑相通,从而完成其主行月经和孕育胎儿的生理作用。

1.1.1.2　Menstruation

Menstruation refers to regular uterine bleeding in women of childbearing age, a manifestation of the normal activity of the reproductive function of women. Normal menstruation occurs once a month. But sometimes under normal conditions menstruation may occur once every other month known as bimonthly menstruation or once three months known as tri-monthly menstruation, or even once a year known as yearly menstruation. If menstruation never occurs in the whole life of a woman, it is called latent menstruation. In some cases menstruation may occur regularly in the first three months of pregnancy without affecting the fetus, it is called menstruation in pregnancy. Such changes in menstruation are regarded as normal phenomena, not morbid.

Menstruation is discharged from the uterus, but its production is in close relation with the normal functions of the viscera, exuberance of qi and blood as well as smooth circulation of meridians. Among these factors, blood is one of the substantial bases for menstruation. But blood is produced from the cereal nutrient transformed by the viscera and transported to the uterus by the meridians.

The production of menstruation is related to the viscera, meridians, qi and blood, especially to the sufficiency of kidney qi and normal functions of the thoroughfare

二、月经

月经是育龄女性周期性子宫出血的生理现象,是女性生殖功能正常活动的表现,所以每月一次,周而复始,故称之为月经。中医古代文献也有称为月事、月使、月水,月候、月信,或经水、经候、经事的。正常的月经是每月一行,但亦偶有身体无病而月经周期异于一般正常人的,如2个月行经一次的称为"并月";3个月行经一次的称为"居经"或"季经";甚至还有一年经行一次的,称为"避年";一生始终不行月经而仍能受孕者,被称为"暗经"。还有女性怀孕后,在早期妊娠期间(妊娠3个月内)仍能按月行经而不影响胎儿者,称为"激经"(亦名盛胎或垢胎)。这些都属于生理上的个别现象,不属病态。

月经虽从子宫排出,但它的产生与脏腑功能正常、气血旺盛、经络通畅有密切关系。其中血是产生月经的基本物质,但血又是水谷之精气经脏腑气化而生成,通过经络转输血海,才能成为月经产生的物质基础之一。

月经的产生,与脏腑、经络、气血相关,与肾气的充盛、冲任二脉的通盛与否关系更

and conception vessels. Kidney qi is key to the physiological development of women all through the life. According to Neijing, at the age of 7 female is gradually rich in kidney qi, starting to change teeth and growing long hair; at the age of 14, reproductive substance has well developed, conception vessel is smooth in circulation, thoroughfare vessel is in predomination, menstruation occurs regularly and pregnancy is possible; at the age of 27, her kidney qi is sufficient and she has reached the age of bearing baby; at the age of 28, her body has perfectly developed; but at the age of 35, yangming meridian begins to decline and her face starts to change and her hair begins to lose; at the age of 42, her body declines further, her face becomes withered and her hair starts to turn grayish; at the age of 49, the conception vessel becomes deficient, the thoroughfare vessel declines, reproductive substance has been exhausted and menstruation stops. At this period, woman is changed in physical building, declines in sex glands and loses reproductive ability.

为密切,其中肾气的充盛与否对女性一生的成长起着决定性的作用。《内经》将肾气的充盛与否对男女生长发育的影响作了详尽的阐述,指出女性在 7 岁以后,肾气逐渐充盛,促使生殖器官开始发育,同时更换乳齿。14 岁左右,天癸开始成熟。由于天癸的作用,使任脉畅通,冲脉充盛,随之月经便开始初潮,具备了受孕生育的能力。但月经初潮的来临并不标志着身体及生殖功能已经完全发育成熟,而是刚刚开始,还要随着肾气的不断充盛渐趋成熟,所以要到 28 岁左右才发育到极盛时期,这时筋骨坚壮,身体旺盛,生殖机能的发育也趋于成熟。而到 49 岁左右,肾气逐渐衰退,天癸的作用也逐渐消失,冲任脉亦虚衰,月经停止,不再能受孕,便丧失生殖能力。《内经》系统地阐述了女性一生的生长发育和各个阶段的生理变化过程,从这些特征上完全可以说明肾、天癸、冲任与月经的关系。肾主藏精,是人体生长发育和生殖的根本,故肾为先天之本,元气之根,肾又系胞,女性肾气盛,先天之精才能发育成熟,并在冲任通盛的健康状况下月经才能来潮。因此,月经的产生,肾气的充盛是起了主导作用的。

1. 1. 1. 3   Leukorrhea

Leukorrhea refers to a little whitish or transparent and odorless secretion in the vagina of healthy women for moistening the vagina. Usually leukorrhea is profuse after menstruation or in the period between two cycles of menstruation or during pregnancy. This is physiological leukorrhea and is regarded as normal. Normal leukorrhea is a yin fluid in the body derived from cereal nutrients which are transformed by the spleen and stomach, stored in the kidney, governed by the conception vessel, controlled by the belt vessel and distributed continuously in the uterus.

1. 1. 1. 4   Pregnancy and puerperium

After the occurrence of menarche, woman is still underdeveloped in the body and genitals, but she is able to get pregnant. The organ for pregnancy and delivery is the uterus. The mechanism of pregnancy lies in the combination of the essence from a man and a woman. If a woman is well developed in kidney essence with free flow of the conception vessel and fullness of the thoroughfare vessel, she will be easy to get pregnant when she has sexual intercourse with a man. The development and growth of fetus in the uterus were vividly described in some of the ancient medical canons.

After pregnancy, qi and blood accumulate in the thoroughfare vessel and conception vessel for providing nourishment for the fetus. That is why menstruation stops. But at the early stage of pregnancy, the uterus only stores essence and never excretes. Since the fetus is growing in the uterus and blood and qi are accumulating in the uterus, qi in the thoroughfare vessel is easy to flow

三、带下

健康妇女的阴道内有少量白色或透明无臭的分泌物,以润湿阴道,一般在月经后或两次月经之间及妊娠期较多,这是生理性白带。属正常现象。正常的白带属于人体的阴液,来源于饮食的精微部分,经脾胃的运化而成,封藏于肾(肾主五液),由任脉主司,受带脉约束,不断敷布于胞中,津润于阴道,以保护和润泽阴道,发挥其正常生理功能。

四、妊娠和产褥

女性在月经初潮以后,身体和生殖器官虽未发育成熟,但已有了生育能力。怀孕和分娩的器官是子宫,而受孕的机理则在两性之精的结合。女性由于肾气盛,肾中所藏生殖之精发育成熟,任脉通,冲脉盛,生殖之精施泄,若此时两性相交,两精结合,就能受孕。

受孕以后,对胎儿在子宫内的生长发育,古代医学也有粗略的认识。怀孕以后,由于要供给胎儿的营养,气血聚于冲任以养胎,故月经停止来潮。但妊娠早期,子宫只藏不泻,胚胎内置,血聚气实,冲气

upwards. If the liver blood in gravida is insufficient, it will lead to relative deficiency of liver yin, relative hyperactivity of liver yang because blood accumulates in the uterus to nourish the fetus. The liver governs thoroughfare vessel, simultaneous upward flow of liver qi and thoroughfare vessel qi frequently leads to attack on the stomach. That is why at the early stage of pregnancy there are morning dizziness, lassitude, somnolence, preference for sour taste, nausea and vomiting which are physiological changes and usually disappear in three months. Since blood accumulates in the uterus to nourish the fetus, it is already deficient during pregnancy. Hemorrhage during delivery further worsens blood deficiency. Asthenia of yin fails to keep yang inside and leads to leakage of yang, bringing about such symptoms like slight fever, aversion to cold and spontaneous sweating which will disappear automatically after yin and yang are balanced. Besides, blood asthenia and profuse sweating may cause constipation because the consumption of body fluid will deprive the intestines of proper moistening.

After delivery, there will be secretion of milk. Usually during the pregnancy, the breasts are gradually enlarged, the areola of mamma is deepened and foremilk is secreted. The milk is transformed from blood and produced by gastric qi. Since blood, propelled by lung-qi, is transformed into milk and stops flowing into the uterus, there is no menstruation during breast feeding period.

易于上逆,若孕妇肝血不足,血聚养胎,则肝阴偏虚,肝阳偏旺,常易横逆犯胃,故妊娠早期多有晨起头晕、倦怠嗜卧、择食酸味、恶心呕吐等现象,这是生理上的暂时变化,并非病理状态,一般在 3 个月后可自然消失。妊娠期中,血聚养胎,血已偏于不足,分娩时的出血,造成阴血更虚,阴虚不能守阳,则阳气外泄,因此产后常有轻微的发热、恶寒、自汗等阳不固密的现象,一般不需治疗,阴阳和则自愈。此外,由于血虚多汗,津液亏耗,不能濡润肠道,大便易于秘结。

分娩以后,产妇就有乳汁分泌。通常在妊娠期,乳房即逐渐发生变化,如乳房胀大、乳晕加深,出现初乳等。乳汁为血所化,赖胃气而生。由于分娩之后养胎之血在肺气的作用下上化为乳汁,故哺乳期一般不来月经。

1.1.1.5　Viscera, qi, blood, meridians and their relations with physiological activities of women

1.1.1.5.1　Viscera

Physiologically the viscera in women mainly function

五、脏腑、气血、经络和女性生理的关系

(一)脏腑

在女性生理方面,脏腑的

to produce essence and transform qi and blood. The heart governs the blood, the liver stores the blood, the spleen commands the blood and is also the source of the blood; the lung controls qi and qi moves the blood; the kidney stores the essence, and the essence and blood share the same origin. The zang-organs and fu-organs, interiorly and exteriorly related to each other, together control the production, storage and regulation of the essence, qi and blood, also closely related to menstruation, leukorrhea, pregnancy and childbirth. Among the zang-organs and fu-organs, the kidney, liver and spleen (stomach) are the most important ones.

The main function of the kidney lies in kidney qi composed of kidney yin and kidney yang which depend on each other and restrain each other. It is the key factor for maintaining vital functions and visceral physiological activities. The conditions of kidney qi is directly related to the physical development and reproduction of woman. When kidney qi becomes exuberant, the tiangui, reproductive essence, in the kidney will be fully developed, the conception vessel will transport qi freely and the thoroughfare vessel will be abundant in content. Under such a condition menstruation occurs regularly and pregnancy is possible.

The kidney-qi functions to consolidate and astringe, and the kidney is connected with the uterine collaterals. After pregnancy, the fetus in the uterus depends on the nourishment of kidney yin and warmth of kidney yang to develop normally.

The kidney also governs water as well as opening and closing activities. If the kidney is abundant in qi and

作用主要是生精化气化血。其中心主血,肝藏血,脾统血,又是血的生化之源;肺主气,气运血;肾藏精,精血又同源;腑与脏为表里,同司精、气、血的生化、贮存、统摄、调节等,与经、带、胎、产均有密切关系,其中又以肾、肝、脾(胃)的作用更为重要。

肾 肾的主要功能体现为肾气,包括肾阴和肾阳。肾阴亦称真阴、元阴,肾阳亦称元阳、真阳,二者相互依存,相互制约,是维持机体生命机能及各脏腑生理活动的本源。因此,肾气的盛衰,与人体的生长发育、衰老和生殖能力有直接关系。女性在肾气充盛后,肾中所藏生殖之精——天癸逐渐成熟,任脉乃通,冲脉乃盛,月事以时下,而能受孕生育。

肾气有固摄作用,肾脉与胞宫络脉相连通,故能维系胞胎;受孕之后,胚胎在子宫中须依赖肾阴的滋养和肾阳的温煦,才能正常发育。因此,肾对胚胎的发育也起着极其重要的作用。

肾还主水,司开阖,肾气充沛,开阖有度,则阴液不断

normal in closing and opening, yin fluid will constantly flow into the conception and belt vessels to lubricate the vagina and produce physiological leukorrhea.

　　The liver stores blood and governs distribution and conveyance of qi and blood, pertaining to yin physically and to yang functionally. Blood stored in the liver nourishes all viscera and skeleton and also flows into the thoroughfare vessel. That is why it is said that "the liver governs the thoroughfare vessel" and "the liver is the congenital base of life for women". The liver also plays an important role in the production of menstruation. The storage, circulation and regulation of blood in the liver depend on the distribution and conveyance of liver qi. Only when the distribution and conveyance functions of the liver is normal can sufficient blood flow into the uterus regularly. Besides, the liver meridian starts from the big toe and moves upwards along the inner line of the lower limbs to the genitals and lower abdomen, connected with the liver, gallbladder and diaphragm, distributing over the hypochondria and rib-side, finally reaching the vertex. Liver qi is also significant in distributing and conveying gastrosplenic qi and bile. The normal distribution and conveyance functions of liver qi are prerequisite to the reception and digestion of food by the stomach, the normal transformation and production of essence by the spleen, smooth transportation of bile from the gallbladder and constant production of qi and blood. The dysfunction of the liver in distribution and conveyance affects the normal functions of the spleen, stomach and gallbladder, leading to epigastric oppression, hypochondriac pain, bitter taste in the mouth, anorexia, abdominal distension and loose stool which are commonly encountered in gynecology. Since the liver meridian distributes over the breasts, lower abdomen and genitals, the functions of liver qi and the

输入于任、带二脉,津津常润于阴道,成为生理性白带。

　　肝　肝藏血,主疏泄,体阴而用阳。肝所藏之血,营养脏腑百骸,下注于冲脉,冲为血海,肝为血脏,故又有"肝司血海"和"女子以肝为先天"之说。因此,在月经的化生方面,肝也有重要作用,肝又主条达疏泄,肝血的贮存、流通、调节需依赖肝气的疏泄作用,肝气的疏泄功能正常,则血海盈满如期。另外,肝的经脉由足大趾经下肢内侧上行,绕前阴,抵少腹,夹肾属肝,络胆,上贯膈,布胁肋(在此经过乳头)……上至巅,与胆、胃、乳房均有一定关系。肝气还有疏泄脾胃和胆汁的功能。肝气疏达,则胃的受纳、腐熟,脾的运化、生精,胆汁的输出正常,则气血的生化有源。若肝失疏泄,可以影响脾、胃、胆的正常功能,而发生脘闷、胁痛、口苦、纳呆、腹胀、便溏等肝脾及肝胃、肝胆失调的证候,这种情况在妇科也是常见的。由于肝的经脉经过乳头、少腹、阴部等部位,因此,肝气的疏泄和肝血旺盛,与乳汁的通调和阴部的滋养等也有密切关联。

conditions of liver blood are closely related to states of lactation and the nourishment of the genitals.

The spleen and the stomach function to transform food and transport cereal nutrients, known as the postnatal base of life and the source of qi and blood. Menstruation, nourishment of the fetus and production of milk all depend on the spleen and stomach to transform and transport cereal nutrients to nourish qi and blood. The spleen also controls blood to flow inside the vessels. Normal functions of the spleen ensure normal production, transportation and command of blood which are key to menstruation, pregnancy, delivery and breast-feeding.

The spleen also governs the distribution of body fluid and transformation of water and dampness. Normal functions of the spleen will maintain normal distribution and conveyance of body fluid which ensure constant production of leukorrhea and lubrication of the vagina. On the contrary, dysfunction of the spleen affects the distribution and conveyance of body fluid, leading to the production of phlegm due to accumulation of fluid and leukorrhagia due to infusion of fluid into the conception and belt vessels.

The stomach, a fu organ characterized by sufficient qi and blood, governs reception and digestion of food and manages blood and qi production with the spleen. The stomach meridian moves downward to meet with the thoroughfare vessel at Qijie. Only when food and water in the stomach is sufficient can blood in the thoroughfare vessel and uterus be full enough to produce menstruation. Since the stomach meridian distributes downwards through the middle line of breast, the stomach influences the production of milk. So only when stomach qi is sufficient can blood and qi be abundant and the production of milk be

脾(胃)　脾主运化水谷,输布精微,为后天之本,气血生化之源。经之所以能行,胎之所以得养,乳之所以生化,无不赖脾之运化水谷,滋养气血的功能。脾又主统血摄血,血能正常运行于脉内,而不致流散,赖脾气之统摄。脾气健运,则血的生化、运行、统摄有常,而这正是女性月经、胎产、哺乳等生理变化所必需的条件。

脾还主输布津液,运化水湿。如脾气健运,则津液输布正常,而能营养肌肉,濡泽皮肤,活络关节,泽润孔窍,保证女性白带的津津常润,同时也起到滑泽阴道的作用。反之,脾失健运,则津液失于输布,聚而为湿为痰;下注任带,则发为带下病证。

胃主受纳腐熟水谷,为水谷之海,与脾同司气血生化之源,又为多气多血之腑。足阳明经下行,与冲脉会于气街,故有“冲脉隶于阳明”之说,胃中水谷盛,则冲脉之血亦盛,血海满盈,月事以时下。因此,胃在月经的正常来潮上也有重要的作用。而且,胃的经脉在胸部经乳中线下行,故乳房属胃所司,乳汁的分泌与胃

constant.

Both the heart and the lung are located in the upper energizer, the former controls blood and the latter governs qi, both playing an important role in the transportation, circulation and regulation of blood. Menstruation, pregnancy, delivery and lactation in women are all related to qi and blood. The heart governs blood and vessels, the propelling of which depends on heart qi. Sufficiency of heart blood and smooth circulation of heart qi will enable blood to flow into the uterus to produce menstruation. The lung governs qi, connecting with all vessels and distributing cereal nutrients down to the uterus to influence menstruation. The heart governs the mind, the liver manages strategy, the spleen controls contemplation and the kidney stores conscience. Such mental activities also play an role in the regulation of menstrution.

Apart from direct influence on menstruation, leukorrhea, fetus and delivery, the kidney, liver, spleen, heart and lung are also connected with the twelve meridians through the relations of the meridians with zang and fu organs, uniting the viscera, qi, blood and meridians into an integrity to maintain and regulate the physiological functions of woman.

1.1.1.5.2　Qi and blood

Blood is the essential base of life for woman because menstruation is transformed from blood, fetus depends on blood to nourish and milk relies on blood to produce. As to the relation between qi and blood, blood depends on qi to

气的作用也有密切关系。胃气充盛,则气血充足,乳汁分泌旺盛。

心与肺　心肺同居上焦,一主血,一主气,在血的输布、运行、调节方面均有重要作用。妇女的经、孕、产、乳,无不与气血相关。心主血,其充在血脉,也就是说,心有推动血液在经脉内运行的作用。而心的这种功能全赖心气,若心血旺盛,心气宣通,血脉流畅,则月事如常。肺主气,居上焦,朝百脉而输精微,如雾露之溉,下达胞宫而参与月经的生理活动。

此外,由于心主神明,肝主谋虑,脾主思虑,肾主藏志,这些脏腑功能及其精神活动的正常与否,对月经的调节也有至关重要的影响。

肾、肝、脾、心、肺五脏,除了与经、带、胎、产有直接作用外,还通过其生克制化的联系,互相依存、互相制约,并借助于经络系统的广泛联系,使脏腑、气血、经络构成一个有机的整体,共同维持和调节女性的生理功能。

(二) 气血

女性以血为本,月经为血所化生,妊娠需血以养胎,胎儿娩出后,血化为乳,以供养婴儿。可见血在经、孕、产、乳

produce, circulate and control, while qi relies on blood to nourish and protect. That is why it is said that qi is the commander of blood and blood is the mother of qi.

1.1.1.5.3 Meridians

Meridians refer to the routes along which qi and blood flow. The meridians that are closely related to the physiological activities of woman are the thoroughfare, conception, governor and belt vessels in the eight extraordinary vessels. The functions of the extraordinary vessels in the human body are to store the qi and blood transported by the twelve meridians and to send out qi and blood for the nourishment of the twelve meridians and viscera. Among the thoroughfare, conception, governor and belt vessels, the thoroughfare and conception vessels are most important in the physiological functions of the reproductive system of women.

The thoroughfare vessel originates from the uterus and moves together with the kidney meridian to the lower abdomen and upward along the navel. It is the region where qi and blood converge, that is why it is called "sea of the twelve meridians", "sea of blood" and "sea of five zang and six fu organs". When woman is well developed, the thoroughfare vessel will be abundant in content and qi and blood from the viscera will flow into the uterus to produce menstruation. The thoroughfare vessel moves upward to connect with the stomach meridian at Qichong(ST 30). So it also governs the production of milk. It is obvious that the thoroughfare vessel is closely related to menstruation, pregnancy and lactation in woman.

方面均有重要的作用。血依赖气的生化、运行和统摄，气依靠血的滋养和固护，二者相互依存，不可分离，故有气为血帅，血为气母之说。

（三）经络

经络又称经脉，是运行气血的通路。人体的经络，由正经、奇经、经别、络脉、经筋等构成，其中与女性生理有密切联系的，是奇经中的冲、任、督、带四脉。

冲、任、督、带是奇经八脉的重要组成部分。奇经在人体的作用，既能贮存十二经脉所运行的气血，又能随时加以调节，以供十二经脉和脏腑活动之需。而冲、任、督、带四脉，与女性生殖功能有密切关系，其中又以冲任二脉最为重要。

冲脉　起于胞中，并足少阴肾经，经下腹部，夹脐上行，为十二经气血汇聚之所，故被称之为"十二经之海"、"血海"，又称为"五脏六腑之海"。女性在身体发育成熟后，冲脉太盛，脏腑气血下注血海，血海满溢而为月经。冲脉上行出于足阳明经的气冲穴，与胃的经脉相通，同司乳汁的生化。因此，冲脉在女性的生理中，与月经、妊娠、乳汁等均有密切关系。

The conception vessel starts from the uterus, moving out from perineum and upward along the middle line of abdomen to connect with all yin meridians. The conception vessel governs essence, blood and body fluid. It is the base of pregnancy. That is why it governs pregnancy. The smooth circulation of qi and blood in the conception vessel, in combination with the thoroughfare vessel, is responsible for menstruation and pregnancy.

The governor vessel also starts from the uterus, moving out from the perineum and posteriorly upward along the middle line of the spine to the vertex. It is connected with the spinal cord, brain and all yang meridians. So it is called "the sea of yang meridians". Its branch moves anteriorly and posteriorly from the genitals. The anterior branch is connected with the conception vessel from Changqiang (GV 1) point and the posterior branch is connected with the kidney meridian at the end of sacrum and continues to move upward in the spine. The thoroughfare, conception and governor vessels all start from the uterus, the thoroughfare vessel is the sea of blood and the conception vessel governs uterus and fetus. The governor vessel controls all yang meridians and the conception vessel controls all yin meridians. The balance of yin and yang as well as smooth circulation of qi and blood together maintain normal conditions of menstruation, pregnancy, delivery and lactation.

The belt vessel starts from the hypochondria and moves around the waist like a belt. Its function is to control the meridians moving upward and downward so as to strengthen the connections of meridians. It is significantly related to the thoroughfare, conception and governor vessels which all start from the uterus, together constituting a system in direct relation with the physiological functions

任脉　与冲脉同起于胞中,出于会阴,上至前阴沿腹部正中线上行,在循行过程中与各阴经相联系,为阴脉之总纲,故称"阴脉之海"。人体的精、血、津、液,都属任脉总司,又为妊养之本,故主胎孕。任脉通畅,与冲脉相协同,能导致月经来潮和受孕育胎。

督脉　亦起于胞中,出于会阴,向后循脊柱正中线上行,至巅顶。在循行过程中,与脊髓、脑和各阳经经脉相联系,是阳经经脉的总纲,因此又称"阳脉之海"。其别络循阴器而分行前后,其前行者自长强走任脉与任脉并,其后行者在骶首端与少阴会,并脊里上行,其气通于肾。冲、任、督三脉皆起于胞中,冲为血海,任主胞胎,督司诸阳,任司诸阴,阴阳平衡,气血调畅,共同维持月经、妊孕、分娩、乳汁的正常。

带脉　起于季胁之端,环绕腰部一周,如带束腰状,故称为带脉。它的作用是约束全身上走下行的经脉,加强经脉间的联系。其中与冲、任、督三脉的联系更为密切。带脉与冲、任、督三脉相通,而三

of woman. Such a system, in cooperation with the activities of the viscera, not only influences menstruation and pregnancy, but also plays an important role in leukorrhea and lactation.

脉皆出于胞中,这样就使冲、任、督、带四脉共同构成与女性生理功能有直接关系的一个系统。这个系统与脏腑相合,协调作用,不仅对月经、胎孕有直接关系,同时在带下、乳汁等方面也起到重要作用。

1.1.2 Pathological characteristics

1.1.2.1 Cause of disease

TCM believes that the pathogenic factors include six exogenous pathogenic factors, seven emotions, improper diet, overstrain, excessive sexual intercourse, incised wound and wound due to insects and animals attack. The pathogenic factors responsible for woman diseases are also included in the factors mentioned above. Among these pathogenic factors, some are very easy to cause gynecological diseases.

1.1.2.1.1 Six exogenous pathogenic factors

Wind, cold, summer-heat, dampness, dryness and fire are the normal climatic changes in the four seasons. If they are excessive, insufficient or appear in the season that they should not exist, they become exogenous pathogenic factors. In gynecology, cold, heat and dampness frequently lead to woman diseases.

Cold is either exogenous or endogenous. Exogenous cold, one of the six exogenous pathogenic factors, pertains to yin and tends to contract and coagulate by nature, often affecting the circulation of qi and blood. In gynecological diseases, the attack by cold is usually due to sudden

第二节 病理特点

一、病因

中医学认为,致病因素不外六淫、七情、饮食、劳倦、房室、金刃、虫兽等。妇科疾病的致病因素亦包括在此范围,但也有一定的特点,即某些致病因素极其容易引起妇科疾病。

(一)外感六淫

风、寒、暑、湿、燥、火称为六气,是指自然界一年四季的正常气候变化。如太过、不及或不应时而见,就形成了外感致病因素,称为"六淫"。在妇科病的致病因素中,以寒、热、湿为常见。

寒 亦有外寒、内寒之分。外寒为六淫之一,属于阴邪,性主收引凝滞,易伤阳气而影响气血的运行。在妇科病中感寒的诱因,多由经期、

catching of wind and rain during menstruation and after delivery or due to work in cold water or excessive intake of uncooked and cold food, leading to invasion of cold into the body. The invasion of cold will stagnate qi and blood as well as impair the thoroughfare and conception vessels, resulting in delayed menstruation, scanty menstruation, dysmenorrhea, amenorrhea and abdominal mass, etc. Endogenous cold is usually caused by weakness of the body and asthenia of spleen and kidney yang which fail to warm the viscera and lead to insufficiency and unsmooth circulation of qi and blood.

Heat is either exogenous or endogenous. Exogenous heat means exogenous pathogenic heat and fire. Heat, fire and summer-heat are of the same nature. Heat pertains to yang pathogenic factors and tends to develop upwards, accelerating the circulation of blood. If pathogenic heat impairs blood and drives blood to flow abnormally, the thoroughfare and conception vessels will be weakened, leading to such problems like early menstruation, profuse menorrhea, metrorrhagia and metrostaxis, reddish leukorrhea, uterine bleeding during pregnancy and lochiorrhea. Endogenous heat is usually caused by excessive intake of hot or pungent foods, or by yin asthenia and blood heat that drive blood to flow abnormally and damage the thoroughfare and conception vessels, resulting in the symptoms mentioned above.

Dampness is a pathogenic factor of yin nature. It is heavy, turbid, greasy and stagnant by nature, tending to stagnate qi. Dampness is caused by attack of exogenous pathogenic dampness or asthenia of spleen and kidney yang which fails to transform and transport water and dampness. Since dampness is stagnant, it is difficult to be eliminated. Dampness tends to mix up with other pathogenic factors. It may mix up with heat or transform into

产后骤遇风雨,或在冷水中作业,或过食生冷寒凉,致寒邪乘虚入侵,凝滞气血,损伤冲任,则可发生月经后期、经量过少、痛经、闭经、癥瘕等病。内寒多因素体虚弱,脾肾阳虚,不能温养脏腑,使气血不足,运行不畅,亦可出现以上病症。

热 亦分外热和内热。外热即外感火热之邪。热、火、暑是同一属性的。热为阳邪,其性炎上,易使血流加速。若热邪伤血,迫血妄行,使冲任不固,可引起月经先期、经量过多、崩漏、赤白带下、胎漏、恶露不绝等。内热多由过食辛热或辛辣之品,或阴虚血热所致,均可迫血妄行,损伤冲任而发病。

湿 湿为阴邪,其性重浊腻滞,易于阻滞气机。可由外感湿邪或因脾肾阳虚,不能运化水湿而成。由于湿性濡滞,常致缠绵不已;湿邪亦易与他邪相合,如与热相并,或郁而化热,则为湿热;与寒相结,则为寒湿;湿聚生痰,则为痰湿,

heat due to stagnation, leading to damp-heat; it may mix up with cold and produce cold-dampness; it may accumulate into phlegm and cause phlegm-dampness. If damp-heat attacks qi and blood or damages the thoroughfare and conception vessels, it will lead to profuse menorrhea, metrorrhagia and metrostaxis as well as lochiorrhea; when it attacks the conception and belt vessels or the liver meridian, it may lead to leukorrhagia and pudendal pruritus. If cold-dampness attacks the thoroughfare and conception vessels, it stagnates qi and blood, leading to dysmenorrhea, amenorrhea and sterility. When phlegm-dampness stagnates in the thoroughfare and conception vessels, it may lead to amenorrhea, leukorrhea and sterility, etc.

Wind is the leading factor in causing diseases. Wind is either endogenous or exogenous. Exogenous wind, one of the six exogenous pathogenic factors, often combines with other pathogenic factors to cause diseases, such as wind-cold and wind-heat. Wind pertains to yang and tends to change. In gynecology, wind often mixes up with cold to damage the thoroughfare and conception vessels and causes various diseases. Clinically gynecological diseases due to wind and cold attacking qi and blood as well as damaging the thoroughfare and conception vessels are also commonly encountered. Endogenous wind refers to a series of symptoms during the course of a disease, such as tremor of limbs, convulsion, dizziness, distorted face, coma and abnormal sensation of skin that are caused by dysfunction of the viscera, adverse flow of qi and blood or deficiency of liver blood. Such symptoms are known as interior disturbance of liver wind, interior stirring of wind or generation of wind due to blood asthenia. The problems caused by endogenous are dizziness during pregnancy, premonitory signs of eclampsia gravidarum and eclampsia gravidarum as well as numbness of limbs and formication

如湿热搏于气血或伤于冲任，则可发生月经过多、崩漏、恶露不绝；伤于任带或肝经，则可发生带下、阴痒。寒湿伤及冲任，凝滞气血，可导致痛经、闭经、不孕。痰湿阻滞冲任，则引起闭经、带下、不孕等症。

其他如风，乃为百病之长，有外风和内风之分。外风指风邪，为六淫之一，常与其他病邪结合而致病，如风寒、风热等。风邪在妇科致病，常与寒邪相合，损伤冲任而为病。临床上由于风寒搏于气血，损伤冲任，引起的妇科病亦属常见。内风，是指病变中出现的肢体振颤、抽搐、眩晕、口眼㖞斜、昏厥以及皮肤感觉异常等一类证候，是疾病发展过程中脏腑功能失调、气血逆乱或肝血亏虚所引起，称为肝风内动、风气内动或血虚生风。妊娠眩晕、先兆子痫和子痫、经绝期诸证出现的肢体发麻、皮肤蚁行感、阴痒等，就是由内风而引起。

over skin and pudendal pruritus during menopause.

1.1.2.1.2　Damage by seven emotional factors

Seven emotions refer to joy, anger, anxiety, contemplation, sorrow, fright and terror, excessive changes of which may lead to imbalance of yin and yang, disharmony between qi and blood as well as dysfunction of the viscera. In clinical treatment, hematemesis, hemorrhage and dizziness during pregnancy are commonly encountered. These problems are usually caused by blood circulating upward with the adverse flow of liver due to impairment of the liver by rage. Excessive contemplation impairs the spleen. If spleen qi is stagnated, transformation and transportation cannot be properly carried out, leading to insufficiency of transformation and deficiency of blood in the uterus, consequently resulting in delayed menstruation, scanty menstruation and amenorrhea.

1.1.2.1.3　Intemperance in life

Apart from the seven emotional factors, gynecological diseases may be caused by intemperance in life which affects the normal functions of the viscera, the thoroughfare and conception vessels as well as qi and blood. The following are some of the most commonly encountered ones.

Improper habit in taking food: Excessive intake of pungent, hot and yang-invigorating foods accumulates heat in the thoroughfare and conception vessels and drives blood to flow abnormally, leading to profuse menstruation, metrorrhagia and metrostaxis. Excessive intake of cold foods may coagulate blood or impair spleen yang, accumulate dampness into phlegm and obstruct the thoroughfare and conception vessels, resulting in dysmenorrhea, amenorrhea and leukorrhagia. Crapulence or hunger or partiality to certain kind of food may damage the viscera and lead to disorder of qi and blood as well as disturbance

（二）内伤七情

七情是指因喜、怒、忧、思、悲、恐、惊等精神情绪变化的刺激,可引起人体阴阳失调、气血不和、脏腑功能失常而发生疾病。其特点是易伤于气、影响脏腑功能。此外,在临床上亦常见因郁怒伤肝,肝气上逆,血随气上行发生经行吐衄,妊娠眩晕。因思虑伤脾,脾气结而不行,使运化失常,化源不足,血海不得充盈,引起月经后期、量过少、闭经等病症。

（三）生活失慎

妇科疾病除了由外感和内伤因素所致外,还与生活失慎等因素有关,从而导致脏腑、冲任的紊乱,招致疾病发生。常见者有以下几种:

饮食不慎　饮食的过冷过热、过饥过饱、择食偏嗜,都会损伤脾胃、气血而引起疾病。如过食辛热助阳之品,可使冲任蕴热,迫血妄行导致月经过多、崩漏等。过食寒凉,或使血为寒凝,或使脾阳受损,聚湿生痰,冲任受阻,而发生痛经、闭经、白带等。过饥过饱,择食偏嗜,使脏腑受损,气血失调,冲任功能紊乱,亦

of the thoroughfare and conception vessels which further lead to gynecological diseases.

Uneven allocation of work：Proper physical work is helpful for strengthening constitution and preventing diseases. However, woman should be careful about the allocation of work during menstruation, pregnancy and breast-feeding, avoiding heavy physical work lest profuse menstruation, metrorrhagia and metrostaxis, abortion, premature labor and prolapse of the uterus be caused. So during menstruation, pregnancy and breast-feeding, woman should properly rest but also take appropriate activities, because excessive rest affects the circulation of qi and blood and gives rise to the occurrence of various diseases. And therefore to do some proper physical work is beneficial to health.

Multiparity and excessive coitus：Frequent delivery or sexual activity during menstruation or after delivery tends to consume qi and blood, impair the liver and kidney as well as damage the thoroughfare and conception vessels, consequently leading to menstruation disorder, leukorrhea problems, abortion, premature delivery and prolapse of uterus. Early marriage and multiparity not only impairs the physique of gravida, but also affects the development of fetus. So proper sexual life and family planning are important measures for preventing woman disease.

The factors mentioned above are just one part of the causes of woman disease. The onset of woman disease also lies in the conditions of healthy qi in the body. Physical training and increasing of health level are key to the prevention of diseases.

1.1.2.2 Pathogenesis

Menstruation, pregnancy, delivery, childfeeding and

能造成妇科疾病。

劳逸失常 适当的体力劳动,对增强体质,防治疾病是必要的。由于妇女有经、孕、产、乳等生理特点,在此期间便应注意劳逸结合,避免过重的体力劳动,防止发生月经过多、崩漏、流产、早产、子宫脱垂等疾病。经、孕、产、乳期间,应注意适当的休息,但也要有一定的活动,不可过逸,过逸则气血运行不畅,也易产生疾病。因此,在不影响健康的情况下,参加一定的劳动,对身体是有益的。

多产房劳 妇女生育过多、过频,或经期产后不禁性生活,易耗伤气血,伤及肝肾,损伤冲任,是引起月经病、带下病、流产、早产、子宫脱垂等的原因之一。特别是早婚、多产,不仅影响产妇的体质,而且影响下一代的健康成长。所以,适度、适时地过好性生活,节制产育,也是预防妇产科病的重要措施。

二、病机

女性的经、孕、产、乳、带,

leukorrhea are all related to the viscera and meridians. Thus, visceral dysfunction, disorder of qi and blood, as well as damage to the thoroughfare vessel, conception vessel, governor vessel and belt vessel due to invasion of pathogenic factors may all lead to gynecological disease.

1.1.2.2.1 Dysfunction of the viscera

Blood, essential to the health of woman, is transformed by the spleen and stomach, governed by the heart, stored in the liver and distributed by the lung to the whole body. The disorder of one viscus or the attack of any pathogenic factors on the viscera may lead to woman disease.

The kidney is essential to life, the base of primordial qi and connected with the uterine collaterals. Insufficiency of kidney qi or asthenia of kidney yin or declination of kidney yang inevitably leads to woman disease. Deficiency of kidney yin and asthenia of both essence and blood cause delayed menstruation, scanty menstruation or amenorrhea. Relative hyperactivity of asthenia fire in the kidney will drive blood to flow abnormally, eventually resulting in early menstruation, profuse menstruation, metrorrhagia and metrostaxis, uterine bleeding during pregnancy and restless movement of fetus. Blood dryness due to heat may bring about amenorrhea. Insufficiency of kidney yang will lead to interior exuberance of cold, giving rise to sterility, leukorrhagia, abortion and premature delivery, etc.

The liver prefers free action and detests depression. Liver depression and qi stagnation may lead to delayed menstruation, irregular menstruation, dysmenorrhea, amenorrhea and various symptoms before menstruation. Deficiency of liver yin and hyperactivity of liver yang generate endogenous wind and lead to premonitory signs of eclampsia gravidarum or eclampsia gravidarum. Impairment of the liver may drive liver qi to flow adversely

与脏腑、经络相关。因此,致病因素的侵袭而导致脏腑功能的失常,气血的失调,或冲、任、督、带的损伤,都可以发生妇科疾病。

(一)脏腑功能失常

女性以血为本。血生化于脾胃,总属于心,藏受于肝,宣布于肺,施泄于肾。如某一脏或腑的功能失常,或某种病因素影响脏腑功能,都可以引起妇科疾病。

肾为生命之本,元气之根,胞脉又系于肾。如肾气不足,或肾阴亏损,或肾阳衰微,均能影响冲任而发生妇科疾病。肾阴不足,精血双亏,则可导致月经后期、经量过少或闭经;或虚火偏亢,热迫血行,可导致月经先期、经量过多、崩漏、胎漏和胎动不安等病;热灼血枯,又可引起闭经。肾阳不足,阴寒内盛,可导致不孕、带下、流产、早产等妊娠疾病。

肝性喜条达而恶抑郁。如肝郁气结,可发生月经后期、月经先后无定期、痛经、闭经、经前期诸证等;肝阴不足,肝阳偏亢,肝风内动,可引起先兆子痫和子痫;怒气伤肝,肝气上逆,血随气逆,可发生经行吐衄;肝气犯胃,胃失和

upward and lead to hematemesis and epistaxis. Attack of liver qi on the stomach may bring about morning sickness.

The spleen (stomach) is the source of transformation and commands blood. Impairment of the spleen and stomach may result in delayed menstruation, scanty menstruation, amenorrhea, sterility and hypogalactia. Asthenia of spleen qi may cause abnormal circulation of blood and lead to profuse menstruation and metrorrhagia and metrostaxis. Sinking of gastrosplenic qi may result in prolapse of the uterus. Failure of spleen yang to transport cereal nutrients may give rise to dampness accumulation, fluid retention, production of phlegm and downward migration of dampness which, in turn, lead to leukorrhagia. Retention of fluid in the muscular interstices causes edema during pregnancy. Accumulation of dampness into phlegm obstructs the thoroughfare and conception vessels and leads to amenorrhea and sterility.

Besides, the heart governs blood and the lung governs qi. Overstrain of the heart may lead to deficiency of heart yin, hyperactivity of heart fire and consumption of blood by fire and heat, eventually resulting in amenorrhea. Asthenia of pulmonary qi or obstruction of pulmonary qi affects blood circulation and causes amenorrhea.

Since there exist relations of mutual promotion, restraint and dependence among the viscera, the disorder of one viscus may involve the others. For example, liver is being promoted by the kidney, so kidney disease may involve the liver. Similarly the kidney is being promoted by the lung, the disorder of the lung will involve the kidney, leading to disorder simultaneously involving the liver and kidney as well as the lung and kidney. Besides, there exists a mutual promoting relationship between yin and yang among the zangfu-organs. Because of such a relationship, the disorder of one zang-organ or fu-organ may

降，可引起妊娠恶阻。

脾（胃），为生化之源，又主统血。脾胃损伤，化源不足，可导致月经后期、经量过少、闭经、不孕、乳汁缺乏等病症；脾气虚弱，统摄无权，致使血不循经，则可发生月经过多、崩漏等病；中气下陷，则可发生子宫脱垂；脾阳不运，不能输布精微，则聚湿、停水、生痰；湿邪下注任带，则可发生带下；水停肌腠，可发生妊娠水肿；湿聚生痰，阻滞冲任，则可导致闭经、不孕等病症。

此外，心主血，如因劳心过度，致心阴不足，心火偏亢，火热耗血，可致闭经。肺主气，贯心脉而运血。如肺气虚损，或气不宣通，亦能影响血的运行而致闭经。

由于脏腑之间有五行生克制化的相互依存、相互制约的关系，因而在某一脏或腑受病时，由于这种联系而相互影响。例如，因肝为肾之子，肾病可以通过相生的关系而影响到肝；同样，肾为肺之子，肺病亦可以通过相生的关系而影响肾，形成肝肾、肺肾同病。此外，脏腑之间还有阴阳水火相承相济的关系，也可在某脏

affect the other. For example, failure of kidney-yang to warm spleen-yang and failure of kidney-yin to coordinate with heart-yin may result in simultaneous disorder of the spleen and kidney as well as the heart and kidney. The disorders of viscera caused by other individual organs also follow such an order. Such an interaction among the viscera is different in principal and secondary symptoms, so the pathological conditions may vary from one disease to another.

Apart from the influence of mutual promotion and restraint among the viscera, visceral dysfunction may gradually transmit and change during the course of a disease. For example, improper diet, overstrain or impairment of the spleen by excessive contemplation may affect the functions of transformation, transportation and distribution of the spleen, leading to abdominal fullness, epigastric distress, loose stool and severe palpitation followed by poor appetite, asthenia of both the spleen and stomach, insufficiency of transformation and emptiness of the uterus, eventually resulting in amenorrhea. Asthenia of both the spleen and stomach and lack of proper moistening and nutrition in the lung will bring about cough, dyspnea and shortness of breath. If the lung fails to nourish the kidney due to asthenia and causes exhaustion of qi in the upper and loss of essence in the lower, the pathological condition will be critical. The disorder or dysfunction of any viscus will consequently result in abnormal changes in menstruation, leukorrhea, pregnancy and delivery. However, the disorder or dysfunction of viscera that is most likely to cause woman disease is that of the kidney, heart, liver or spleen.

1.1.2.2.2　Disorder of qi and blood

Blood is essential to woman and is easy to be consumed by menstruation, pregnancy, delivery and breast-feeding, eventually leading to relative hyperactivity of qi due to deficiency of blood. So the invasion of pathogenic

或腑受病时，由于这种联系而相互影响。如脾可因肾阳不温脾阳、心可因肾阴不得上济心阴而为脾肾、心肾同病。其余各脏均可以此类推。当然，这种影响还有着标本缓急的不同，其具体病理则根据有关病症而有不同的情况。

脏腑功能失常，除因生克制化关系可以并病之外，还能在发病过程中逐步传变。例如，饮食劳倦或忧思伤脾，使运化、输布功能失常，始则腹满便溏，食少脘闷，继则心悸怔忡，脾胃俱虚，化源不足，血海无余，则月经不行；脾胃皆虚，肺失滋养，则咳嗽、喘息、短气；肺虚不能养肾，气竭于上，精亏于下，病则危险。任何一脏或一腑的功能失常，最终都有可能造成经、带、孕、产的病态，但是关系密切，最易或较常导致妇科疾患的是肾、心、肝、脾脏的功能失常，千万不可忽视。

（二）气血失调

女性以血为本，经、孕、产、乳期间又极易于耗血，致使其处于血不足而气偏盛的状态。因此一旦遭受病邪的

factors is likely to affect qi and blood and cause disease. For example, invasion of exogenous pathogenic heat or excessive intake of pungent and hot foods tends to generate heat, the struggle between heat and blood drives blood to flow abnormally and lead to such problems like early menstruation, profuse menstruation, metrorrhagia and metrostaxis, hematemesis and epistaxis during menstruation, abortion and puerperal fever. Invasion of exogenous pathogenic cold or excessive intake of cold and uncooked foods generates cold, the struggle between cold and blood coagulates blood and leads to delayed menstruation, dysmenorrhea, amenorrhea, puerperal abdominal pain, abdominal mass and sterility, etc. Invasion of exogenous pathogenic dampness, or dampness due to spleen asthenia, accumulation of dampness into phlegm and struggle between damp-heat and blood in the meridians and vessels may bring about leukorrhagia, amenorrhea and sterility, etc. Transformation of heat from dampness stagnation and struggle between accumulating damp-heat and blood may result in profuse menstruation, yellowish vaginal discharge and multi-colored vaginal discharge. Dampness accumulation and fluid retention in the muscular interstices may cause edema during menstruation. Besides, blood asthenia due to prolonged duration of disease, dysfunction of the viscera and insufficiency of transformation may give rise to delayed menstruation, scanty menstruation, dysmenorrhea, amenorrhea, sterility and hypogalactia, etc.

Other factors responsible for profuse menstruation, metrorrhagia and metrostaxis as well as hematemesis and epistaxis are consumption of qi by pathogenic heat and abnormal flow of blood due to leakage of qi caused by heat. Invasion of pathogenic cold stagnates qi and blood, consequently leading to oligomenorrhea, dysmenorrhea and amenorrhea. Invasion of pathogenic dampness prevents qi

侵袭,气血容易受损而为病,如外感热邪或过食辛热容易生热,热搏于血,迫血妄行,可致月经先期、经量过多、崩漏、经行吐衄、流产、产后发热等。外感寒邪或过食生冷寒凉,寒搏于血,血为寒凝,运行不畅,可致月经后期、痛经、闭经、产后腹痛、癥瘕、不孕等。外感湿邪,或脾虚生湿,湿聚生痰,湿痰与血相结,阻滞经脉,可为白带、闭经、不孕等;或湿郁化热,湿热蕴结,与血相搏,可致月经过多、黄带、赤白带;湿聚水停,浸渍肌腠,可致妊娠水肿。另外,久病或多产伤血,或脏腑功能失常,生化之源不足而致血虚,可引起月经后期、经量过少、痛经、闭经、不孕、乳汁缺乏等,都是血分病变所常见的。

其他如热邪伤气,热则气泄,气泄则血亦随之而泄,可致月经过多、崩漏、经行吐衄。寒邪伤气,寒则气收,气收则闭而不通,血亦随之阻滞,可致月经量少、痛经、闭经。湿邪伤气,阻滞气机,亦可致妊

from normal flowing and results in swelling and distension during pregnancy.

The manifestations caused by seven emotional factors are upward flow of qi, slack flow of qi, exhaustion of qi, sinking of qi, disorder of qi, stagnation of qi and consumption of qi which impair the viscera and cause various woman diseases. Qi commands and controls blood. Consumption of qi due to prolonged illness or overstrain will make it unable to command and control blood, leading to profuse menstruation, early menstruation, metrorrhagia and metrostaxis as well as abortion. Sinking of qi usually fails to hold the viscera in the original location e. g. the prolapse of the uterus.

1.1.2.2.3 Impairment of the thoroughfare, conception, governor and belt vessels

Impairment of the thoroughfare, conception and governor vessels is the main pathological change in gynecological diseases. The thoroughfare vessel is the sea of blood and is closely related to menstruation. The conception vessel is responsible for providing nutrition during pregnancy and is closely related to pregnancy. The governor vessel governs yang and is connected with the conception vessel. Altogether they maintain a relative balance between yin and yang and are responsible for pregnancy. The belt vessel manages all the meridians and regulates the reproductive system together with the thoroughfare, conception and governor vessels. The disorder of the thoroughfare vessel may lead to irregular menstruation, metrorrhagia and metrostaxis, amenorrhea and abortion; the disorder of the conception vessel may result in leukorrhagia due to downward migration of fluid, sterility due to malnutrition during pregnancy and abdominal mass due to stagnation of qi and blood; the disorder of the governor vessel may affect the function of yang-qi and cause sterili-

娠肿胀等。

七情所伤,常导致气上、气缓、气消、气下、气乱、气结、气耗等病变,如损伤脏腑功能,亦可引起妇科疾病。气又能帅血、摄血。如久病或劳倦伤气,以致气虚不能摄血,可致月经过多、月经提前、崩漏、流产;如气虚下陷,不能升举内在脏器,亦可见子宫脱垂等病症。

(三) 冲、任、督、带损伤

冲、任、督、带的损伤,是妇科病的主要病理变化,冲为血海,与月经密切相关。任主妊养,与孕育密切相关。督司诸阳,与任脉循环往复,共同维持脉气阴阳的相对平衡,与孕育亦有关系。带脉约束诸脉,与冲、任、督共同调节生殖系统的功能。冲脉受病,血海蓄溢失常,可发生月经失调、崩漏、闭经、流产等。任脉受病,或致阴液不固而为带下,或妊养失司而为不孕,或气血积滞而为癥瘕。督脉为病,阳气失调,可致不孕。带脉为病,约束无权,可致带下、子宫脱垂等。导致这些经脉损伤的原因,可为间接损伤,也可为直接损伤。

ty; the disorder of the belt vessel may bring about leukorrhagia and prolapse of the uterus. The impairment of
these meridians and vessels may be direct or indirect.

Indirect impairment is caused by disorder of the viscera, qi or blood. For example, insufficiency of kidney qi
and deficiency of the thoroughfare vessel may lead to primary amenorrhea; migration of dampness due to spleen
asthenia into the conception and belt vessels may result in
leukorrhea and pudendal pruritus; weakness of the thoroughfare and conception vessels due to qi asthenia and
sinking may bring about profuse menstruation, metrorrhagia and metrostaxis as well as prolapse of the uterus; abnormal flow of blood due to heat and weakness of the thoroughfare and conception vessels may cause profuse menstruation, metrorrhagia and metrostaxis, etc.

Improper sterilization during delivery, abortion and
vaginal operation, or lack of proper care or sexual activity
during menstruation and after delivery may lead to invasion of pathogenic factors into the uterus and result in
such problems like irregular menstruation, dysmenorrhea,
puerperal fever, lochiorrhea, leukorrhea, abdominal mass
and sterility which can be regarded as the direct impairment of the thoroughfare and conception vessels. Generally speaking, only direct or indirect impairment of the
thoroughfare, conception, governor and belt vessels, especially the thoroughfare and conception vessels, can lead
to disorders of menstruation, leukorrhagia, pregnancy and
delivery.

Though the diseases caused by dysfunction of the viscera, disorders of qi and blood as well as impairment of
the thoroughfare, conception, governor and belt vessels
are different in pathogenesis, they also affect each other
in pathology. So in the analysis of diseases, trials must be
made not only in determining which organs or meridians

由脏腑或气血功能失常，
影响冲、任、督、带功能的，为
间接损伤。如肾气未充，冲任
未盛，可致原发性闭经；脾虚
生湿，湿注任带，任带不固，可
致带下、阴痒；气虚下陷，冲任
不固，可致月经过多、崩漏、子
宫脱垂；血热妄行，冲任不固，
可致月经过多、崩漏等病症。

由于分娩、流产或阴道手
术时消毒不严，或经期、产后
不洁，或不禁房事，以致病邪
乘虚侵袭，诸如月经不调、痛
经、产后发热、恶露不尽、带
下、癥瘕、不孕等，均可视为冲
任的直接损伤。一般来说，只
有在直接或间接损伤冲、任、
督、带，特别是损伤冲任两脉
的情况下，才能发生经、带、胎
产等妇女特有的疾病。

脏腑功能失常，气血失
调，冲、任、督、带损伤，虽各有
不同的病机，但它们之间又可
互相影响。因此，无论病变起
于任何经脉、任何脏腑，还是
在气、在血，其病理反应总是

are invaded by pathogenic factors and whether qi or blood is impaired, but also in analyzing the interaction between them. Such a comprehensive analysis is essential to recognizing the nature and taking proper treatment of the disease in question.

有关联的。所以在分析病情的时候,既要了解病邪侵入何经何脉,病变在何脏何腑,是伤气还是伤血,更要了解它们的相互关系,才能从复杂的证候中分清标本传变,抓住实质而进行治疗。

1.2 Diagnostic methods and key points for syndrome differentiation of gynecological diseases

The diagnostic methods and key points for syndrome differentiation of gynecological diseases are, though similar to those of the diseases in internal medicine, unique in some aspects. The general conditions of the patient are studied first with the four diagnostic methods. Then the cause and location of disease, the relation between the pathogenic factors and healthy qi as well as the development and variation of the principal and secondary aspects of disease can be correctly differentiated. The diagnosis and syndrome differentiation in gynecology mainly focus on the aspects of menstruation, leukorrhea, pregnancy and delivery of child.

1.2.1 Diagnostic methods

1.2.1.1 Inquiry

Inquiry in gynecology includes the following aspects:

Inquiry of menstruation: Inquiry of menstruation includes age of menarche, cycle, duration, quantity, color and nature of menstruation; whether there is blood clot and foul odor; whether there are such symptoms like distension and pain in the lower abdomen, waist and sacrum, chest and hypochondria as well as breast before and during

第二章 妇科疾病的中医诊断方法与辨证要点

妇科病的诊断方法一般与内科相同,运用四诊和辨证的方法,但又有一定的特点。总的说来,就是通过四诊掌握疾病的全部症象,然后再运用有关病因、脏腑、气血、经络、病机等概念,结合经、带、胎、产的变化进行分析、判断,寻找出疾病的病因、病位和正邪消长、标本传变等变化,作出正确的诊断。妇科病的四诊和辨证,着重于有关经、带、胎、产的四诊和辨证特点。

第一节 诊断方法

一、问诊

妇科问诊必须包括以下内容。

问月经 应问初潮年龄、周期、经期、经量、经色及经质,有无血块及臭气。经前、经期、经后有无下腹、腰骶、胸胁、乳房作胀或疼痛,有无经期以外的出血,末次月经

menstruation; the date of last menstruation and the date of menstruation before the last period; whether there are dizziness, lassitude, nausea, vomiting and partiality in food as well as distension and pain in the waist, sacrum and lower abdomen in the case of amenorrhea.

Inquiry of leukorrhea: Including quantity, color, thick or thin texture and odor of leukorrhea.

Inquiry of pregnancy and delivery: Inquiry of pregnancy and delivery includes whether there are pregnancy, delivery, abortion (including artificial abortion), times of delivery, the last deliver and abortion date; whether there are dystocia, operation, massive postpartum hemorrhage, lactation after delivery, puerperal fever and abdominal pain as well as the quantity, color, nature and odor of lochia; whether there is contraception and what kind of measures are taken; months or weeks of pregnancy and morning sickness as well as whether there are symptoms of edema, dizziness and headache should be inquired when inquiring a pregnant woman.

1.2.1.2　Inspection

Complexion: Pale or bright-whitish complexion indicates qi asthenia or yang asthenia; sallow complexion indicates blood asthenia or spleen asthenia; grayish complexion or blackish periorbit indicates decline of kidney qi; blackish spots on the forehead, nose bridge and upper lip are known as pregnant macules that are not pathological.

Lips and tongue: Bright-reddish color indicates asthenia heat; light-reddish color indicates blood asthenia; purplish color or petechiae on the tongue indicates blood stasis; and light, tender and blackish color indicates yang asthenia.

的日期,必要时应追询末次以前的一次月经的日期。如系停经,应问停经时间,有无头晕、倦怠、恶心、呕吐、择食等症状以及腰骶、下腹胀痛等伴随症状。

问白带　应问白带的多少、颜色、质清或稠、有无臭气等。

问胎产　已婚妇女,应问是否妊娠、生育、流产(包括人工流产)和分娩次数,末次分娩及流产的日期。有无难产和手术史,有无产后大出血,产后有无乳汁,产后有无发热、腹痛以及恶露的量、色、质、气味等。是否采取避孕措施以及采用何种避孕方法。如是孕妇应问妊娠月份或周数,恶阻情况,有无水肿、头晕、头痛等症状。

二、望诊

面色　苍白或㿠白为气虚或阳虚;萎黄为血虚或脾虚;灰黯或眶黯多为肾气虚衰。妊娠期前额、鼻柱、上唇出现黯色、斑点,称为妊娠斑,不是病态。

唇、舌　色鲜红为虚热,淡红为血虚,紫黯或舌有瘀点为内有瘀血,舌淡胖为阳虚。

Menstruation, leukorrhea and lochia: Cares should be taken to differentiate the changes in the quantity, color and nature.

1.2.1.3   Listening and olfaction

Listening to voice is the same as that in the other clinical specialties. Smelling of odor is mainly for understanding the special odor of menses, leukorrhea and lochia to confirm what the patient has described.

1.2.1.4   Pulse taking

Pulse in woman is usually feebler and softer than that in man, which is normal. In menstruation, leukorrhagia, pregnancy and delivery, there are some special pulse conditions.

1.2.1.4.1   Menstruation pulse

Before or during menstruation, if pulse over the cun region is floating and full or floating and slippery without the symptoms of fever, headache and bitter taste in the mouth, it is normal pulse in menstruation. If the pulse is taut and rapid or slippery, rapid and powerful, it indicates accumulation of heat in the thoroughfare and conception vessels, usually seen in early menstruation, profuse menstruation and metrorrhagia and metrostaxis. Deep and slow or thin and slow pulse indicates interior cold due to yang asthenia and insufficiency of the thoroughfare and conception vessels, usually seen in delayed menstruation and scanty menstruation. Thin and scattered pulse indicates interior heat due to yin asthenia, usually seen in profuse menstruation and dripping vaginal bleeding. Thin and unsmooth pulse indicates asthenia of both the liver and kidney as well as deficiency of essence and blood, often seen in scanty menstruation and dysmenorrhea. Taut and

月经、白带及恶露　应注意量、色、质的改变。

三、闻诊

闻诊包括听声音和嗅气味。听声音与临床各科相同。嗅气味主要是了解月经、白带、恶露的特殊臭气。用以证实患者自述的情况。

四、切诊

女性正常脉通常弱于男性,脉象略沉静而柔软。在经、带、胎、产期间,也有一些常见的特殊脉象。

(一) 月经脉

在月经将来或行经期,出现无身热、头痛、口苦等外感或里热现象,而寸脉浮洪或浮滑,是经期的常脉;如脉见弦数或滑数有力,常为冲任蕴热,可见月经先期、经量过多、崩漏等症;沉迟或细迟,常为阳虚内寒,冲任不足,可见于月经后期、经量过少;脉细而散,多为阴虚内热,可见于月经量多、漏下淋漓;脉细而涩,多为肝肾两虚,精血不足,可见于经量过少、痛经;脉弦而涩,则为气滞血瘀,可见于月经后期或痛经。经闭不行,若证实非孕,脉细而涩,多为血虚不足;脉滑而断续不匀,多

unsmooth pulse indicates qi stagnation and blood stasis, frequently seen in delayed menstruation or dysmenorrhea. Thin and unsmooth pulse in amenorrhea without pregnancy indicates blood asthenia. Slippery and uneven pulse signifies blood sthenia and qi stagnation.

1.2.1.4.2　Leukorrhea pulse

Profuse leukorrhea with taut and slippery or deep and scattered pulse may indicate internal accumulation of damp-heat; slippery and powerful pulse may signify interior retention of phlegm-dampness; deep and slow or weak pulse over the chi region on both hands may suggest insufficiency of kidney yang; soft and slow pulse may be the sign of downward migration of pathogenic dampness due to spleen asthenia.

1.2.1.4.3　Pregnancy pulse

Preference for sour taste and vomiting 2 or 3 months after amenorrhea, accompanied by moderate pulse conditions over the six regions, or with slippery chi pulse or slippery cun pulse, may suggest pregnancy. After pregnancy, deep and thin or short and unsmooth pulse over the six regions or weak pulse over the chi region may indicate deficiency of qi and blood or insufficiency of kidney qi, cares should be taken to prevent abortion.

1.2.1.4.4　Pulse after delivery

The pulse just after delivery is usually short and immediately turning into moderate and smooth due to sudden asthenia of blood and predomination of yang-qi. If the pulse under such a condition is large, or accompanied by fever and headache, it indicates failure of blood to be restored or invasion of exogenous pathogenic factors.

In general, the data collected by using the four diagnostic methods should be comprehensively analyzed in clinical treatment. For some special cases, syndrome differentiation has to be made according to the conditions

为血实气滞。

（二）带下脉

白带过多,脉见弦滑或沉散有力,应考虑湿热内蕴;滑大有力,要注意痰湿内停;两尺沉迟或微弱,当重视肾阳不足;脉濡而缓,需想到脾虚湿邪下注。

（三）妊娠脉

停经二三月,思酸作呕,六脉和缓,或尺脉滑利,或寸脉滑动,则妊娠可能性较大。怀孕以后,六脉沉细或短涩,或尺脉微弱,多为气血亏虚或肾气不足,应防流产。

（四）产后脉

新产之初,因阴血骤虚,阳气偏盛,脉可偏数,但多短暂,后即转为缓和平脉。如反见大数,或兼有身热、头痛,常示阴血未复或感受外邪。

总之,在临证时,通常都应四诊合参,色、脉、证结合起来分析,但个别情况,也不排除舍脉从证或舍证从脉的辨

of the pulse other than the syndrome or vice versa.

1.2.2 Key points for syndrome differentiation

1.2.2.1 Syndrome differentiation of menstruation disorders

In light of the cycle, early menstruation is usually due to blood heat or qi asthenia; delayed menstruation is often due to blood asthenia or blood cold; irregular menstruation is frequently caused by liver stagnation or kidney asthenia; prolonged menstruation is often caused by qi asthenia or blood heat; shortened duration of menstruation is usually caused by blood asthenia or asthenia cold. In light of the quantity, profuse menstruation is usually seen in blood heat or qi asthenia; scanty menstruation is frequently caused by blood asthenia or blood cold. In light of the color, bright reddish or purplish menses is due to heat; blackish menses is due to cold, light-reddish menses is due to asthenia and light-blackish menses like smoke-dust is due to asthenia cold. In light of the texture, thick menses is due to heat and sthenia, thin menses is due to asthenia and cold, and menstruation with blood clot is due to stasis. In light of odor, menstruation with foul odor is due to heat, menstruation without odor indicates cold, menstruation with stinking and foul smell signifies blood stasis and putrefaction. In light of pain, palpable abdominal pain during menstruation is asthenia; unpalpable abdominal pain is sthenia; abdominal pain alleviated with warmth is due to cold; abdominal pain aggravated with warmth is due to heat; pain appearing before or during menstruation is sthenia; pain appearing after menstruation is asthenia;

证分析,而这些都应当在临证时仔细权衡。

第二节　辨证要点

一、月经病的辨证

月经情况,应着重月经的期、量、色、质、气味以及下腹部的胀满或疼痛等来分析。以经期而论,一般周期提前,多为血热或气虚;周期延后,多为血虚或血寒;周期先后无定,多为肝郁或肾虚;经期延长,多为气虚或血热;经期缩短,多为血虚或虚寒。以月经量而论,量多者,以血热或气虚常见;量少者,以血虚或血寒较多。以经色而论,色鲜红或紫红者属热,黯红者属寒,淡红者为虚,黯淡如烟灰色者为虚寒。以月经性状而论,稠粘者属热属实,清稀者属虚属寒,瘀块者属瘀。再如气味臭秽者多热,无臭者多寒,恶臭难闻者属瘀血败浊为患,病多险恶。经期腹痛,喜按为虚,拒按为实;得热痛减为寒,得热反剧为热;痛在经前或经期为实,经后为虚。平时下腹作痛,经期加重多属湿热蕴结,气血瘀滞;经期下腹胀满不舒

frequent lower abdominal pain with aggravation during menstruation is due to accumulation of damp-heat and stagnation of qi and blood; lower abdominal distension and fullness during menstruation is due to qi stagnation.

多属气滞。

1.2.2.2　Syndrome differentiation of leukorrhea disorders

Syndrome differentiation of leukorrhea disorders should be made from the aspects of color, texture and odor of leukorrhea. Usually yellowish and sticky menses indicates sthenia and heat syndromes; whitish and thin menses indicates asthenia and cold syndromes; menstruation with foul odor indicates sthenia-heat; menstruation with stinking odor indicates asthenia-cold; yellowish or yellowish and bluish sticky menses like pus with foul odor is due to accumulation of damp-heat; whitish menstruation like snivel, or accompanied by lassitude or complicated by poor appetite, is due to downward migration of spleen dampness; dripping leukorrhea mingled with blood is due to yin asthenia and intrinsic heat complicated by dampness; profuse and thin menorrhea, or accompanied by lumbago and weakness, is due to insufficiency of kidney yang; grayish, whitish and turbid menses, or mingled with abnormal color and with foul odor, is due to putrid blood and stasis of turbid substance.

1.2.2.3　Syndrome differentiation of pregnant diseases

If woman of childbearing age and normal menstruation has the manifestations of amenorrhea, accompanied by lassitude, preference for sleep, anorexia, food partiality, preference for sour taste, vomiting and slippery pulse, it is probable that she is pregnant. As to vaginal bleeding after pregnancy due to movement of fetus, light-

二、带下病的辨证

带下病的辨证,应从白带的色、质、气味来分析。一般以色黄、稠粘为实证、热证;色白、清稀为虚证、寒证。其气臭秽为实热,其气腥臭为虚寒。如色黄或黄绿如脓,粘稠,有臭秽气味,多属湿热蕴结。色白或状如涕,或伴有精神疲倦,或兼饮食减少,多属脾湿下注。白带夹血,淋漓不净,多属阴虚内热挟湿。清稀量多,或伴腰痛无力,多属肾阳不足。色灰白浑浊,或杂见异色,有恶臭,多属败血瘀浊。

三、妊娠病的辨证

育龄期月经正常的女性出现停经,并伴有倦怠喜睡、厌食择食、思酸作呕、脉滑症状者,应考虑早期妊娠;怀孕后,胎动下血,色淡质清或伴神倦气短或脉弱者,属气血两

colored and thin blood or accompanied by lassitude, shortness of breath or weak pulse is due to asthenia of both qi
and blood; vaginal bleeding accompanied by aching and
weakness of loins and prolapsing sensation in the lower
abdomen is due to kidney asthenia; deep-red blood or accompanied by dysphoria, dry mouth and slippery-rapid
pulse is due to blood heat. Morning sickness, vomiting,
anorexia or slow, slippery and weak pulse are due to asthenia of spleen and stomach qi; vomiting of bitter fluid or
sour fluid, or accompanied by taut and slippery pulse is
due to adverse flow of liver and stomach qi; vomiting of
sputum or saliva, distension or accompanied by soft and
slippery pulse is due to retention of phlegm-dampness in
the middle energizer; edema or lassitude or epigastric distension, or accompanied by deep, slippery and weak
pulse, is due to spleen asthenia; aching in loins and sacrum or aversion to cold as well as deep or slow pulse are
due to insufficiency of kidney yang; dizziness, headache,
blurred vision, chest distress and vomiting in the late
stage of pregnancy are premonitory signs of eclampsia
gravidarum and measures should be taken to prevent eclampsia gravidarum.

1. 2. 2. 4 Syndrome differentiation of puerper-
al diseases

In the ancient times there were so called "three examinations" of puerperal diseases. One is to examine
whether there is pain in the lower abdomen so as to decide
whether there is lochiostasis; another is to examine
whether defecation is smooth in order to make sure
whether body fluid is sufficient or deficient; the third is to
examine whether lactation is smooth or not and whether
appetite is normal or abnormal for the purpose of deciding
whether gastric qi is sufficient or deficient. Besides,

虚;兼见腰酸无力,小腹下坠
者,属肾虚;血色深红或伴心
烦口干或色红,脉滑数者,属
血热。妊娠恶阻,呕吐厌食或
脉缓滑无力者,多为脾胃气
虚;呕吐苦水或酸水,或伴脉
弦滑者,多为肝胃气逆;呕吐
痰涎,作胀或兼脉濡滑者,为
痰湿中阻。妊娠水肿或倦怠
或脘胀,或兼脉沉滑无力者,
属脾虚;兼见腰骶酸痛或畏寒
怯冷,脉或沉迟者,属肾阳不
足。妊娠晚期,出现头晕、头
痛、眼花、胸闷作呕等,为先兆
子痫,应积极处理,预防发展
为子痫。

四、产后病的辨证

凡孕妇产后,古有"三审"
之说,一审下腹痛与不痛,以
辨有无恶露停滞;二审大便通
与不通,以验津液的盛衰;三
审乳汁行与不行以及饮食多
少,以查胃气的强弱。另外,
还应注意恶露的量、色、质、气
味,以及有无发热等。如恶露
量多、秽臭,下腹疼痛拒按,甚

cares should be taken to examine the quantity, texture, color and odor of lochia as well as whether there is fever. Profuse lochia with foul odor, unpressable lower abdominal pain, or even fever, headache, thirst, reddish tongue with yellowish fur and full and rapid pulse are the signs of virulent heat invading the uterus and damaging the thoroughfare and conception vessels. Scanty lochia lingering for days with purplish color and blood clot as well as unpressable lower abdominal pain are signs of blood stasis; light-colored and thin lochia indicates insufficiency of qi and blood. Lack of milk after delivery, distension, hardness and pain of breast as well as poor appetite are signs of liver qi stagnation; softness of breasts without distending pain and scanty and thin milk are due to asthenia of qi and blood.

The characteristics of syndrome differentiation above are described according to the commonly-encountered symptoms of menstruation, leukorrhagia, pregnancy and childbirth. In clinical application, syndrome differentiation must be done in view of the physical condition, vitality, complexion, pulse and general symptoms; with the four diagnostic methods and eight principles; and synthetic analysis of the cause, viscera, qi, blood and meridians.

或身热、头痛、渴欲饮冷、舌红、苔黄、脉洪数者,多为热毒直犯胞宫,损伤冲任。量少而多日不净,色紫黯,有小血块,下腹痛而拒按,多为瘀血停滞;色淡质清,多为气血不足。产后乳少,乳房胀硬而痛,胸胁胀满,胃纳不佳,多为肝气郁滞。如乳房柔软,无胀痛,乳汁少而清稀,多为气血虚弱。

以上辨证特点,是根据经、带、胎、产的常见证候来叙述的。临床运用时,还应结合患者的形、气、色、脉以及全身症状,运用四诊八纲的方法,通过对病因、脏腑、气血、经络等基本理论综合分析,作出准确的辨证结论。

1.3 Therapeutic principles for gynecological diseases

The therapeutic methods for gynecological diseases are basically the same as those for the diseases of other clinical specialties. Pathologically gynecological diseases are mainly related to the kidney, liver, spleen, stomach, qi and blood as well as the thoroughfare and conception vessels. In terms of the causes, gynecological diseases are usually caused by cold, heat, dampness and emotional factors. So therapeutically, differentiation must be made of the external and internal, cold and heat, asthenia and sthenia as well as yin and yang in order to decide whether the disease in question is due to the disorder of the kidney, liver, spleen, heart or qi and blood. Only by making such a careful analysis can proper treatment, prescription and use of herbs be made.

1.3.1 Invigorating the kidney

The kidney is the prenatal base of life, source of reproduction and connected with the thoroughfare and conception vessels. Only when kidney qi is sufficient, can menstruation come, the conception vessel be free in circulation and the thoroughfare vessel keep predominant. Such a condition is also essential to the physiological activities of menstruation, pregnancy, delivery and breast-feeding. Insufficiency of kidney qi or consumption of kidney yin or decline of kidney yang or asthenia of both yin and yang will prevent tiangui from occurring or lead to senilism and disturbance of the thoroughfare and conception

第三章 妇科疾病的治疗原则

妇科疾病的治法,与临床其他各科基本相同,但由于妇科病的特殊病理反应主要集中在肾、肝、脾胃和气血、冲任等方面,而病因又以寒、热、湿及七情内伤等为多见,因此在治法上,也应根据四诊八纲,分清表里、寒热、虚实、阴阳,着重辨其属肾、属肝、属脾、属心和在气、在血,并按标本缓急进行辨证论治,方能收到应有的效果。现将妇科的几种常用治法介绍于下:

一、补肾

肾为先天之本,天癸之源,冲任之脉皆系于肾。女性肾气充沛,然后天癸至,任脉通,冲脉盛,才有经、孕、产、乳的生理功能活动。如肾气不足,或肾阴亏耗,或肾阳衰少,或阴阳俱虚,不能协调充盛,以致天癸不至或早竭,冲、任通盛失调,就能导致经、带、胎、产、乳等方面的疾病。所以,补肾应为妇科的根本治

vessels, consequently resulting in disorders related to menstruation, leukorrhea, pregnancy, delivery and lactation. So kidney-invigorating is the basic therapeutic method in treating gynecological diseases, especially for the treatment of young woman whose kidney qi is not sufficient yet. Kidney-invigorating methods include warming kidney to reinforce yang, nourishing kidney to enrich yin, fostering yin to suppress yang or nourishing both yin and yang that are selected according to the pathological conditions.

The kidney and the liver are all located in the lower energizer; the kidney essence and liver blood share the same origin. So kidney yin can nourish liver yin and prevent liver yang from becoming hyperactive. Liver blood and kidney essence are closely related to menstruation, pregnancy, delivery and breast-feeding. Clinically deficiency of kidney yin may lead to asthenia of both liver and kidney yin, eventually resulting in irregular menstruation or even amenorrhea and menopausal syndrome; deficiency of kidney yin fails to nourish wood and leads to hyperactivity of liver fire, consequently bringing about profuse menstruation, metrorrhagia and metrostaxis, or even dizziness during menstruation due to liver yang transforming into wind; failure of the liver to convey and disperse may lead to consumption of yin by stagnant fire with the involvement of the kidney, frequently resulting in liver stagnation and kidney asthenia which bring about scanty menstruation, delayed menstruation, amenorrhea and dysmenorrhea. Such disorders should be treated by regulating both the liver and the kidney.

法,特别对肾气未充的青年女子尤为重要。其补益方法,则应根据病情,酌选温肾助阳、滋肾养阴、育阴潜阳、阴阳双补等法。

肾与肝同居下焦,肾精与肝血有乙癸同源、相互资生的关系,由于有这种"精血同源"、"肝肾同源"的相互联系,所以肾阴可以滋养肝阴,使肝阳不至于亢奋。肝血、肾精与经、孕、产、乳有直接关系,临床上有因肾阴不足,导致肝肾阴虚,或见月经不调,乃至闭经,或经断前后诸证;或因肾阴不足,水不涵木,致肝火偏旺,见月经过多、崩漏,甚而肝阳化风,出现经行眩晕症;亦有因肝失疏泄,郁火伤及肾阴而致肝郁肾虚,常见月经过少、月经后期、闭经、痛经等,这些均宜肝肾共同进行调治。

肾与心也有相互协调的关系,心火下交于肾,以温养肾阳,肾水上济于心,以滋养心阴。在正常情况下,心阳和肾阴相互升降,上下交通,保持相对平衡,也即是所谓的"水火既济",从而达到"阴平阳秘"。如肾阴亏损,或心火炽盛,就会出现阴虚火旺的心烦、怔忡、失眠、潮红、潮热、盗汗等心肾不交证候,这在崩漏、闭经、经断前后诸证中经常见到。临证当采用滋阴降火、交通心肾的方法予以治疗。

1.3.2　Regulating the liver

The liver is significant in storing blood, controlling blood sea, maintaining close contact with the thoroughfare vessel and managing conveyance and dispersion. The liver physically pertains to yin and functionally to yang. It prefers free action and detests depression. Dysfunction of the liver in conveyance, or stagnation of qi transforming into fire, or stimulation of liver fire due to rage may consume liver yin and lead to hyperactivity of liver yang, or asthenia of yin and hyperactivity of yang which will all affect the thoroughfare vessel and bring about such disorders like irregular menstruation, metrorrhagia and metrostaxis, dysmenorrhea, amenorrhea, morning sickness and eclampsia gravidarum. So regulation and nourishment of the liver is also one of the important therapeutic methods for the treatment of gynecological diseases. In the middle-aged women, menstruation, pregnancy, delivery and breast-feeding frequently impair blood and tend to result in asthenia of liver blood and exuberance of liver qi. So regulation and nourishment of the liver is especially important for the treatment of middle-aged woman. However, in actual treatment, the therapeutic method should be selected according to the conditions of the patient. For example, failure of the liver to convey should be treated with dispersing therapy; liver depression transforming in-

二、调肝

肝为藏血之脏,司血海,与冲脉相通,肝又主疏泄,体阴而用阳,喜条达而恶郁滞。如肝之疏泄失调,或气郁化火,或怒动肝火,使肝阴亏损,或肝阳偏亢,或阴虚阳亢,均能影响冲脉,而致月经不调、崩漏、痛经、闭经、恶阻、子痫等病症。因此,调肝养肝亦为妇科病的重要治法之一。中年妇女由于经、孕、产、乳等数伤于血,易致肝血偏虚、肝气偏盛,调肝养肝就更为必要。具体的治疗方法应视病情而定。肝失疏泄者,宜疏之散之;肝郁化火或怒动肝火者,宜清之泻之;肝阴亏损或肝血不足者,宜柔之养之;肝阳偏亢者,又当平潜之。总之,应使肝气平和,肝血充足为要。

to fire or liver fire due to rage can be treated by clearing and purgative therapy; consumption of liver yin or deficiency of liver blood can be treated by softening and nourishing therapy; hyperactivity of liver yang can be treated by suppressing therapy. In a word, the purpose of regulating the liver is to balance liver qi and make liver blood sufficient.

1.3.3　Invigorating the spleen

The spleen is the postnatal base of life and the source of qi and blood. The spleen manages transformation and transportation as well as commanding blood. The stomach that is internally and externally in relation with the spleen governs reception of food and is an organ with sufficient qi and blood. The thoroughfare vessel also pertains to yangming meridian. Normal functions of the spleen and stomach in woman ensure sufficient blood in the uterus for normal menstruation and pregnancy. Dysfunction of the spleen and stomach, weakness in reception, transformation and transportation may lead to either insufficiency of the source for transformation, or failure in commanding blood, or retention of dampness, which may further impair the thoroughfare and conception vessels and lead to such disorders like irregular menstruation, metrorrhagia and metrostaxis, amenorrhea, leukorrhagia, morning sickness, edema during pregnancy and prolapse of uterus. So strengthening the spleen and harmonizing the stomach is also one of the important therapeutic methods in treating gynecological diseases. Such a treatment is especially important for the treatment of menopausal syndrome in the aged women whose kidney qi has declined and both qi and blood have become asthenic. Since these women mainly depend on cereal nutrients, spleen-invigorating therapy for promoting transformation is essential to them.

三、健脾

脾为后天之本，气血生化之源，脾主运化，又主统摄；与之互为表里的胃又主受纳，为多气多血之腑，而冲脉又隶属于阳明。女性脾胃功能强健，则血海满而月经如期，胎孕正常；脾胃失调，受纳运化功能减弱，或致生化之源不足，或统摄无权，或水湿停滞，若进而损及冲任，则可导致月经失调、崩漏、闭经、带下、妊娠恶阻、妊娠水肿、子宫脱垂等病，故健脾和胃亦为妇科病重要治法。特别是围绝经期（更年期）女性在经断前后，肾气已衰，气血俱虚，全赖水谷滋养，此时补脾以资化源，就显得尤为重要。但具体治法，应本虚者补之、滞者行之、寒者温之、热者清之、陷者升之、逆者平之等施治原则，同时还应注意温寒无过于辛燥，清热无过于苦寒，养阴无过于滋腻，以免辛燥伤阴、滋腻伤阳或苦寒克伐而重伤脾胃。

The general therapeutic principles are nourishing therapy
for the asthenia syndrome, promoting therapy for the
stagnation syndrome, warming therapy for the cold syndrome, clearing therapy for the heat syndrome, elevating
therapy for the sinking syndrome and soothing therapy for
the adverse syndrome. Cares should be taken to avoid
using warming therapy with excessive acrid and dry herbs
to treat cold syndrome, clearing therapy with excessive
herbs of bitter taste and cold nature to treat heat syndrome and nourishing therapy with excessive tonic herbs
to nourish yin lest yin be consumed by acridness and dryness, yang be damaged by tonic elements and the spleen
be restrained by herbs of bitter taste and cold nature.
Such errors in using herbs will all seriously impair the
spleen and stomach.

The functions of the stomach and spleen in reception, digestion, transformation and transportation are in
close relation with the conveyance of liver qi and warming
function of kidney yang. Failure of the liver in conveyance
and dispersion may affect the functions of the spleen in
transformation and transportation and the function of the
stomach in reception, leading to chest oppression, vomiting, epigastric and abdominal distension and hypochondriac distension and pain due to disharmony between the liver
and spleen or disharmony between the liver and stomach.
Such dysfunctions are commonly seen in irregular menstruation and morning sickness. Such disorders should be
treated by soothing the liver, regulating the spleen or
suppressing the liver and harmonizing the stomach. If fire
in mingmen (gate of life) declines and fails to warm the
spleen to promote transformation and transportation, it
may lead to diarrhea and edema during menstruation and
edema during pregnancy or thin leukorrhagia which should
be treated by warming and nourishing the spleen and kidney.

脾胃的受纳、腐熟、运化功能,与肝气的疏泄和肾阳的温煦作用有密切关系。如肝失疏泄,可以影响脾的运化或胃的受纳,出现胸闷纳呆、呕吐、脘腹作胀、两胁胀痛等肝脾不和或肝胃不和的症状,这在月经失调、妊娠恶阻中也是常见的。对此,又须疏肝理脾或抑肝和胃。再如命门火衰,不能暖脾以助运化,或有经行泄泻、经行浮肿,妊娠水肿或带下清稀者,又宜温补脾肾法。

The spleen and the heart are closely related to each other. The heart governs blood and the spleen produces blood, both of which depend on the spleen to transform and transport cereal nutrients. The function of heart yang in transporting blood in the vessels relies on the spleen qi to command. Insufficiency of transformation may lead to deficiency of heart blood, and resulting in palpitation, insomnia, or scanty menstruation and amenorrhea. Failure of the spleen in commanding blood may lead to profuse menstruation, metrorrhagia and metrostaxis which consume blood and cause palpitation and insomnia. So asthenia of both the spleen and the heart is common in disorders of menstruation and should be treated by nourishing both the heart and the spleen.

1.3.4　Regulating qi and blood

Blood is essential to woman, but menstruation, pregnancy, delivery and breast-feeding tend to consume blood and damage qi, eventually leading to gynecological diseases. So regulating of qi and blood is also one of the main therapeutic methods used to treat gynecological diseases. In syndrome differentiation, it must be made sure whether the diseases involves qi or blood and whether they are of cold or heat, or of asthenia or sthenia. Qi and blood depend on each other, so qi must be regulated together with blood and vice versa. If the disease mainly involves qi, the treatment focuses on regulating of qi supplemented by balancing blood. The asthenia syndrome is treated by reinforcing therapy and the stagnation syndrome is treated by promoting therapy with the supplementation of nourishing blood or activating blood. If the disease mainly involves blood, the treatment mainly concentrates on regulating of blood with the supplementation of harmonizing qi. Blood asthenia syndrome is treated by supplementing

脾与心也有密切联系。心主血,脾生血,赖脾之运化水谷精微;而心阳之运血行于脉中,亦须赖脾气之统摄。若化源不足,可致心血衰少,发生怔忡、不寐,或见经少、经闭。若统摄无权,或致经多、崩漏,耗伤阴血,亦可见心悸失眠。故月经病心脾两虚者并非少见。对此,则又当治以补益心脾法。

四、调理气血

妇女以血为本,但经、孕、产、乳每易耗血伤气,因此调理气血亦为治疗妇科病的一个重要治法。惟在辨证时,必须分清病之在气、在血,属寒、属热、属虚、属实,以为立法的依据。气与血相互依存,不可分割,故调气必兼理血,理血亦必兼调气,但应各有侧重。病在气者,以调气为主,佐以理血,虚者补之,滞者行之,并佐以养血或活血。病在血者,以理血为主,并佐以调气,虚者补血养血,血瘀者活血祛瘀,血热者清热凉血,血寒者温经散寒,出血多或日久不止者固涩止血。若气血同病,则宜参考上述方法,适当配合运

blood and nourishing blood; blood stasis is treated by activating blood and resolving stasis; blood heat is treated by clearing away heat and cooling blood; blood cold is treated by warming meridians to disperse cold; massive bleeding or continuous bleeding is treated by astringing blood to stop bleeding. If diseases involve both qi and blood, they should be treated by proper application of the therapeutic methods mentioned above. For the asthenia of both qi and blood, it should be treated by nourishing both qi and blood; for the disorder of qi asthenia and blood stasis, it can be treated by supplementing qi combined with activating blood and resolving stasis; for the disorder of blood asthenia and qi stagnation, it may be treated by supplementing blood combined with regulating qi and dredging stagnancy. In such a way, the supplementation of asthenia will not lead to stagnation of pathogenic factors and the attack on pathogenic factors will not damage qi.

1.3.5 Regulating the thoroughfare and conception vessels

Gynecological diseases are mainly caused by impairment of the thoroughfare and conception vessels. So regulating the thoroughfare and conception vessels is one of the basic treatments for gynecological diseases. However, in the past dynasties, the treatment of gynecological disease usually focused on the treatment of the heart, liver, kidney, spleen and stomach, though the impairment of the thoroughfare and conception vessels is emphasized. This is due to the fact that qi, blood, essence and fluid in the thoroughfare and conception vessels all come from the heart, liver, kidney and spleen. Obviously the kidney, liver, spleen and stomach meridians are closely related to the thoroughfare and conception vessels. That is why the treatment of the kidney, liver, spleen and stomach is

用。如气血两虚者,则宜气血双补;气虚血瘀者,则宜于补气中佐以活血祛瘀;血虚气滞者,又当在补血中佐以理气行滞。如此,则补虚而不致滞邪,攻邪也不致伤正,总之,以气血充盛和畅为度。

五、调理冲任

妇科病多系损伤冲任而作。故调理冲任是妇科病的重要治法之一。不过考之历代医籍,对妇科病虽很强调冲任损伤,但其治法又多重在心、肝、肾、脾、胃。这是因为冲任所受之气、血、精、液均来自于心、肝、肾、脾、胃等脏腑,而肾、肝、脾、胃之经脉与冲任二脉有紧密联系,故调治肾、肝、脾、胃大多兼有调治冲、任之效。从中药的归经来看,部分入肾、肝、脾、胃的药,能兼入冲、任,尤以入肝、肾两经的

effective in regulating the thoroughfare and conception vessels. As to the relation of drugs with the meridians, some of the drugs working on the kidney, liver, spleen and stomach meridians also act on the thoroughfare and conception vessels, especially the drugs working on the liver and kidney meridians. That is why doctors in the past dynasties usually used drugs working on the liver and kidney meridians to treat the disorders of the thoroughfare and conception vessels. Regulating the thoroughfare vessel, stabilizing the thoroughfare vessel, strengthening the thoroughfare vessel and warming the thoroughfare vessel are the therapeutic methods for regulating the thoroughfare and conception vessels developed by Zhang Xichun in the early 20th century based on the characteristics of gynecology.

药兼入冲、任者居多,所以历代医家每取入肝、肾之药来调治冲、任之病,如近代名医张锡纯根据妇科特点,创理冲、安冲、固冲、温冲等系列方药,专供调理冲任之用。

2 Specific Discussions

2.1 Menstruation diseases

2.1.1 Irregular menstruation

Irregular menstruation refers to abnormal changes of the cycle and quantity of menstruation. The changes of cycle manifest early menstruation, delayed menstruation, irregular menstruation and menostaxis, etc.; the changes of quantity manifest profuse menstruation and scanty menstruation.

Irregular menstruation is usually due to emotional factors, or attack by exogenous cold, heat and dampness that impair the thoroughfare and conception vessels and affect the functions of the viscera and the balance between qi and blood as well as that between yin and yang. Clinically changes of cycle and quantity usually appear simultaneous in irregular menstruation, though there is difference between the change of cycle and the change of quantity. For example, early menstruation is usually profuse and delayed menstruation is often scanty. Scanty early menstruation and profuse delayed menstruation are either of asthenia or of sthenia, and due to either cold or heat. Syndrome differentiation of irregular menstruation for deciding treatment should be done according to the period, quantity, color and nature of menses as well as the conditions of the tongue and pulse.

The therapeutic methods for the treatment of irregular

各 论

第一章

月经病

第一节 月经失调

月经失调是指月经的周期和经量的异常。以周期改变为主的,有月经先期、月经后期和月经先后无定期及经期延长等病变;以经量改变为主的,则有月经过多和月经过少等。

月经失调多由内伤七情,或外感寒、热、湿邪,以致冲、任二脉损伤,脏腑功能紊乱,气血阴阳失调而发生疾病。临床上,月经失调,虽有期和量的不同变化,但两者又常并见,如月经先期常伴经量过多,月经后期常伴经量过少,也有先期量少或后期量多的,均有属虚属实、属寒属热的不同。临床上应根据月经周期、量、色、质的改变,结合舌、脉诸证,审证求因,辨证论治。

月经失调的治疗,有调理

menstruation are regulating qi and blood, nourishing the kidney, strengthening the spleen and dispersing stagnation of liver qi. For the regulating qi and blood, the key point is to differentiate whether the disorder involves qi or blood. Menstruation comes from the kidney, so nourishing the kidney qi can stabilize the uterus and supplementing the kidney is essential to the regulation of menstruation. Nourishing the spleen and stomach can promote the production of blood and dispersing stagnant liver qi can promote the flow of qi, which may ensure timely sufficiency of blood in the thoroughfare and conception vessels as well as the uterus.

Besides, treatment should concentrate on either the root aspect or branch aspect in clinical treatment according to the occurrence of disorder before menstruation, or during menstruation or after menstruation. Usually routine treatment focuses on the root aspect, treatment during menstruation concentrates on the branch aspect and treatment after menstruation emphasizes on the regulation of the spleen and stomach as well as that of qi and blood. Cares should be taken in using drugs of warm and dry nature to disturb blood before and during menstruation and drugs of cold and cool nature during menstruation. Regulation of menstruation should be done according to whether irregular menstruation occurs before or after disease. If disease occurs after irregular menstruation, the treatment should focus on the regulation of menstruation; if disease occurs before irregular menstruation, the treatment should concentrate on dealing with the disease. Moreover the treatment is carried out according to the age of the patient.

气血、补肾、扶脾、疏肝之异。调理气血,首先应辨清在气在血,分别论治;月经源于肾,养肾气以安血室,以为调经之要;补脾胃以资血之源;疏肝以条达气机,冲、任血海按时盈满,则月经渐趋正常。

此外,临证尚需按经前、经期和经后的不同,分别采取着重治标或治本的调治方法,一般以平时治本、经期治标、经后调养脾胃气血最为常用。调经还需分清先病后病,经不调而后生病者,当先调经,先生病而后经不调者,当先治疗其病。此外,还要照顾各年龄阶段的特点进行治疗,注意经前、经期慎用温燥动血之药,经期慎用寒凉之药。

2.1.1.1 Early menstruation

月经先期

Menstruation occurring 7 - 10 days earlier than usual

月经周期提前 7 天以上,

is called early menstruation. If it occurs 3 - 5 days earlier than usual or just occasionally occurs earlier, it is not morbid. Continuous occurrence of early menstruation for three cycles is regarded as morbid.

Early menstruation is usually due to blood heat and qi asthenia. Blood heat is due to frequent predominance of yang, or five emotions transforming into fire due to extreme emotional changes, or excessive intake of acrid and hot foods, or attack by exogenous heat which lead to accumulation of heat in blood and the thoroughfare and conception vessels, driving blood to flow abnormally; it may be caused by frequent deficiency of yin or intemperance in sexual life or serious and prolonged disease which consumes body fluid and disturbs the uterus; it may result from weakness of the thoroughfare and conception vessels.

[Key points for diagnosis]

(1) Menstruation occurs over 7 days earlier than usual.

(2) Early menstruation accompanied by profuse discharge of menses may lead to metrorrhagia and metrostaxis.

(3) Menstruation more than 10 days earlier than usual with vaginal bleeding should be differentiated from intermenstrual bleeding.

(4) No organic changes in the pelvis are found in gynecologic examination.

[Syndrome differentiation and treatment]

For early menstruation, syndrome differentiation concentrates on days of earlier occurrence and the changes of quantity, color and texture in combination with the conditions of physical conditions, facial expressions and pulse states so as to make sure whether it is of asthenia or of heat syndrome. For the treatment of asthenia

甚至 10 余天一行者,称为月经先期。若仅超前 3～5 天,或偶有提前者,一般不作先期而论,一般月经连续提前 3 个周期以上者可诊断为本病。

本病以血热、气虚证多见。血热可因素体阳盛,或七情过极,五志化火,或过食辛热,或外感热邪,致血分蕴热,伏于冲任,迫血妄行;也可因素体阴虚,或纵欲无度,或大病久病,阴液耗伤,冲任不固所致。

【诊断要点】

(1) 月经周期提前 7 天以上。

(2) 本病若伴经量过多则可发展为崩漏。

(3) 月经若提前 10 余天见有阴道出血者,应与经间期出血鉴别。

(4) 妇科检查盆腔无器质性改变。

【辨证论治】

月经先期的辨证,重点在于周期的提前,经量、经色、经质的改变,结合形、气、色、脉的情况,辨其属虚、属热之不同;治疗以虚则补之,或补中气,或固肾气;热则清之,实热

syndrome, the therapeutic method is either reinforcing method, or supplementing gastrosplenic qi, or strengthening kidney qi, or clearing away heat. For the treatment of heat syndrome, the therapeutic method should be clearing away heat. For the treatment of sthenia-heat, the therapeutic method is mainly clearing away heat and cooling blood; for the treatment of asthenia-heat, the therapeutic method is mainly nourishing yin and clearing away heat.

(1) Blood heat syndrome

1) Syndrome of liver stagnation and blood heat

Main symptoms: Early menstruation, increased quantity, purplish, reddish and sticky menses, distension of hypochondria and breasts as well as mental depression, restlessness, susceptibility to rage, bitter taste in the mouth, dry throat, yellow urine, dry stool, red tongue with yellow fur, wiry and fast pulse.

Therapeutic methods: Soothing the liver, clearing away heat and regulating menstruation.

Prescription and drugs: Modified Danzhi Xiaoyao San composed of 10g of Mudanpi (*Cortex Moutan Radicis*), 6g of Zhizi (*Fructus Gardeniae*), 6g of Chaihu (*Radix Bupleuri*), 10g Danggui (*Radix Angelicae Sinensis*), 10g of Baishaoyao (*Radix Paeoniae Alba*), 10g of Baizhu (*Rhizoma Atractylodis Macrocephalae*), 10g of Fuling (*Poria*), 6g of Bohe (*Herba Menthae*) (to be decocted later), 12g of Guya (*Fructus Oryzae*) and 3g of Gancao (*Radix Glycyrrhizae*).

Modification: For profuse menorrhea, 15g of Xianhecao (*Herba Agrimoniae*) and 12g of Diyu (*Radix Sanguisorbae*) are added; for profuse menorrhea with blood stasis, 15g of Yimucao (*Herba Leonuri*) and 3g of Shen-

者清热凉血为主,虚热者又当养阴清热为主。

一、血热证

(一)肝郁血热证

主要证候　月经提前,经量增多,经色紫红,经质粘稠,胁胀乳胀,精神忧郁,烦躁易怒,口苦咽干,小便色黄,大便干结,舌质红苔黄,脉弦数。

治　法　舒肝清热调经。

方　药　丹栀逍遥散加减:牡丹皮10g,栀子6g,柴胡6g,当归10g,白芍药10g,白术10g,茯苓10g,薄荷(后下)6g,谷芽12g,甘草3g。

加　减　若经量特多者,加仙鹤草15g,地榆12g;量多兼瘀者,加益母草15g,参三七3g;胀痛甚者,加川楝子6g,

sanqi (*Radix Notoginseng*) are added; for severe distension and pain, 6g of Chuanlianzi (*Fructus Toosendan*)
and 10g of Yanhusuo (*Rhizoma Corydalis*) are added;
for severe fever, 6g of Xiakucao (*Spica Prunellae*) and
10g of Huangqin (*Radix Scutellariae*) are added; for
transmission of liver disease into the spleen with epigastric oppression and anorexia, 6g of Houpo (*Cortex Magnoliae Officinalis*), 6g of Chenpi (*Pericarpium Citri
Reticulatae*) are added; for greasy tongue fur, 6g of Cangzhu (*Rhizoma Atractylodis*) and 6g of processed Banxia
(*Rhizoma Pinelliae*) are added.

2) Syndrome of predominant yang and blood heat

Main symptoms: Early menstruation with profuse,
deep-red colored and sticky menses, flushed face and dry
lips, dysphoria, thirst with preference for drinking,
yellow urine, dry feces, reddish tongue with yellowish
fur, and rapid pulse.

Therapeutic methods: Clearing away heat, cooling
blood and regulating menstruation.

Prescription and drugs: Modified Qingjing San composed of 10g of Mudanpi (*Cortex Moutan Radicis*), 10g
of Digupi (*Cortex Lycii*), 10g of Baishaoyao (*Radix Paeoniae Alba*), 10g of Shengdihuang (*Radix Rehmanniae*), 6g of Huangbai (*Cortex Phellodendri*), 6g of Qinghao (*Herba Artemisiae Annuae*), 10g of Zhimu (*Rhizoma Anemarrhenae*) and 10g of Fuling (*Poria*).

Modification: For profuse menorrhea or menostaxis, 15g of Xianhecao (*Herba Agrimoniae*) and 10g of
Huaihua (*Flos Sophorae*) are added; for severe fever
with thirst, 15g of Shigao (*Gypsum Fibrosum*) (to be
decocted first) is added; for blood stasis due to heat accompanied by lower abdominal pain, 15g of Yimucao
(*Herba Leonuri*) and 10g of Puhuang (*Pollen Typhae*)

延胡索10 g;热重者,加夏枯草
6 g,黄芩10 g;肝病传脾而脘
闷纳呆者,可酌加厚朴6 g,陈
皮6 g;苔腻者,加苍术6 g,制
半夏6 g。

(二) 阳盛血热证

主要证候 月经提前,经
量增多,经色深红,经质粘稠,
面红唇干,心胸烦躁,口渴喜
饮,小便色黄,大便干结,舌质
红苔黄,脉数。

治 法 清热凉血调经。

方 药 清经散加减:
牡丹皮10 g,地骨皮10 g,白芍
药10 g,生地黄10 g,黄柏6 g,
青蒿6 g,知母10 g,茯苓10 g。

加 减 若经量多或经
期延长者,加仙鹤草15 g,槐花
10 g;热甚烦渴者,酌加生石膏
(先煎)15 g;因热致瘀而伴少
腹疼痛者,酌加益母草15 g,蒲
黄(另包)10 g。若见苔黄腻、
胸闷纳呆、带下色黄等症,挟

(wrapped separately) are added; for accompanied damp-heat syndrome with greasy and yellowish tongue fur, chest distress, anorexia, and yellowish leukorrhea etc. , prescriptions like Longdan Xiegan Tang can be used to clear away heat and eliminate dampness first.

3) Syndrome of yin asthenia and blood heat

Main symptoms: Early menstruation with scanty, sticky and purplish menses, feverish sensation over palms and soles, frequent tidal fever and night sweating, rest-lessness and insomnia, yellowish urine, oral erosion and ulceration, reddish tongue with scanty fluid, thin and yellow-ish tongue fur or without fur as well as thin and rapid pulse.

Therapeutic methods: Nourishing yin, clearing away heat and regulating menstruation.

Prescription and drugs: Modified Liangdi Tang composed of 10g of Shengdihuang (*Radix Rehmanniae*), 10g of Xuanshen (*Radix Scrophulariae*), 10g of Mai-mendong (*Radix Ophiopogonis*), 10g of Digupi (*Cortex Lycii*), 10g of Ejiao (*Colla Corii Asini*) (to be melted) and 10g of Baishaoyao (*Radix Paeoniae Alba*).

Modification: For hyperactivity of liver yang with dizziness or tidal fever and tinnitus, 10g of Zhiguiban (Vinegar-fried *Plastrum Testudinis*), 20g of Sheng-longgu (*Os Draconis*) and 15g of Wuzeigu (*Os Sepiae*) are added; for insomnia due to asthenic heat, 6g of Zhizi (*Fructus Gardeniae*) and 10g of Suanzaoren (*Semen Ziziphi Spinosae*) are added; for pain due to blood stasis, 15g of Yimucao (*Herba Leonuri*) and 10g of Yanhusuo (*Rhizoma Corydalis*) are added.

(2) Qi asthenia syndrome

Main symptoms: Early menstruation with prolonged duration and profuse, light-colored and thin menses, anorexia, loose stool, empty prolapsing sensation in the

湿热证,须清热化湿,可选龙胆泻肝汤之类方药。

(三)阴虚血热证

主要证候 月经提前,经量较少,经质稠,经色紫红,手足心发热,时有潮热盗汗,心烦不眠,小便黄少,有口糜舌烂,舌质红,苔薄黄少津或无苔,脉细数。

治 法 养阴清热调经。

方 药 两地汤加减:生地黄10 g,玄参10 g,麦门冬10 g,地骨皮10 g,阿胶(烊化)10 g,白芍药10 g。

加 减 若肝阳上亢证兼见眩晕或潮热、耳鸣者,酌加炙龟版10 g,生龙骨20 g,乌贼骨15 g;虚热不眠者,加栀子6 g,酸枣仁10 g;有瘀痛者,加益母草15 g,延胡索10 g。

二、气虚证

主要证候 月经提前,经期延长,经量较多,经色淡,质清稀,纳呆便溏,小腹空坠,舌

lower abdomen, light-colored tongue with thin and whitish fur, as well as thin and slow pulse.

Therapeutic methods: Nourishing qi and supplementing the spleen, controlling blood circulation and regulating menstruation.

Prescription and drugs: Modified Buzhong Yiqi Tang composed of 10g of Huangqi (*Radix Astragali*), 10g of Dangshen (*Radix Codonopsis Pilosulae*), 6g of Chenpi (*Pericarpium Citri Reticulatae*), 6g of Shengma (*Rhizoma Cimicifugae*), 6g of Chaihu (*Radix Bupleuri*), 10g of Danggui (*Radix Angelicae Sinensis*), 10g of Baizhu (*Rhizoma Atractylodis Macrocephalae*) and 3g of Gancao (*Radix Glycyrrhizae*).

Modification: For yang asthenia accompanied by cold syndrome with blackish, thin and scanty menses, abdominal pain with preference for warmth, moist and whitish tongue fur, 10g of Xiangfu (*Rhizoma Cyperi*) and 6g of Aiye (*Folium Artemisiae Argyi*) are added; for spleen asthenia and dampness obstruction with whitish and greasy tongue fur, 10g of Zisugeng (*Caulis Perillae*) and 5g of Sharen (*Fructus Amomi*) are added; for insufficiency of kidney qi, body chills, profuse urination at nights and light-colored tongue with whitish fur as well as deep and thin pulse, 10g of Chuanxuduan (*Radix Dipsaci*) and 10g of Duzhong (*Cortex Eucommiae*) are added for warming the kidney and regulating menstruation.

[**Other therapeutic methods**]

(1) Chinese patent drugs

1) Guipi Pill: 6g each time and three times a day, applicable to the treatment of qi asthenia syndrome.

2) Gujing Pill: 6g each time and three times a day, applicable to the treatment of blood heat syndrome.

(2) Empirical and folk recipes

1) 30g of Shengdihuang (*Radix Rehmanniae*) is

质淡,苔薄白,脉细缓。

治　法　益气补脾,摄血调经。

方　药　补中益气汤加减:黄芪10 g,党参10 g,陈皮6 g,升麻6 g,柴胡6 g,当归10 g,白术10 g,甘草3 g。

加　减　若阳虚兼寒,症见经色黯黑,质薄量少,腹痛喜暖,苔白而润者,加香附10 g,艾叶6 g;脾虚湿滞,舌苔白腻者加紫苏梗10 g,砂仁(后下)5 g;若肾气不足,周身畏寒,夜尿增多,舌质淡,苔白,脉沉细,加川续断10 g,杜仲10 g。

【其他疗法】

1. 中成药

(1) 归脾丸　每次6 g,1日3次,适用于气虚证。

(2) 固经丸　每次6 g,1日3次,适用于血热证。

2. 单验方

(1) 生地黄30 g,粳米

washed, cut into slices and decocted into 100ml decoction which is mixed up with porridge made of 60g of Jingmi (*Fructus Oryzae Sativae*) for oral taking, applicable to the treatment of heat syndrome.

2) 15g of Dangshen (*Radix Codonopsis Pilosulae*), 15g of Huangqi (*Radix Astragali*), 20 pieces of Dazao (*Fructus Jujubae*), 60g of Bailianmi (*Semen Nelumbinis*). Dangshen and Bailianmi with 1,000ml of water are decocted into 200ml of decoction. After removal of the residue, the decoction is added with Dazao and Bailianmi to decoct into porridge for oral taking. One dose is for one day and it continues for one week.

2.1.1.2　Delayed menstruation

Delayed menstruation means that menstruation occurs over seven days later than usual or occurs once 40 - 50 days. However, occasional delayed menstruation is regarded as normal. Only delayed menstruation occurring for consecutive three times is considered morbid.

Delayed menstruation is either asthenia or sthenia. The former is due to consumption of blood after prolonged disease or delivery or frequent asthenia of yang and endogenous asthenia-cold; the latter is due to exogenous cold attack and endogenous cold generated by interior injury leading to stagnation of cold in the meridians and vessels, or due to mental depression or qi stagnation and blood stasis.

[Key points for diagnosis]

(1) Menstruation occurs seven days later than usual continuously for three cycles.

(2) Excluding pregnancy in diagnosing woman of childbearing age.

60 g,生地黄洗净后切片,煎熬成100 ml,粳米煮粥与汁混合,连服数日,用于热证。

（2）党参15 g,黄芪15 g,大枣 20 枚,白莲米60 g,先以党参、黄芪加水1 000 ml,煎至200 ml去渣,入大枣和白莲米共煮成粥,1 日 1 料,连用1 周。

月经后期

月经周期延后 7 天以上者,称为月经后期。若偶见延后,且无其他病象出现,不作后期而论。一般月经连续延后 3 个周期以上者诊断为本病。

月经后期有虚实之分：虚者因久病、经产、营血亏损,或素体阳虚、虚寒内生；实者因感受外寒、内伤生冷、寒凝经脉,或性情抑郁,气滞血瘀而致。

【诊断要点】

（1）月经经期延后 7 天以上,连续 3 个月经周期以上者。

（2）育龄期应排除妊娠。

(3) Excluding hemorrhagic disease if menstruation with mild vaginal bleeding occurs half a month later than usual accompanied by abdominal pain.

[Syndrome differentiation and treatment]

The key point for syndrome differentiation is to differentiate between asthenia and sthenia in light of the quantity, color and texture of menses as well as the conditions of the tongue and pulse. According to the therapeutic principles of supplementing the asthenia and purging the sthenia, the treatment should concentrate on nourishing blood to regulate menstruation and activating blood to remove stasis. The drugs are selected according to the differentiation of the organs involved.

(1) Blood asthenia syndrome

Main symptoms: Delayed menstruation with scanty, light-colored and thin menses or accompanied by lower abdominal pain, sallow or pale complexion, lusterless skin, dizziness, lassitude, palpitation, insomnia, light-colored tongue and thin pulse.

Therapeutic methods: Supplementing blood, nourishing qi and regulating menstruation.

Prescription and drugs: Modified Dabuyuan Jian composed of 15g of Dangshen (*Radix Codonopsis Pilosulae*), 15g of Shanyao (*Rhizoma Dioscoreae*), 10g of Shudihuang (*Rhizoma Rehmanniae Praeparata*), 12g of Danggui (*Radix Angelicae Sinensis*), 12g of Baishaoyao (*Radix Paeoniae Alba*), 10g of Duzhong (*Cortex Eucommiae*), 10g of Shanzhuyu (*Fructus Corni*), 10g of Danshen (*Radix Salviae Miltiorrhizae*), 10g of Xiangfu (*Rhizoma Cyperi*) and 3g of crude Gancao (*Radix Glycyrrhizae*).

Modification: For asthenia-heat due to consumption

（3）以往周期正常,此次经期延后 15 天以上,阴道少量出血,伴腹痛者,应排除妊娠出血性疾病。

【辨证论治】

月经后期的辨证要点,重在结合经期的延后,详查经量、经色、经质及舌、脉诸证,辨其虚实。依照虚者补之,实者泄之的原则,治则当以养血调经,活血行滞,根据在肝、在肾、在脾之不同,选用适当方药。

一、血虚证

主要证候 月经后期,月经量少,色淡质薄,或有少腹疼痛,面色萎黄或苍白,皮肤不泽,头昏倦乏,心悸失眠,舌质淡,脉细。

治 法 补血益气调经。

方 药 大补元煎加减:党参15 g,山药15 g,熟地黄10 g,当归12 g,白芍药12 g,杜仲10 g,山茱萸10 g,丹参10 g,香附10 g,生甘草3 g。

加 减 病久伤阴,致生

of yin by prolonged disease accompanied by flushed cheeks and tidal fever as well as feverish sensation over the palms, soles and chest, 10g of Digupi (*Cortex Lycii*) and 10g of Zhimu (*Rhizoma Anemarrhenae*) are added; for palpitation and insomnia, 15g of Yejiaoteng (*Caulis et Folium Polygoni Multiflori*) and 10g of Suanzaoren (*Semen Ziziphi Spinosae*) are added.

(2) Asthenia-cold syndrome

Main symptoms: Delayed menstruation with scanty, thin and blackish or grayish menses, aching pain in the loins and sacrum, frequent urination in the night, loose stool, light-colored tongue with whitish fur and deep-slow pulse.

Therapeutic methods: Supporting yang, eliminating cold and regulating menstruation.

Prescription and drugs: Modified Aifu Nuangong Wan composed of 6g of Aiye (*Folium Artemisiae Argyi*), 10g of Xiangfu (*Rhizoma Cyperi*), 12g of Danggui (*Radix Angelicae Sinensis*), 5g of Wuzhuyu (*Fructus Evodiae*), 10g of Danshen (*Radix Salviae Miltiorrhizae*), 10g of Shengdihuang (*Radix Rehmanniae*), 6g of Rougui (*Cortex Cinnamomi*), 10g of Mudanpi (*Cortex Moutan Radicis*), 10g of Huangqi (*Radix Astragali*) and 10g of Chuanduan (*Radix Dipsaci*).

Modification: For clear urine and severe loose stool, 10g of Buguzhi (*Fructus Psoraleae*) and 10g of Baizhu (*Rhizoma Atractylodis Macrocephalae*) are added; for insufficiency of yang-qi with phlegm and dampness, 10g of Cangzhu (*Rhizoma Atractylodis*) and 15g of Yiyiren (*Semen Coicis*) are added.

(3) Blood cold syndrome

Main symptoms: Delayed menstruation with blackish and scanty menses or with blood clot, or abdominal pain that

虚热,证兼颧红潮热、五心烦热者,加地骨皮 10 g,知母 10 g;若心悸、失眠者,加夜交藤 15 g,酸枣仁 10 g。

二、虚寒证

主要证候　经期延后,经量少而质薄,经色黑或暗淡,腰骶酸痛,夜尿频多,大便溏薄,舌质淡苔白,脉沉迟。

治　法　扶阳祛寒调经。

方　药　艾附暖宫丸加减:艾叶 6 g,香附 10 g,当归 12 g,吴茱萸 5 g,丹参 10 g,生地黄 10 g,肉桂 6 g,牡丹皮 10 g,黄芪 10 g,川断 10 g。

加　减　若小便清,大便溏薄,加补骨脂 10 g,白术 10 g;气阳不足,兼痰湿者,加苍术 10 g,薏苡仁 15 g。

三、血寒证

主要证候　经期延后,经色黯而量少,或有瘀块,或小

can be alleviated with warmth, cold limbs, aversion to cold, blackish tongue with whitish fur and deep-tense pulse.

Therapeutic methods: Warming meridians to dispel cold and regulating menstruation.

Prescription and drugs: Modified Wenjing Tang composed of 12g of Renshen (*Radix Ginseng*), 5g of Chuanxiong (*Rhizoma Chuanxiong*), 10g of Danggui (*Radix Angelicae Sinensis*), 10g of Baishaoyao (*Radix Paeoniae Alba*), 5g of Guizhi (*Ramulus Cinnamomi*), 5g of Wuzhuyu (*Fructus Evodiae*), 10g of Mudanpi (*Cortex Moutan Radicis*), 10g of Niuxi (*Radix Achyranthis Bidentatae*), 10g of Ezhu (*Rhizoma Curcumae*) and 3g of Gancao (*Radix Glycyrrhizae*).

Modification: For severe abdominal pain, 10g of Wuyao (*Radix Linderae*) and 10g of Yanhusuo (*Rhizoma Corydalis*) are added; for unpressable abdominal pain with blood clot in menses, 10g of crude Puhuang (*Pollen Typhae*) and 10g of Wulingzhi (*Faeces Trogopterorum*) are added; for cold phlegm, 6g of Shichangpu (*Folium Acori Tatarinowii*) and 6g of Ganjiang (*Rhizoma Zingiberis*) are added.

(4) Qi stagnation syndrome

Main symptoms: Delayed menstruation with deep-red and scanty menses or with blood clot, mental depression, or lower abdominal distension and pain, or breast distension and hypochondriac pain, thin and yellowish tongue fur and taut pulse.

Therapeutic methods: Regulating qi and eliminating stagnation combined with activation of blood.

Prescription and drugs: Modified Chaihu Shugan San composed of 6g of Chaihu (*Radix Bupleuri*), 10g of Zhike (*Fructus Aurantii*), 10g of Baishaoyao (*Radix*

腹疼痛,得热减轻,肢冷畏寒,舌质黯苔白,脉沉紧。

治　法　温经散寒调经。

方　药　温经汤加减:人参12 g,当归10 g,川芎5 g,白芍药10 g,桂枝5 g,吴茱萸5 g,牡丹皮10 g,牛膝10 g,莪术10 g,甘草3 g。

加　减　腹寒痛甚者,加乌药10 g,延胡索10 g;腹痛拒按,时下血块,加生蒲黄10 g,五灵脂10 g;寒痰者加石菖蒲6 g,干姜6 g。

四、气郁证

主要证候　经期延后,经色暗红或有块,经量较少,精神抑郁,或少腹胀痛,或乳胀胁痛,舌苔薄黄,脉弦。

治　法　理气开郁,佐以活血。

方　药　柴胡疏肝散加减:柴胡6 g,枳壳10 g,白芍药10 g,甘草3 g,香附10 g,川芎

Paeoniae Alba）, 3g of Gancao (*Radix Glycyrrhizae*),
10g of Xiangfu (*Rhizoma Cyperi*), 5g of Chuanxiong
(*Rhizoma Chuanxiong*), 10g of Niuxi (*Radix Achyran-*
this Bidentatae), 10g of Yanhusuo (*Rhizoma Coryda-*
lis) and 10g of Danshen (*Radix Salviae Miltiorrhizae*).

Modification: For qi stagnation transforming into
fire with bitter taste in the mouth and yellowish tongue
fur, 10g of Mudanpi (*Cortex Moutan Radicis*), 6g of
Zhizi (*Fructus Gardeniae*) and 10g of Huangqin (*Radix*
Scutellariae) are added; for unpressable abdominal pain
with blood clot in menses, 15g of Yimucao (*Herba Le-*
onuri) and 5g of Sanqi (*Radix Notoginseng*) are added.

[Other therapeutic methods]

(1) Chinese patent drugs

1) Danggui Pill: 8 pills each time and three times a
day, applicable to the treatment of blood asthenia or blood
stasis syndrome.

2) Aifu Nuangong Pill: 8 pills each time and three
times a day, applicable to the treatment of cold syndrome.

(2) Empirical and folk recipes

1) 6g of Shengjiang (*Rhizoma Zingiberis Recens*),
6g of Aiye (*Folium Artemisiae Argyi*) and 15g of brown
sugar are decocted. The decoction is taken orally twice a
day, and applicable to the treatment of blood cold syndrome.

2) 10g of Danshen (*Radix Salviae Miltiorrhizae*),
10g of Xiangfu (*Rhizoma Cyperi*), 6g of Aiye (*Folium*
Artemisiae Argyi), 6g of Gancao (*Radix Glycyrrhizae*)
and 15g of Yimucao (*Herba Leonuri*) are decocted. The
decoction is taken orally.

2.1.1.3 Irregularity of menstrual cycle

Menstruation occurs over seven days earlier or later

5 g,牛膝10 g,延胡索10 g,丹
参10 g。

加 减 若气郁化火,口
苦、苔黄者,加牡丹皮10 g,栀
子6 g,黄芩10 g;腹痛拒按,经
血有块者,加益母草15 g,三七
5 g。

【其他疗法】
1. 中成药
（1）当归丸 每次 8 丸,
1 日 3 次,适用于血虚或血
瘀证。
（2）艾附暖宫丸 每次 8
丸,1 日 3 次,适用于寒证。
2. 单验方
（1）生姜6 g,艾叶6 g,红
糖15 g,煎煮为饮,1 日 2 次,
适用于血寒证。

（2）丹参10 g,香附10 g,
艾叶6 g,甘草6 g,益母草15 g,
煎煮为饮。

月经先后无定期

月经周期时或提前、时或

than usual is called irregularity of menstrual cycle which is often caused by mental depression, stagnation of liver qi; or by frequent asthenia of the kidney, lack of proper care after prolonged illness, multiparity and excessive sexual life which consume kidney qi. Prolonged duration of the illness may lead to metrorrhagia and metrostaxis.

[Key points for diagnosis]

(1) Menstruaton occurs seven days earlier or later than usual for three continuous cycles.

(2) Menstruation is not prolonged and menses is not profuse. Cares should be taken to differentiate it from metrorrhagia and metrostaxis.

[Syndrome differentiation and treatment]

The main symptom is irregular menstrual cycles. Syndrome differentiation should be done in light of the quantity, color and texture of menses as well as the conditions of pulse. Clinically irregular menorrhea due to disturbance of liver qi and dysfunction of kidney qi is commonly encountered. Regulation of the liver or treatment of the kidney should focus on harmonizing qi, nourishing blood and regulating the thoroughfare vessel.

(1) Liver stagnation syndrome

Main symptoms: Irregular menstrual cycle, scanty or profuse menorrhea, purplish menses and unsmooth menstruation, dysphoria, susceptibility to rage, preference for sighing, hypochondriac distension and pain, breast distension, epigastric oppression and anorexia, thin and yellowish tongue fur as well as taut pulse.

Therapeutic methods: Soothing the liver and regulating qi, nourishing blood and regulating menstruation.

Prescription and drugs: Modified Xiaoyao San composed of 6g of Chaihu (*Radix Bupleuri*), 10g of Danggui

落后 7 天以上,称为月经先后无定期。本病主要由于情怀不畅,肝气郁滞,或素体肾虚,久病失养,多产房劳,肾气亏损所致。若病延日久,也可转为崩漏病。

【诊断要点】

(1) 月经周期不定,时或提前、时或落后 7 天以上,反复 3 个月经周期者。

(2) 本病经期不长,经量不多,应注意与崩漏区别。

【辨证论治】

经来先后无定期是本病的主证,但应结合经量、经色、经质及脉证辨证论治。临床以肝气失调和肾气失司证较为多见。无论调肝或治肾,总宜注重气机的调顺和养血调冲。

一、肝郁证

主要证候   月经周期不定,经量或多或少,经色紫红,经行不畅,心烦易怒,时欲叹息,两胁胀痛,乳胀,脘闷纳少,舌苔薄黄,脉弦。

治   法   疏肝理气,养血调经。

方   药   逍遥散加减:柴胡 6 g,当归 10 g,白术 10 g,

(*Radix Angelicae Sinensis*), 10g of Baizhu (*Rhizoma Atractylodis Macrocephalae*), 10g of Baishaoyao (*Radix Paeoniae Alba*), 10g of Fuling (*Poria*), 5g of Bohe (*Herba Menthae*) (to be decocted later), 6g of Jingjie (*Herba Schizonepetae*) and 3g of Gancao (*Radix Glycyrrhizae*).

白芍药10 g，茯苓10 g，薄荷（后下）5 g，荆芥6 g，甘草3 g。

Modification： For blood stasis due to qi stagnancy, lower abdominal distending pain during menstruation and menorrhea with blood clot, 12g of Danshen (*Radix Salviae Miltiorrhizae*), 15g of Yimucao (*Herba Leonuri*), 10g of Yanhusuo (*Rhizoma Corydalis*) and 10g of Puhuang (*Pollen Typhae*) (to be wrapped for decocting) are added; for profuse, reddish and thick menses due to heat transformed from liver stagnation, 10g of Mudanpi (*Cortex Moutan Radicis*) and 6g of Zhizi (*Fructus Gardeniae*) are added.

加　减　因气郁致瘀，经期小腹胀痛，经血有块者，加丹参12 g，益母草15 g，延胡索10 g，蒲黄（包煎）10 g；肝郁化热而经多、色红、质稠者，加牡丹皮10 g，栀子6 g。

（2）**Kidney asthenia syndrome**

二、肾虚证

Main symptoms： Irregular menstrual cycle with light-colored, scanty and thin menses, aching pain in the loins and sacrum, dizziness and tinnitus, frequent urination in the night, light-colored tongue with thin fur and deep-weak pulse.

主要证候　经来先后无定，经色淡，经量少而质薄，腰骶酸痛，头晕耳鸣，夜尿频多，舌淡苔薄，脉沉弱。

Therapeutic methods： Nourishing the kidney and harmonizing the spleen, nourishing blood and regulating menstruation.

治　法　补肾和脾，养血调经。

Prescription and drugs： Modified Guishen Wan composed of 10g of Tusizi (*Semen Cuscutae*), 10g of Duzhong (*Cortex Eucommiae*), 10g of Gouqizi (*Fructus Lycii*), 10g of Shanzhuyu (*Fructus Corni*), 10g of Danggui (*Radix Angelicae Sinensis*), 10g of Shudihuang (*Rhizoma Rehmanniae Praeparata*), 15g of Shanyao (*Rhizoma Dioscoreae*) and 10g of Fuling (*Poria*).

方　药　归肾丸加减：菟丝子10 g，杜仲10 g，枸杞子10 g，山茱萸10 g，当归10 g，熟地黄10 g，山药15 g，茯苓10 g。

Modification： For simultaneous disease of the liver

加　减　若肝肾同病者，

and kidney, both the liver and kidney should be treated with Dingjing Tang composed of 6g of Chaihu (*Radix Bupleuri*), 10g of Danggui (*Radix Angelicae Sinensis*), 10g of Baishaoyao (*Radix Paeoniae Alba*), 10g of Shudihuang (*Rhizoma Rehmanniae Praeparata*), 15g of Shanyao (*Rhizoma Dioscoreae*), 10g of Tusizi (*Semen Cuscutae*) and 6g of Jingjiesui (*Spica Schizonepetae*).

[Other therapeutic methods]

(1) Chinese patent drugs

1) Xiaoyao Pill: 5g each time and three times a day, applicable to the treatment of qi stagnation.

2) Yueju Pill: 5g each time and three times a day, applicable to the treatment of phlegm stagnation.

(2) Empirical and folk recipes

1) Slices of 30g of Xiangfu (*Rhizoma Cyperi*) and 15g of Danggui (*Radix Angelicae Sinensis*) are steeped in millet wine. After three days the wine is drunk twice a day and 15ml each time, applicable to the treatment of liver stagnation syndrome.

2) 15g of Gouqizi (*Fructus Lycii*), 20g of Xianjuye (*fresh Folium Citri Reticulatae*), 10g of Zisugeng (*Caulis Perillae*) and 15g of brown sugar are steeped in boiling water for 15-20 minutes. The decoction is taken orally as tea, applicable to the treatment of kidney asthenia and liver stagnation syndrome.

2.1.1.4 Profuse menorrhea

Profuse menorrhea means that the quantity of menses obviously increases or menstruation lasts for over seven days.

Profuse menorrhea is usually caused by failure of qi to control blood due to asthenia, or by heat driving blood

应肝肾同治,用定经汤。柴胡6 g,当归10 g,白芍药10 g,熟地黄10 g,山药15 g,菟丝子10 g,荆芥穗6 g。

【其他疗法】

1. 中成药

(1) 逍遥丸 每次5 g,1日3次;适用于气滞之证。

(2) 越鞠丸 每次5 g,1日3次;适用于痰滞之证。

2. 单验方

(1) 香附30 g,当归15 g,黄酒250 g,前两药切片泡酒,3日后可饮用,1日2次,每次15 ml,适用于肝郁证。

(2) 枸杞子15 g,鲜橘叶20 g,紫苏梗10 g,红糖15 g,置保温杯中,加开水泡15~20分钟,频作茶饮,适用于肾虚肝郁证。

月经过多

月经量较以往明显增多,或经期持续超过7天不净,月经总量增加者,称为月经过多。

本病的发病机理,多由气虚统摄无权,或血热妄行、冲

to flow abnormally, or by weakness of the thoroughfare and conception vessels.

[Key points for diagnosis]

(1) Menorrhea increases noticeably but stops after a certain period of time.

(2) Profuse menorrhea usually appears together with early menstruation or delayed menstruation.

(3) Fulminant profuse menorrhea or incessant menorrhea or irregular menstrual cycle indicates metrorrhagia and metrostaxis.

[Syndrome differentiation and treatment]

Profuse menorrhea is characterized by increase of menstrual flow in quantity. Clinically profuse menorrhea may appear together with abnormal changes in menstrual cycle. In some cases, the menstrual cycle is normal, and only menorrhea has increased. Increased quantity and thin texture are usually the characteristics for syndrome differentiation. If menses is not fresh, it is due to qi asthenia; if menses is profuse, thick and fresh or purplish light, it is due to blood heat. Treatment focuses on stopping bleeding during menstruation and on stabilizing the thoroughfare vessel and strengthening body resistance in normal times. Drugs of warm and dry nature should be avoided lest blood be disturbed.

(1) Qi asthenia syndrome

Main symptoms: Profuse menorrhea or prolonged menorrhea with light color and thin texture menses, indolence, somnolence, empty prolapsing sensation in the lower abdomen, dull cold pain in the loins and abdomen, bright-whitish complexion, light-colored and tender tongue with thin fur, asthenic and floating or weak pulse.

Therapeutic methods: Invigorating qi and lifting the sinking, controlling blood and strengthening the thor-

任不固所致。

【诊断要点】

一、月经量明显增多，但在一定时间内能自行停止。

二、本病常与月经先期、月经后期同时出现。

三、经量特多，暴下如注，或经血日久不止，或有周期紊乱者，则为崩漏。

【辨证论治】

经量增多，是本病的特征。但临床有与周期异常同时出现的，如月经先期量多证；也有周期正常，仅经量增多的。月经量多质薄、经色偏淡属气虚；量多质稠、经色鲜红或紫亮属血热。行经期治疗以止血为主，平时则应安冲固本。临证用药，以少用温燥之品为宜，以免动血。

一、气虚证

主要证候　月经量多或经期延长，经色淡，经质稀薄，怠惰思睡，少腹空坠，腰腹隐隐冷痛，面色㿠白，舌质淡嫩，苔薄，脉虚浮或无力。

治　法　益气升陷，摄血固冲。

oughfare vessel.

Prescription and drugs: Modified Juyuan Jian composed of 12g of Dangshen (*Radix Codonopsis Pilosulae*), 10g of Huangqi (*Radix Astragali*), 10g of Baizhu (*Rhizoma Atractylodis Macrocephalae*), 6g of Shengma (*Rhizoma Cimicifugae*) and 3g of Gancao (*Radix Glycyrrhizae*).

Modification: Profuse menorrhea during menstrual course, 6g of Aiyetan (*Carbonized Folium Artemisiae Argyi*), 15g of Wuzeigu (*cuttlefish bone*) and 15g of Xueyutan (*Crinis Carbonisatus*) are added; for prolonged menstruation or even dripping menstruation, 10g of Puhuang (*Pollen Typhae*) (to be wrapped) and 15g of Yimucao (*Herba Leonuri*) are added; for cold pain in the loins and abdomen, 10g of Xuduan (*Radix Dipsaci*) and 6g of Aiye (*Folium Artemisiae Argyi*) are added.

(2) Blood heat syndrome

Main symptoms: Profuse menorrhea or prolonged menstruation with purplish red or bright-red color and thick and sticky texture menses or blood clot, lower abdominal pain, or hypochondriac pain, or fever, dysphoria, thirst, scanty and yellowish urine, constipation, reddish tongue with yellowish fur and slippery and rapid pulse.

Therapeutic methods: Clearing away heat and cooling blood, nourishing yin and stopping bleeding.

Prescription and drugs: Modified Gujing Wan composed of 6g of Huangbai (*Cortex Phellodendri*), 10g of Huangqin (*Radix Scutellariae*), 10g of Baishaoyao (*Radix Paeoniae Alba*), 10g of Guiban (*Plastrum Testudinis*) (to be decocted first), 15g of Chungenpi (*Cortex Toonae Sinensis*), 10g of Xiangfu (*Rhizoma Cyperi*), 10g of Ejiao (*Colla Corii Asini*) (to be melted separately) and 10g of Digupi (*Cortex Lycii*).

方　药　举元煎加减：党参12 g，黄芪10 g，白术10 g，升麻6 g，甘草3 g。

加　减　正适经期量多者，加艾叶炭6 g，乌贼骨15 g，血余炭15 g；经期过长，甚至淋漓不断者，加生蒲黄（包煎）10 g，益母草15 g；腰腹冷痛者，加续断10 g，艾叶6 g。

二、血热证

主要证候　月经量多或过期不止，经色紫红或鲜红，经质稠粘，或有小血块，小腹胀痛，或有胁痛，或有发热，心烦口渴，小便短黄，大便秘结，舌红，苔黄，脉滑数。

治　法　清热凉血，养阴止血。

方　药　固经丸加减：黄柏6 g，黄芩10 g，白芍药10 g，龟版（先煎）10 g，椿根皮15 g，香附10 g，阿胶（另烊）10 g，地骨皮10 g。

Modification: If menorrhea continues to increase or menstruation is prolonged, 20g of Wuzeigu (*Os Sepiae*), 15g of Qiangentan (*Carbonized Rhizoma Rubiae*), 15g of Xianhecao (*Herba Agrimoniae*) and 12g of Xiaoji (*Herba Cephalanoploris*) are added; if exogenous pathogenic heat transforms into fire and changes into toxin with the symptoms of fever, aversion to cold and unpressable lower abdominal pain and hardness, 12g of Baijiangcao (*Herba Patriniae*), 15g of Hongteng (*Caulis Sargentodoxae*), 12g of Pugongying (*Herba Taraxaci*) and 10g of crude Puhuang (*Pollen Typhae*) are added; the prescription can be used together with Shengmai San to treat asthenia of both qi and yin due to prolonged illness with the symptoms of profuse menorrhea, shortness of breath, palpitation, feverish sensation over palms, soles and chest, tinnitus, insomnia and dizziness.

[Other therapeutic methods]

(1) Chinese patent drugs

1) Gujing Pill: 10g each time and twice a day, applicable to the treatment of blood heat syndrome.

2) Xue'an: 4 tablets each time and three times a day, applicable to the treatment of stagnation syndrome.

(2) Empirical and folk recipes

1) 62g of crude Diyu (*Radix Sanguisorbae*) is ground into powder. Each time 6g of the powder is decocted in sweet wine for oral taking. Such a recipe is applicable to the treatment of blood heat syndrome.

2) 60g of Renshen (*Radix Ginseng*) and 500g of Huangqi (*Radix Astragali*) are decocted for three times. After the removal of residue, 500g of Yitang (*malt sugar*) is added into the decoction. Each time 10g of extract is taken, twice a day. This recipe is applicable to the treatment of qi asthenia syndrome.

加　减　若经血量多不减或经期延续过长者,加乌贼骨20 g,茜根炭15 g,仙鹤草15 g,小蓟12 g;若外感热邪化火成毒,证见发热恶寒,少腹硬痛拒按者,加败酱草12 g,红藤15 g,蒲公英12 g,生蒲黄(包煎)10 g;病久见气阴两虚证,如经量多,气短心悸,五心烦热,耳鸣失眠,头晕者,可与生脉散合用。

【其他疗法】

1. 中成药

(1) 固经丸　每次10 g,1日2次;适用于血热之证。

(2) 血安　每次4片,1日3次;适用于瘀滞之证。

2. 单验方

(1) 生地榆62 g,甜酒适量,地榆研末,每次6 g,甜酒煎服,适用于血热之证。

(2) 人参60 g,黄芪500 g,饴糖500 g,前两药反复煎熬3次,去渣后入饴糖,出膏,每次10 g,1日2次,适用于气虚之证。

2.1.1.5 Scanty menstruation

Scanty menstruation means that menorrhea is obviously reduced and the menstrual cycle is less than two days.

The cause of scanty menstruation is similar to that of delayed menstruation and is either asthenia or sthenia. Asthenia syndrome is due to constitutional blood asthenia or kidney asthenia which leads to deficiency of essence and blood, asthenia of nutrient blood and insufficiency of blood in the uterus. Sthenia syndrome is due to stagnation of exogenous cold in the meridians and vessels; or due to qi stagnation and unsmooth circulation of blood that blocks the thoroughfare and conception vessels and the uterus, preventing the occurrence of menorrhea; or due to internal retention of phlegm and dampness that hinders the uterine collaterals and leads to scanty menorrhea.

[Key points for diagnosis]

(1) Menstrual cycle is basically normal, but menses is scanty or even just a little.

(2) Cares should be taken to exclude scanty menses due to contraceptives in women of childbearing age.

(3) Menstruation in early pregnancy is different from the problem mentioned above.

[Syndrome differentiation and treatment]

Scanty menses is the basic characteristic of this syndrome. Clinically it may exist together with delayed menstruation. In some cases the menstrual cycle is normal, and only menorrhea is reduced. The asthenia and sthenia syndromes can be differentiated according to the color and texture of menses as well as whether there is abdominal pain or not. Usually light-colored and clear menses without abdominal distending pain is of asthenia

月经过少

月经量明显减少,或经期缩短少于 2 天者,称为月经过少。

本病的发病机理基本上与月经后期类同,分虚实两证:虚者因素体血虚或肾虚,以致精血不足,营血亏虚,血海不充而月经过少;实者可由感寒,寒凝经脉,或气滞经血不畅,致冲任胞宫瘀阻,经血下行不畅;或痰湿内阻,胞脉不畅而月经过少。

【诊断要点】

(1) 月经周期基本正常,经量很少,甚或点滴即净。

(2) 注意排除育龄女性因服用避孕药而致经量过少。

(3) 注意早孕而有激经者应与本病区别。

【辨证论治】

经量过少是本证的特征,临床可与月经后期同时存在,也有周期正常而仅经量减少者。应从经色、经质及有无腹痛以辨虚实。一般以色淡、质清、腹无胀痛为虚;色紫暗夹血块,腹痛拒按者,为血瘀;色淡红、质粘如痰者为痰湿。本

syndrome; menstruation with purplish and blackish blood clot and unpressable abdominal pain signifies blood stasis; light-reddish and sticky menses like sticky sputum suggests phlegm-dampness. The treatment of this syndrome should concentrate on nourishing essence and blood. Since asthenia syndrome appears more frequently than sthenia syndrome, cares must be taken in using purgative and drastic herbs lest qi and blood be impaired and menstruation be difficult to be restored. Scanty menstruation accompanied by delayed menstruation may turn into amenorrhea.

(1) Blood asthenia sydnorme

Main symptoms: Scanty menses, even just several drops of menses with light color and thin texture, dizziness, palpitation, sallow complexion, empty prolapsing sensation in the lower abdomen, light-reddish tongue and thin pulse.

Therapeutic methods: Nourishing blood, invigorating qi and regulating menstruation.

Prescription and drugs: Modified Zixue Tang composed of 12g of Dangshen (*Radix Codonopsis Pilosulae*), 15g of Shanyao (*Rhizoma Dioscoreae*), 12g of Fuling (*Poria*), 10g of Shudihuang (*Radix Rehmanniae Praeparata*), 10g of Danggui (*Radix Angelicae Sinensis*), 10g of Baishaoyao (*Radix Paeoniae Alba*), 5g of Chuanxiong (*Radix Chuanxiong*) and 10g of Huangqi (*Radix Astragali*).

Modification: For asthenia heat, 10g of Digupi (*Cortex Lycii Radicis*) and 10g of Xuanshen (*Radix Scrophulariae*) are added; for insomnia and palpitation due to blood asthenia, 15g of Yejiaoteng (*Caulis et Folium Polygoni Multiflori*) and 5 g of Wuweizi (*Fructus Schisandrae*) are added; if it is accompanied by liver depression with hypochondriac distension or breast disten-

病治法当重在濡养精血。因虚多实少，慎不可恣投攻破之品，以免重伤气血，使经血难复。月经过少而常伴后期者，可发展为闭经。

一、血虚证

主要证候　经量过少，甚至点滴即净，色淡质薄，头晕眼花，心悸怔忡，面色萎黄，小腹空坠，舌质淡红，脉细。

治　法　补血益气调经。

方　药　滋血汤加减：党参12 g，山药15 g，茯苓12 g，熟地黄10 g，当归10 g，白芍药10 g，川芎5 g，黄芪10 g。

加　减　若虚热者加地骨皮10 g，玄参10 g；血虚而失眠，心悸加夜交藤15 g，五味子5 g；兼肝郁有胁胀或乳胀作痛者，加柴胡5 g，香附10 g，川楝子6 g。

ding pain, 5g of Chaihu (*Radix Bupleuri*), 10g of Xiang-fu (*Rhizoma Cyperi*) and 6g of Chuanlianzi (*Fructus Meliae Toosendan*) are added.

(2) Kidney-deficiency syndrome

Main symptoms: Scanty, thin, light-colored or grayish menstruation, even just several drops of menses, dizziness and tinnitus, flaccid and weak waist and knees, pain in the heel, cold sensation in the lower abdomen, profuse urine in the night, light-colored tongue, deep and slow pulse.

Therapeutic methods: Reinforcing the kidney, nourishing blood and regulating menstruation.

Prescription and drugs: Modified Guishen Wan composed of 10g of Duzhong (*Cortex Eucommiae*), 10g of Tusizi (*Semen Cuscutae*), 10g of Shudihuang (*Rhizoma Rehmanniae Preparata*), 10g of Danggui (*Radix Angelicae Sinensis*), 15g of Shanyao (*Rhizoma Dioscoreae*), 10g of Fuling (*Poria*), 10g of Shanzhuyu (*Fructus Corni*) and 10g of Gouqizi (*Fructus Lycii*).

Modification: For deficiency of kidney-yang, herbs for warming the kidney can be added, such as 10g of Yinyanghuo (*Herba Epimedii*), 10g of Bajitian (*Radix Morindae Officinalis*) and 10g of Xianmao (*Rhizoma Curculigini*); for deficiency of kidney-yin, 10g of Shengdihuang (*Radix Rehmanniae*), 12g of Nüzhenzi (*Fructus Ligustri Lucidi*) and 10g of Xuanshen (*Radix Scrophulariae*) are added; for severe internal heat, 10g of Danpi (*Cortex Moutan Radicis*), 6g of Zhizi (*Fructus Gardeniae*) and 10g of Zhimu (*Rhizoma Anemarrhenae*) are added.

(3) Blood stasis syndrome

Main symptoms: Scanty and blackish menses with

二、肾虚证

主要证候　经量过少,甚至点滴即净,色淡红或黯红,质薄,头晕耳鸣,腰膝酸软,足跟痛,小腹觉冷,夜尿多,舌质淡,脉沉迟。

治　法　补肾养血调经。

方　药　归肾丸加减:杜仲10 g,菟丝子10 g,熟地黄10 g,当归10 g,山药15 g,茯苓10 g,山茱萸10 g,枸杞子10 g。

加　减　若偏于肾阳虚者,酌加温肾药,如淫羊藿10 g,巴戟天10 g,仙茅10 g;偏于肾阴虚者,加生地黄10 g,女贞子12 g,玄参10 g;内热甚的,加牡丹皮10 g,栀子6 g,知母10 g。

三、血瘀证

主要证候　经量过少,经

blood clot, unpalpable distending pain in the lower abdomen which is alleviated after blood clot being discharged.

Therapeutic methods: Activating blood to resolve stasis and nourishing blood to regulate menstruation.

Prescription and drugs: Modified Taohong Siwu Tang composed of 10g of Taoren (*Semen Persicae*), 12g of Honghua (*Flos Carthami*), 10g of Danggui (*Radix Angelicae Sinensis*), 5g of Chuanxiong (*Rhizoma Chuanxiong*), 10g of Baishaoyao (*Radix Paeoniae Alba*), 10g of Shudihuang (*Rhizoma Rehmanniae Preparata*), 12g of Zelan (*Herba Lycopi*), 10g of Wulingzhi (*Faeces Trogopterori*), 12g of Danshen (*Radix Salviae Milti*) and 3g of Gancao (*Radix Glycyrrhizae*).

Modification: For qi stagnation and blood stasis, 10g of Xiangfu (*Rhizoma Cyperi*) and 10g of Wuyao (*Radix Linderae*) are added; for blood stasis due to cold coagulation, 6g of Guizhi (*Ramulus Cinnamomi*) and Wuzhuyu (*Fructus Evodiae*) are added.

(4) Phlegm-dampness syndrome

Main symptoms: Scanty, light-colored and sticky menses, heavy body, chest oppression and nausea, sticky leukorrhea, weakness of the four limbs, light-colored tongue with whitish greasy coating, and slippery pulse.

Therapeutic methods: Resolving phlegm, drying dampness and regulating menstruation.

Prescription and drugs: Modified Cangfu Daotan Wan composed of 10g of Cangzhu (*Rhizoma Atractylodis*), 10g of Xiangfu (*Rhizoma Cyperi*), 12g of Fuling (*Poria*), 10g of Fabanxia (*Rhizoma Pinelliae*), 10g of Chenpi (*Pericarpium Citri Reticulatae*), 3g of Gancao (*Radix Glycyrrhizae*), 10g of Danxing (*Arisaema cum Bile*), 10g of Zhike (*Fructus Aurantii*), 12g of Liuqu

色紫黑,有血块,小腹胀痛拒按,血块排出后胀痛减轻,舌紫黯,脉细涩。

治 法 活血化瘀,养血调经。

方 药 桃红四物汤加减:桃仁10g,红花12 g,当归10 g,川芎5 g,白芍药10g,熟地黄10 g,泽兰12 g,五灵脂10 g,丹参12 g,甘草3 g。

加 减 若气滞血瘀者,加香附10 g,乌药10 g;若为寒凝血瘀者,加桂枝6 g,吴茱萸6 g。

四、痰湿证

主要证候 月经量少,色淡红,质粘腻如痰,形体肥胖,胸闷泛恶,带多粘腻,四肢倦怠,舌质淡,苔白腻,脉滑。

治 法 化痰燥湿调经。

方 药 苍附导痰丸加减:苍术10g,香附10g,茯苓12 g,法半夏10 g,陈皮10 g,甘草3 g,胆星10 g,枳壳10 g,六曲12 g,生姜3 片。

(*Massa Medicata Fermentata*) and 3 slices of Shengjiang (*Rhizoma Zingiberis Recens*).

Modification: For delayed scanty menses or gradual onset of amenorrhea, 12g of Danggui (*Radix Angelicae Sinensis*), 12g of Zelan (*Herba Lycopi*) and 12g of Chuanniuxi (*Radix Achyranthis Bidentatae*) (*Radix Cyathulae*) are added to nourish and activate blood to regulate menstruation; for profuse phlegm and heavy body, 10g of Shichangpu (*Rhizoma Acori tatarinowii*) and 10g of prepared Yuanzhi (*Radix Polygalae*) are added to resolve phlegm and activate collaterals.

[Other therapeutic methods]

(1) Chinese patent drugs

1) Wuji Baifeng Pill: 10g each time and three times a day, applicable to blood deficiency syndrome.

2) Yimu Bazhen Pill: 10g each time and three times a day, applicable to blood deficiency syndrome.

3) Danggui (*Radix Angelicae Sinensis*) Pill: 10g each time and three times a day, applicable to blood stasis syndrome.

4) Sizhi Xiangfu (*Rhizoma Cyperi*) Pill: 10g each time, three times a day, applicable to phlegm-dampness syndrome.

(2) Empirical and folk recipes

1) 15 charred Chinese roses are taken with millet wine, applicable to qi stagnation and blood stasis.

2) 250g of pig trotters and 20g of Niuxi (*Radix Achyranthis Bidentatae*) are cooked with 20 -50g of millet wine, applicable to kidney deficiency syndrome.

加　减　若月经量少落后或渐闭经者,酌加当归12 g,泽兰12 g,川牛膝12 g以养血活血通经;若痰多,形体肥胖,加石菖蒲10 g,炙远志10 g,以化痰活络。

【其他疗法】

1. 中成药

（1）乌鸡白凤丸　每次10 g,1 日 3 次;适用于阴血虚证。

（2）益母八珍丸　每次10 g,1 日 3 次;适用于血虚证。

（3）当归丸　每次10 g,1 日 3 次;适用于血瘀证。

（4）四制香附丸　每次10 g,1 日 3 次;适用于痰湿证。

2. 单验方

（1）月季花 15 朵,黄酒适量,月季花烧炭,温黄酒送下,适用于气滞血瘀证。

（2）猪蹄250 g,牛膝20 g,炖煮过程中加入米酒 20～50 g,适用于肾虚证。

2.1.2　Intermenstrual bleeding

Intermenstrual bleeding refers to periodic uterine bleeding during ovulation. It does not necessarily occur every time during menstruation. Usually uterine bleeding during ovulation is not profuse and tends to be overlooked. The bleeding usually occurs 12 – 16 days in the menstrual cycle, lasting about 2 – 7 days and generally stopping automatically. The accompanied symptoms is light lumbar or abdominal pain in one side, known as pain during ovulation.

This problem, pertaining to functional uterine bleeding in Western medicine and known as intermenstrual bleeding in TCM, usually occurs among women aging from 20 to 30. It occurs in a time between two menstruations. This period is marked by emptiness of the uterus after discharge of menses, deficiency of the thoroughfare and conception vessels, gradual accumulation of menstrual blood from emptiness to abundance. The period between two menstruations is marked by the development from deficiency to exuberance, exuberance of yin-essence, internal activation of yang-qi and ovulation. If the regulatory function of yin and yang is normal, the body can adapt to such physiological changes. However, uterine bleeding may be caused because of weakness of the thoroughfare and conception vessels due to impairment of yin-collaterals by internal activation of yang-qi during ovulation resulting from weak constitution, deficiency of kidney-essence, or early marriage, excessive sexual intercourse, multiparity, or

第二节　经间期出血

经间期出血又称月经中期出血,是指两次月经期之间,即排卵之时,周期性发作的子宫出血,但不一定每次月经中间期均见。排卵期出血一般流血量较少,常不易引起注意,流血时间多发生在月经周期的第 12～16 天,持续 2～7天,一般多能自止。流血时常伴有轻微的腰部及一侧下腹部疼痛,即所谓排卵期疼痛。

本病多发生于 20～30 岁的女性,多属于西医学功能失调性子宫出血,中医学称之为经间期出血。

本病的发生在两次月经之间,这一时期的特点是月经排净之后,血海空虚,冲任不足,经血逐渐蓄积,由空虚渐至充盛。两次月经之间为由虚至盛的转折,阴精充实,阳气内动,而出现絪缊(排卵)之期。一般体内阴阳调节功能正常,可自行适应这种变化。但若禀赋不足,肾精亏虚,或早婚、房劳、多产,或烦心过度,忧郁恚怒,相火内炽而伤及肾阴,导致肾阴亏虚,阴不恋阳,于絪缊之时,阳气内动,

dysphoria, rage, deficiency of kidney-yin and failure of yin to coordinate with yang due to consumption of kidney-yin by intense kidney-fire. Or it may be caused by invasion of damp-heat due to improper care during menstruation and after delivery. Or it may be caused by accumulation of damp-heat into the uterine collaterals, thoroughfare and conception vessels due to failure of the spleen to transform and transport nutrients that generates dampness and heat. Or it may be caused by blockage of the uterine collaterals due to retention of menses and blood stasis after delivery. Or it may be caused by qi stagnation and blood stasis due to depression.

[Key points for diagnosis]

(1) Regular menstrual cycle, normal menstruation, periodic uternine bleeding between two menstruations obviously less than nomral menses or just several drops of bleeding and stopping automatically after 2 – 7 days, usually accompanied by weakness of the waist, vague pain in the lower abdomen, distending pain in the breasts, profuse transparent leuckorrhea.

(2) BBT appears in bipolar curve and bleeding appears at alternative point between high and low curve or before and after the point.

(3) Type B ultrasonic wave examination indicates that the bleeding occurs in full follicular development or before and after ovulation.

(4) This disease should be differentiated from early menstruation, scanty menses and multi-colored leuckorrhage.

[Syndrome differentiation and treatment]

This disease is mainly marked by kidney-yin deficiency. The syndrome should be differentiated in the light of the

损伤阴络,冲任不固而致出血。或经期、产后调摄不慎,湿热之邪乘虚而入,或因脾失健运,不能运化水谷精微以生精血,反聚而生湿,湿蕴化热,湿热蕴阻于胞络、冲任,细缊之时,阳气内动,引动内热,损伤冲任而致出血。或经、产留瘀,瘀血内停,阻于胞络,或因情志不畅,气滞而血瘀,细缊之时,阳气内动,瘀血与之相搏,损伤胞络而致出血。

【诊断要点】

(1) 临床可见月经周期规律,经量、经期均在正常范围,而于两次月经中间,排卵期前后出现周期性的子宫出血,流血量明显少于正常月经量,或点滴而下,一般在2~7天内即可自止,并可伴有腰酸,小腹作胀隐痛,乳房胀痛,带下量多,色白透明呈蛋清状。

(2) 基础体温(BBT)测定多呈双相型曲线,出血发生于高、低相交替之时或前后。

(3) B超跟踪监测可观察到出血发生于卵泡发育成熟及排卵前后。

(4) 本病应与月经先期、月经量少、赤白带下相鉴别。

【辨证论治】

本病以肾阴虚为主,结合经间期出血的颜色、质地和舌

color and texture of intermenstrual bleeding as well as the conditions of the tongue and pulse. The syndrome of yin deficiency and fire exuberance is marked by earlier, scanty and reddish bleeding without clot. The syndrome of damp-heat is usually mixed up with multi-colored leuckorrhage. The syndrome of blood stasis is usually marked by lower abdominal pain and grayish bleeding with blood clot. Since hemorrhage is scanty, it can be treated by nourishing the kidney to enrich blood in combination of draining dampness and resolving stasis. According to the pathological characteristics of this disease and the states of yin and yang as well as qi and blood, yang should also be reinforced in the supplementation of yin. For that reason, proper herbs can be selected to reinforce yang.

(1) Syndrome of yin deficiency and fire exuberance

Main symptoms: Scanty or slightly profuse intermenstrual bleeding with red color and without blood clot, dizziness and tinnitus, weakness of the waist and knees, dysphoria and insomnia, feverish sensation in the palms and soles, yellowish urine and retention of feces, reddish tongue with scanty coating, thin and rapid pulse.

Therapeutic methods: Nourishing yin and clearing away heat, cooling blood and stopping bleeding.

Prescription and drugs: Modified Erzhi Wan Combined with Liuwei Dihuang Tang composed of 15g of Nüzhenzi (*Fructus Ligustri Lucidi*), 15g of Mohanlian (*Herba Ecliptae*), 10g of Shengdihuang (*Radix Rehmanniae*), Digupi (*Cortex lycii*), 20g of Shanyao (*Rhizoma Dioscoreae*), 10g of Shanzhuyu (*Fructus Corni*), 10g of Xuanshen (*Radix Scrophulariae*), 10g of Maimendong (*Radix Ophiopogonis*), 10g of carbonized Jingjie (*Herba Schizonepetae*) and 3g of crude Gan-

脉辨证论治。阴虚火旺证,一般在此期偏前出血,量少色红,无血块;湿热证,常与带下赤白相杂而下;瘀血证,重在少腹作痛,出血色紫黯,有血块。治疗因本病的出血量很少,应从滋肾养血为主,配合利湿化瘀,注意本病的病理特点及其此期阴阳气血活动的特征,补阴不忘补阳,选择适当的补阳药物。

一、阴虚火旺证

主要证候　经间期出血,量少或稍多,色红无血块,头晕耳鸣,腰膝酸软,心烦少寐,手足心热,溲黄便结,舌红,苔少,脉细数。

治　法　滋阴清热,凉血止血。

方　药　二至丸合六味地黄汤加减:女贞子15 g,墨旱莲15 g,生地黄10 g,地骨皮10 g,山药20 g,山茱萸10 g,玄参10 g,麦门冬10 g,荆芥炭10 g,生甘草3 g。

cao (*Radix Glycyrrhizae*).

Modification: For reddish complexion and headache, 6g of Shanzhi (*Radix Pittospori Glabrati*) and 6g of Chaihu (*Radix Bupleuri*) are added; for dysphoria and insomnia, 10g of Suanzaoren (*Semen Ziziphi Spinosae*) and 10g of Hehuanhua (*Cortex Albiziae*) are added; for severe dizziness, 10g of Gouqizi (*Fructus Lycii*), 10g of Hangjuhua (*Flos Chrysanthemi*) and 12g of Baijili (*Radix Tribuli Album*) are added.

(2) Syndrome of damp-heat accumulation

Main symptoms: Scanty or slightly profuse intermenstrual bleeding in reddish and purplish color and sticky texture, mental lassitude, chest oppression, anorexia, dysphoria, dryness in the mouth without desire for drinking, scanty and reddish urine, lower abdominal pain, frequent yellowish or multi-colored leukorrhea with sticky texture and foul odor, or pruritus vulvae, reddish tongue with whitish greasy or yellowish greasy coating, slippery and rapid pulse.

Therapeutic methods: Clearing away heat and draining dampness, cooling blood and stopping bleeding.

Prescription and drugs: Modified Qinggan Zhilin Decoction composed of 10g of Danggui (*Radix Angelicae Sinensis*), 10g of Chishaoyao (*Radix Paeoniae Rubra*), 10g of Baishaoyao (*Radix Paeoniae Alba*), 10g of Shengdihuang (*Radix Rehmanniae*), 10g of carbonized Danpi (*Cortex Moutan Radicis*), 20g of Yiyiren (*Semen Coicis*), 10g of Jingjiesui (Apex *of Herba Schizonepetae*), 10g of fried Cangzhu (*Rhizoma Atractylodis*), 6g of Huangbai (*Cortex Phellodendri*) and 10g of carbonized Cebai (*Cacumen Platycladi*).

Modification: For excessive heat and thirst, 6g of Shanzhi (*Radix Pittospori Glabrati*) and 10g of Lugen

加　减　若面赤头痛者，加山栀6 g，柴胡6 g；心烦少寐者，加酸枣仁10 g，合欢花10 g；头目眩晕甚者，加枸杞子10 g，杭菊花10 g，白蒺藜12 g。

二、湿热蕴结证

主要证候　经间期出血，量少或稍多，色紫红，质粘稠，神倦乏力，胸闷纳差，心烦口干不欲饮，小便短赤，小腹胀痛，平素带多，色黄或赤白混杂，质稠粘，有臭气，或有阴痒，舌质红，苔白腻或黄腻，脉滑数。

治　法　清热利湿，凉血止血。

方　药　清肝止淋汤加减：当归10 g，赤芍药10 g，白芍药10 g，生地黄10 g，丹皮炭10 g，薏苡仁20 g，荆芥穗10 g，炒苍术10 g，黄柏6 g，侧柏炭10 g。

加　减　若烦热口渴，加山栀6 g，芦根10 g；小腹胀痛，

(*Rhizoma Phragmitis*) are added; for lower abdominal pain, 6g of Chuanlianzi (*Fructus Toosendan*) and 10g of Yanhusuo (*Rhizoma Corydalis*) are added; for chest oppression and greasy taste in the mouth, 10g of Huoxiang (*Herba Agastaches*) and 10g of Peilan (*Herba Eupatorii*) are added; for scanty and reddish stranguria, 6g of Mutong (*Caulis Akebiae*), 12g of Cheqiancao (*Herba Plantaginis*) and 3g of Gancaoshao (*Radix Glycyrrhizae*) are added.

(3) Syndrome of internal retention of blood stasis

Main symptoms: Scanty or slightly profuse intermenstrual bleeding with blackish color and blood clot, distending pain or stabbing pain in both sides of the lower abdomen, chest oppression and dysphoria, thirst without desire for drinking, grayish tongue or with petechiae, thin and taut pulse.

Therapeutic methods: Resolving stasis and stopping bleeding, regulating qi and harmonizing the collaterals.

Prescription and drugs: Modified Zhuyu Zhixue Tang composed of 10g of Shengdihuang (*Radix Rehmanniae*), 10g of Danggui (*Radix Angelicae Sinensis*), 12g of Chishaoyao (*Radix Paeoniae Rubra*), 5g of Dahuang (to be decocted later), 10g of Taoren (*Semen Persicae*), 12g of Mudanpi, 10g of fried Guiban, 10g of Zhike (*Fructus Aurantii*), 10g of Wulingzhi (*Faeces Trogopterori*), 10g of raw Puhuang (to be wrapped for decocting) and 12g of Chenzongtan (*Trachycarpi Carbonisatus*).

Modification: For distending pain and scorching fever in the lower abdomen, 12g of Baijiangcao (*Herba patriniae Cum Radice*), 8g of Chuanlianzi (*Fructus Toosendan*) and 10g of Yanhusuo (*Rhizoma Corydalis*) are added; for lumbago, 12g of Xuduan (*Radix Dipsaci*) and 12g of Sangjisheng (*Herba Taxilli*) are added.

加川楝子6 g,延胡索10 g;胸闷口腻,加藿香10 g,佩兰10 g;小便短赤淋痛,加木通6 g,车前草12 g,甘草梢3 g。

三、瘀血内阻证

主要证候　经间期出血,量少或稍多,色紫黑有血块,少腹两侧胀痛或刺痛,胸闷烦躁,口渴不欲饮,舌质黯或有瘀点,脉细弦。

治　法　化瘀止血,理气和络。

方　药　逐瘀止血汤加减:生地黄10 g,当归10 g,赤芍药12 g,大黄(后下)5 g,桃仁10 g,牡丹皮12 g,炙龟版10 g,枳壳10 g,五灵脂10 g,生蒲黄(包煎)10 g,陈棕炭12 g。

加　减　若小腹胀痛、灼热者,加败酱草12 g,川楝子8 g,延胡索10 g;腰酸,加续断12 g,桑寄生12 g。

[Other therapeutic methods]

(1) Chinese patent drugs

1) Wuji Baifeng Pill: 1 pill each time, twice a day, applicable to the syndrome of kidney-yin deficiency.

2) Fufang Danggui (*Radix Angelicae Sinensis*) Injection: 2 injections each time (2ml/one injection), once a day for 5 days, applicable to syndrome of blood stasis.

3) Gongxuening Capsule: 1 - 2 capsules each time, three times a day, applicable to the syndrome of blood stasis or yin deficiency and fire exuberance.

(2) Empirical and folk recipes

1) 60g of fresh Ou (*Rhizoma Nelumbinis*) and 60g of Cebaiye (*Cacumen Platycladi*) are pounded. The juice is taken orally with wine, applicable to bleeding of damp-heat syndrome.

2) 250g of Tianmendong (*Radix Asparagi*), 250g of Maimendong (*Radix Ophiopogonis*) and 250g of Wuzeigu (*Os Sepiae*) are decocted. After the removal of residue, the decoction is concentrated into paste with honey and is taken 10 - 15ml each time, twice a day and applicable to the syndrome of kidney-yin deficiency.

2.1.3 Metrorrhagia and metrostaxis

Metrorrhagia and metrostaxis refer to sudden profuse discharge or dripping menses, similar to dysfunctional uterine bleeding in modern medicine. It is usually caused by weak constitution, insufficiency of kidney-qi, weakness of the thoroughfare and conception vessels to control menses, or excessive sexual intercourse and multiparity that impair kidney qi. Or it may be caused by spleen-defi-

【其他疗法】

1. 中成药

（1）乌鸡白凤丸　每次1丸,1日2次,适用于肾阴亏虚证。

（2）复方当归注射液　每次2支(2 ml/支),1日1次肌肉注射,连用5天,适用于血瘀证。

（3）宫血宁胶囊　每次1~2粒,1日3次,适用于血瘀证或阴虚火旺证。

2. 单验方

（1）鲜藕60 g,侧柏叶60 g,打碎取汁,陈酒分送服,适用于湿热证出血。

（2）天门冬250 g,麦门冬250 g,乌贼骨250 g,浓煎去渣,炼蜜成膏,每服10~15 ml,1日2次,适用于肾阴亏虚证。

第三节　崩漏

崩漏是指经血非时暴下不止或淋漓不尽,本病属西医学功能失调性子宫出血疾病范畴。

本病多因先天禀赋不足,肾气未充,冲任不盛,或因房劳多产,损伤肾气,致肾虚封

ciency in constitution, or improper diet and overstrain and excessive anxiety that impairs spleen qi and leads to collapse of qi due to deficiency. Or it may be caused by yin-deficiency in constitution, or prolonged illness, hemorrhage, multiparity, excessive sexual intercourse that consumes yin-blood, deficiency of yin and water as well as internal exuberance of asthenia-fire. Or it may be caused by yang-excess in constitution, or invasion of exogenous heat into blood phase, or extreme changes of seven emotions and transformation of five emotions into fire that drives blood to escape the vessels. Or it may be caused by mental depression, stagnation of liver qi, qi stagnation and blood stasis, or internal impairment due to retention of menses or lochia in the thoroughfare and conception vessels.

[**Key points for diagnosis**]

(1) Serious disturbance in menstrual cycle, menstruation and menstrual blood, profuse and sudden menses or scanty and dripping menses, or menstruation first profuse and then scanty or dripping, or menstruation scanty and dripping first and then profuse and sudden, or irregular continuous menses, usually no abdominal pain.

(2) Profuse menses or prolonged menses usually accompanied with symptoms of anemia, coma tending to occur in acute profuse uterine bleeding.

(3) Gynecological examination and other supplementary tests show no organic disorder of the appendages.

(4) Diagnostic uterine curettage examination indicates endometrial changes in proliferative phase and excessive endometrial hyperplasia, or poor action of endometrial secretion, or coexistence of residual secretory endometrium and new endometrium in proliferative phase.

(5) Uterine bleeding during menstrual cycle should

藏失职，冲任不固，不能制约经血。亦有素体脾虚，或饮食劳倦、忧思过度损伤脾气，气虚下陷，升举无权，统摄失司，经血失于制约。或因素体阴虚，或久病、失血、多产、房劳损伤阴血，阴虚水亏，虚火内炽。或素体阳盛，或外感热邪、热入血分，或七情过极，五志化火而迫血妄行。或情怀不畅，肝郁气滞，气滞血瘀，或因经期、产后余血未尽，兼夹外感内伤，瘀血内阻冲任而致经血妄行。

【诊断要点】

（1）月经周期、经期及经量出现严重紊乱，出血量多势急或量少淋漓不断，或先多后少而淋漓不净，或先量少淋漓而后转为暴下量多，或量时多时少，持续不断。一般无腹痛。

（2）出血量多或长时间出血者，多伴有贫血症状；急性大量失血时易发生休克。

（3）妇科检查及其他辅助检查子宫、附件等无明显器质性病变。

（4）诊断性刮宫病理检查示：子宫内膜为增生期变化或子宫内膜增生过长；或子宫内膜分泌反应欠佳；或子宫内膜呈残留的分泌内膜和新生的增殖期内膜相间共存。

（5）本病应与妊娠出血性

be differentiated from uterine bleeding due to pregnancy, metritis, submucosal myoma of uterus endometriosis, and uterine tumor.

(6) Exclude bleeding caused by hematopathy and disturbance of blood coagulation mechanism.

[**Syndrome differentiation and treatment**]

The syndrome should be differentiated according to the quantity, color and texture changes of bleeding in light of the tongue and pulse conditions as well as the duration of disease to decide whether it is of asthenia or sthenia and of cold or heat. Usually metrorrhagia and metrostaxis tend to be of asthenia and heat. The treatment is taken on the basis of the conditions differentiated. Besides, age is also an important factor to be taken into consideration. For example, the patients at puberty are usually due to insufficiency of kidney qi; the patients of childbearing age are frequently due to liver stagnation and blood heat and the patients during perimenopausal period are often due to asthenia of the liver and kidney or asthenia of spleen qi.

There are three therapeutic methods that are usually used to treat metrorrhagia and metrostaxis.

Stopping bleeding: Usually qi-strengthening therapy is applied to control bleeding. If bleeding cannot be stopped, blood transfusion must be taken promptly; if bleeding is alleviated, treatment should be selected according to the conditions of the patient.

疾病、子宫炎性出血、子宫粘膜下肌瘤、子宫内膜异位症，以及子宫肿瘤引起的子宫出血相鉴别。

（6）排除血液病、凝血机制障碍性疾病导致的出血。

【辨证论治】

崩漏的主证是血证，故辨证当根据出血量、颜色和质地的变化，参合舌脉以及发病的久暂，辨其虚、实、寒、热。一般而言，崩漏虚证多而实证少，热者多而寒者少。崩漏有以崩为主的，有以漏为主的，或崩与漏交替出现的，或停经日久而忽然血大下的。久崩多虚，久漏多瘀。"崩为漏之甚，漏为崩之渐"，即崩可转漏，漏可成崩。临证时须审其轻重虚实。此外，患者不同的年龄阶段亦是崩漏辨证的重要参考，如青春期患者多属先天肾气不足，育龄期患者多见肝郁血热，围绝经期患者多因肝肾亏损或脾气虚弱。

治疗崩漏，尚需本着"急则治其标，缓则治其本"的原则，灵活掌握塞流、澄源、复旧三法。

塞流：即是止血之法。暴崩之际，急当止血防脱，一般用固气摄血法。血势不减者，宜输血救急，血势渐缓，则谨守病机，辨证论治。

Finding cause and dealing with the principal aspect: When bleeding is alleviated, treatment is given in light of syndrome differentiation, avoiding simple use of cold or warm or tonic or astringent herbs.

Restoration: Restoration means nourishing the kidney, regulating the liver or strengthening the spleen. Since menstrual disease is usually related to the kidney, the treatment should concentrate on nourishing the kidney, strengthening the thoroughfare vessel and regulating menstruaton.

In clinical treatment, these three therapeutic methods should be used in combination in light of syndrome differentiation. For example, the treatment for the patients during adolescence focuses on nourishing kidney qi and invigorating the thoroughfare and conception vessels; the treatment for the patients of childbearing age concentrates on soothing the liver, nourishing the liver and regulating the thoroughfare and conception vessels; the treatment for the patients during perimenopausal period emphasizes nourishing the kidney, regulating the liver, strengthening the spleen and reinforcing the thoroughfare and conception vessels.

(1) Syndrome of kidney asthenia and loss of consolidation

Main symptoms: Occurrence of menstrual blood not at the due time, or profuse and fulminant blood flow, dripping bleeding, dark red or bright red color menses, accompanied by dizziness, tinnitus, aching sensation and weakness in the loins, grayish complexion, deep and thin or fast pulse.

Therapeutic methods: Nourishing the kidney to replenish essence, nourishing blood to strengthen the thor-

澄源：一般用止血法后，待血势稍缓便须根据不同病证辨证论治，切忌不问原由，概投寒凉或温补之剂，或专事止涩，致犯虚虚实实之戒。

复旧：即固本善后，治法或补肾，或调肝，或扶脾。然月经病之本在肾，故总宜益肾固冲调经。

治崩漏三法不可截然分割，塞流需澄源，澄源当固本。治崩宜升提固涩，不宜辛温行血；治漏宜养血理气，不可偏于固涩。青春期患者，重在补肾气，益冲任；育龄期患者重在舒肝养肝，调冲任；围绝经期患者重在滋肾调肝，扶脾固冲任。

一、肾虚不固证

主要证候　经血非时而下，或量多如注，淋漓不断，色暗红或鲜红，头晕耳鸣，腰酸乏力，面色晦黯，脉沉细或数。

治　法　补肾填精，养血固冲。

oughfare vessel.

Prescription and drugs: Modified Yougui Wan combined with Zuogui Wan composed of 10g of Shudihuang (*Rhizoma Rehmanniae Praeparata*), 10g of Shanzhuyu (*Fructus Corni*), 10g of Gouqizi (*Fructus Lycii*), 12g of Tusizi (*Semen Cuscutae*), 10g of Lujiaojiao (*Colla Cornus Cervi*)(to be melted), 15g of Nüzhenzi (*Fructus Ligustri Lucidi*), 15g of Mohanlian (*Herba Ecliptae*), 12g of Sangjisheng (*Ramulus Taxilli*), 10g of Ejiao (*Colla Corii Asini*) (to be melted) and 10g of Duzhong (*Cortex Eucommiae*).

Modification: For palpitation and shortness of breath, 12g of Dangshen (*Radix Codonopsis Pilosulae*) and 10g of Huangqi (*Radix Astragali*) are added; for dysphoria and insomnia, 10g of Suanzaoren (*Semen Ziziphi Spinosae*) and 15g of Gouteng (*Ramulus Uncariae cum Uncis*) are added; for feverish sensation over palms, soles and chest, 10g of roasted Guiban (*Plastrum Testudinis*) and 10g of Digupi (*Cortex Lycii*) are added; for bright red bleeding, 10g of Diyu (*Radix Sanguisorbae*) and 10g of Cebaiye (*Cacumen Platydadi*) are added; for aversion to cold and cold limbs, 6g of sliced Fuzi (*Radix Aconiti Praeparata*) and 10g of Fupenzi (*Fructus Rubi*) are added; for frequent urination, 10g of Sangpiaoxiao (*Ootheca Mantidis*) and 10g of Yizhiren (*Fructus Alpiniae Oxyphyllae*) are added.

(2) Syndrome of asthenia spleen failing to command blood

Main symptoms: Occurrence of menstrual blood not at the due time, or profuse and fulminant blood flow, or dripping bleeding with thin texture menses, bright-whitish complexion or sallow complexion, edema of limbs, lassitude, cold limbs, lack of qi and no desire to speak, ano-

方　药　右归丸合左归丸加减：熟地黄10 g,山茱萸10 g,枸杞子10 g,菟丝子12 g,鹿角胶（烊化）10 g,女贞子15 g,墨旱莲15 g,桑寄生12 g,阿胶（烊化）10 g,杜仲10 g。

加　减　若心悸气短加党参12 g,黄芪10 g;心烦失寐加酸枣仁10 g,钩藤15 g;手足心热加炙龟版10 g,地骨皮10 g;血色鲜红加地榆10 g,侧柏叶10 g;畏寒肢冷加淡附片6 g,覆盆子10 g;小便频多加桑螵蛸10 g,益智仁10 g。

二、脾虚失统证

主要证候　经血非时而下,或量多如注,或淋漓不断,色淡红,质稀薄,面色㿠白或萎黄不泽,面浮肢肿、倦怠乏力,四肢不温,少气懒言,纳少

rexia and loose stool, empty prolapsing sensation in the lower abdomen, light and bulgy tongue or tooth-printed tongue with thin and white fur, thin and weak pulse.

Therapeutic methods: Nourishing qi to elevate yang and strengthening the spleen to control blood.

Prescription and drugs: Modified Guben Zhibeng Tang composed of 15g of Dangshen (*Radix Codonopsis Pilosulae*), 10g of Huangqi (*Radix Astragali*), 10g of Baizhu (*Rhizoma Atractylodis Macrocephalae*), 6g of roasted Shengma (*Rhizoma Cimicifugae*), 12g of Shan-yao (*Rhizoma Dioscoreae*), 10g of roasted Muxiang (*Radix Aucklaneliae*), 6g of Paojiangtan (carbonized *Rhizoma Zingiberis*), 12g of Chuanxuduan (*Radix Dipsaci*) and 5g of roasted Gancao (*Radix Glycyrrhizae*).

Modification: For profuse bleeding, 20g of calcined Longgu (*Os Draconis*), 20g of calcined Muli (*Concha Ostreae*) and 15g of Chenzongtan (*Trachycarpi Carbonisatus*) are added; for bleeding with blood clot, 10g of roasted Wulingzhi (*Faeces Trogopterorum*) and 10g of Aiyetan (carbonized *Folium Artemisiae Argyi*) are added; for dripping bleeding, 30g of Yimucao (*Herba Leonuri*) and 30g of Qiancao (*Radix Rubiae*) are added; for palpitation, 10g of roasted Yuanzhi (*Radix Polygalae*) and 10g of Shilianrou (*Herba Sinocrassulae*) are added.

(3) Syndorme of abnormal flow of blood due to heat

Main symptoms: Occurrence of menstrual blood not at the due time, or profuse and fulminant blood flow, dripping bleeding, bright-red or deep red color and thin texture menses, accompanied by dysphoria, dry mouth, or fever, yellowish urine, constipation, red tongue with yellow fur, slippery pulse or thin and rapid pulse.

Therapeutic methods: Clearing away heat and con-

便溏,小腹空坠,舌质淡胖或有齿印,苔薄白,脉细弱。

　　治　法　益气升阳,健脾摄血。

　　方　药　固本止崩汤加减:党参15g,黄芪10g,白术10g,炙升麻6g,山药12g,煨木香10g,炮姜炭6g,川续断12g,炙甘草5g。

　　加　减　若量多如崩加煅龙骨20g,煅牡蛎20g,陈棕炭15g;血块多者,加炒五灵脂10g,艾叶炭10g;淋漓不净加益母草30g,茜草30g;心悸怔忡加炙远志10g,石莲肉10g。

三、血热妄行证

　　主要证候　经血非时而下,或量多如注,或淋漓不断,色鲜红或深红,质稠粘,心烦口干,或有发热,小便黄,大便结,舌质红,苔黄,脉滑或细数。

　　治　法　清热固经,凉血

trolling menstruation, cooling blood to stop bleeding.

Prescription and drugs: Modified Qingre Gujing Tang composed of 10g of Huangqin (*Radix Scutellariae*), 6g of stir-baked Shanzhi (*Fructus Gardeniae*), 10g of Shengdihuang (*Radix Rehmanniae*), 12g of Digupi (*Cortex Lycii*), 15g of crude Diyu (*Radix Sanguisorbae*), 10g of Mudanpi (*Cortex Moutan Radicis*), 10g of roasted Guiban (*Plastrum Testudinis*), 10g of Ejiao (*Colla Corii Asini*), 10g of Chenzongtan (*Trachycarpi Carbonisatus*), 10g of Oujietan (*Nodus Nelumbinis Rhizomatis Carbonisatus*) and 5g of crude Gancao (*Radix Glycyrrhizae*) are added.

Modification: For restless fever and thirst, 10g of Zhimu (*Rhizoma Anemarrhenae*), 10g of Maimendong (*Radix Ophiopogonis*) and 10g of Xuanshen (*Radix Scrophulariae*) are added; for bleeding with blood clot, 10g of stir-baked Puhuang (*Pollen Typhae*) and 6g of stir-baked Wulingzhi (*Faeces Trogopterorum*) are added; for dyphoria, tidal fever, flushed cheeks, feverish sensation over palms, soles and chest, red and dry tongue as well as thin and rapid pulse as the main symptoms, Baoyin Jian and 10g of Maimendong (*Radix Ophiopogonis*), 10g of Shashen (*Radix Adenophorae*) and 6g of Qinghao (*Herba Artemisiae Annuae*) are added.

(4) Syndrome of retention of blood stasis

Main symptoms: Occurrence of menstrual blood not at the due time, or profuse and fulminant blood flow, dripping bleeding, or occasional bleeding, purplish red or blackish red color menses, or mingled with blood clot, unpressable lower abdominal pain, purplish tongue or with ecchymosis and unsmooth or taut pulse.

Therapeutic methods: Activating blood to remove stagnation and resolving stasis to stop bleeding.

止血。

方　药　清热固经汤加减：黄芩10 g,炒山栀6 g,生地黄 10 g,地骨皮12 g,生地榆15 g,牡丹皮10 g,炙龟版10 g,阿胶10 g,陈棕炭10 g,藕节炭10 g,生甘草5 g。

加　减　若烦热口渴加知母10 g,麦门冬10 g,玄参10 g;血块多加炒蒲黄10 g,炒五灵脂6 g;若以心烦,潮热颧红,手足心热,舌红而干,脉细数为主症者,用保阴煎加麦门冬10 g,沙参10 g,青蒿6 g。

四、瘀血阻滞证

主要证候　经血非时而下,或量多如注,或淋漓不断,或时来时止,色紫红或黯红或夹有瘀块,小腹胀痛拒按,舌质紫黯或有瘀点,脉涩或弦。

治　法　活血行滞,化瘀止血。

Prescription and drugs: Modified Jiawei Shixiao San composed of 10g of stir-baked Puhuang (*Pollen Typhae*), 10g of stir-baked Wulingzhi (*Faeces Trogopterorum*), 6g of charred Dahuang (*Radix et Rhizoma Rhei*), 12g of stir-baked Danggui (*Radix Angelicae Sinensis*), 12g of Chishaoyao (*Radix Paeoniae Rubra*) and Baishaoyao (*Radix Paeoniae Alba*) respectively, 30g of charred Qiancao (*Radix Rubiae*), 10g of crude Shanzha (*Fructus Crataegi*), 30g of Yimucao (*Herba Leonuri*), 30g of Luxiancao (*Herba Pyrolae*) and 30g of Mabiancao (*Herba Verbenae*).

Modification: For profuse and incessant bleeding, 4g of Shensanqi powder (*Radix Notoginseng*) (to be taken separately) is added; for cold sensation in the lower abdomen, 10g of Aiyetan (carbonized *Folium Artemisiae Argyi*) and 10g of Buguzhi (*Fructus Psoraleae*) are added; for blood clot in the menstrual blood, 12g of charred Guanzhong (*Rhizoma Dryopteris Gassirhizomae*) is added; for lower abdominal distending pain, 10g of roasted Xiangfu (*Rhizoma Cyperi*) and 10g of Yanhusuo (*Rhizoma Corydalis*) are added.

[Other therapeutic methods]

(1) Chinese patent drugs

1) Gujing Pill: 6 -9g each time and three times a day, applicable to the treatment of blood heat syndrome.

2) Bazhen Granulae: One bag each time and twice or three times a day, applicable to the treatment of qi asthenia syndrome.

3) Xuejie Capsule: 4 capsules each time and three times a day, applicable to the treatment of blood stasis syndrome.

4) Erzhi Pill: 6 - 9 pills each time and twice a day, applicable to the treatment of kidney asthenia syndrome.

方　药　加味失笑散加减:炒蒲黄10g,炒五灵脂10 g,大黄炭6 g,炒当归12 g,赤白芍药各12 g,茜草炭30 g,生山楂10 g,益母草30 g,鹿衔草30 g,马鞭草30 g。

加　减　若量多不止者,加参三七粉4 g(另吞);小腹觉冷,加艾叶炭 10 g,补骨脂10 g;经血瘀块较多加贯众炭12 g;小腹胀痛显著者,加制香附10 g,延胡索10 g。

【其他疗法】
1. 中成药
（1）固经丸　每次服6～9 g,1 日 3 次,适用于血热证。
（2）八珍冲剂　每次服1包,1 日 2～3 次,适用于气虚证。
（3）血竭胶囊　每次服4粒,1 日 3 次,适用于血瘀证。
（4）二至丸　每次服6～9 g,1 日 2 次,适用于肾

5) Xue'an: 4 tablets each time and three times a day, applicable to the treatment of metrorrhagia due to spleen asthenia or blood heat.

6) Gongxuening: 1 – 2 pills each time and three times a day, applicable to the treatment of metrorrhagia due to blood stasis.

(2) Empirical and folk recipes

1) 30g of Heimu'er (*Riculariae*) and 30 Chinese dates are decocted for oral taking for several days. This treatment is applicable to blood heat syndrome.

2) 250g of fresh Zhumagen (*Radix Boehmeriae Niveae*) is washed and ground to extract juice which is mixed up with 30g of sugar for oral taking once a day for several days. This treatment is applicable to the treatment of yin asthenia and blood heat.

2.1.4 Dysmenorrhea

Dysmenorrhea refers to lower abdominal pain or other discomforts before, after or during menstruation. Clinically abdominal pain during menstruation starting from menarche is called primary dysmenorrhea and abdominal pain during menstruation after the occurrence of menarche is called secondary dysmenorrhea. Dysmenorrhea usually occurs among women of 15 – 25 years among young women during adolescence, or the unmarried or the married without delivery of child. Serious dysmenorrhea may affect health.

Dysmenorrhea is usually caused by emotional factors, invasion of six exogenous pathogenic factors and stagnation of qi and blood; or by retention of blood in the uterus

虚证。

（5）血安　每次服 4 粒，1 日 3 次,适用于脾虚或血热证漏下者。

（6）宫血宁　每次服 1～2 粒,1 日 3 次,适用于血瘀证漏下者。

2. 单验方

（1）黑木耳30 g,红枣 30 枚,煎汤食服,每日 1 次,连服数日,适用于血热证。

（2）鲜苎麻根250 g,砂糖 30 g,将苎麻根洗净捣绒取汁,砂糖冲服,每日 1 次,连服数日,适用于阴虚血热证。

第四节　痛经

痛经是指妇女在月经来潮前后或行经期间出现小腹疼痛或其他不适,且随月经周期而发作的病症。临床上通常将初潮开始即有行经腹痛者,称为原发性痛经。初潮时无腹痛,以后出现痛经者,称为继发性痛经。发病年龄多在15～25 岁之间,常见于青春期少女、未婚及已婚未产的青年女性,严重者可危及健康。

凡情志所伤、六淫侵袭、气血瘀阻,或肝肾亏虚、气血不足等,皆可发生经行腹痛。

due to liver depression and qi stagnation resulting from emotional upsets; or by cold-dampness attacking the lower energizer and lodging in the uterus due to walking in water during menstruation or sitting on damp ground; or by constitutional deficiency of qi and blood, or consumption of qi and blood due to serious disease and prolonged illness; or by congenital defect or impairment of the liver and kidney, consumption of blood and malnutrition of the uterus due to multiparity and excessive sexual life.

[Key points for diagnosis]

(1) The main clinical symptom is lower abdominal pain during menstruation. It usually occurs 1 - 2 days before menstruation or after menstruation.

(2) The manifestations are paroxysmal spasmodic pain or distending pain in the lower abdomen; the pain may radiate to the lumbosacral region, anus, vagina or medial side of the leg. In serious cases there are pale complexion, cold sweating, cold hands and feet, nausea and vomiting, diarrhea or even syncope. In a few cases, dysmenorrhea may be accompanied by symptoms of irritation sign of bladder, such as frequent urination and urgent urination. The duration of pain lasts from 2 - 3 days. The pain usually reaches its peak on the first day of menstruation and then gradually alleviates or disappears. In the cases of membraniform dysmenorrhea, patches of endometrium exfoliate. Pain may be relieved after the removal of endometrial patches. Functional dysmenorrhea will gradu-

若因情志不舒,肝郁气滞,气不运血,则血行受阻,滞留胞宫,故不通则痛;或在经期冒雨涉水,感寒饮冷,或坐卧湿地,寒湿伤于下焦而客于胞宫,经血为寒湿凝滞,运行不畅而作痛;或因素体气血不足,或大病久病之后,气血亏耗,血行无力,通而不畅;或因先天禀赋不足,或由多产、房劳,以致肝肾亏损,阴血不足,血海空虚,胞宫失于濡养而致小腹虚痛。

【诊断要点】

(1) 本病以伴随月经周期而出现的小腹疼痛为主要临床特征。一般多发生在经前1~2天,或月经来潮后的第1~2天,也有发生在月经将净时或经净后的1~2天。

(2) 主要表现为小腹部阵发性痉挛性疼痛或胀痛、坠痛,疼痛可向腰骶部、肛门、阴道和大腿内侧放射。严重者可伴有面色苍白、出冷汗、手足厥冷、恶心呕吐、腹泻,甚至出现晕厥。少数人也可伴有膀胱刺激症状,如尿频、尿急等,疼痛持续时间长短不一,从数小时到2~3天不等,一般在月经来潮首日疼痛达到高峰,随后逐渐减轻或消失。膜样痛经患者可见有大片子宫内膜脱落,排出后疼痛可得

ally alleviate with the increase of age and improve after marriage or delivery of child.

(3) Basic temperature detection usually indicates ovulation menstrual cycle. Gynecological examination can be done to see whether there are abnormal changes in the shape, location and texture of the uterus and whether there is thickening change of the appendage as well as whether there is mass and tenderness.

(4) Ultrasonic test, pelvic pneumography and peritoneoscopy are made to decide whether dysmenorrhea is functional or organic. Prostaglandin test of menses can suggest whether there is abnormal increase of prostaglandin.

(5) Measures should be taken to differentiate dysmenorrhea from abdominal pain caused by extrauterine pregnancy, rupture of corpus luteum, torsion of ovarian cyst, acute pelvitis, acute cystitis, urinary stones, appendicitis, colitis and acute gastroenteritis, etc.

[Syndrome differentiation and treatment]

Differentiation of syndromes should concentrate on revealing the nature of dysmenorrhea in light of the time, location and degree of pain; the quantity, color and texture of menses; and complications, tongue and pulse conditions. Usually pain occurring before and during menstruation is of sthenia; pain occurring after menstruation is often of asthenia. Unpressable pain is of sthenia; while dull pain with preference for pressure is of asthenia. Pain alleviated with warmth is due to cold, while pain worsened with warmth is due to heat. Pain severer than distension is due to blood stasis, while distension severer than pain is

缓解。功能性痛经可随年龄的增长而症状逐渐减轻,常于结婚后或分娩后好转。

(3)基础体温测定多表现为有排卵型月经周期。妇科检查可了解子宫形态、位置大小、质地等有否异常,两侧附件有无增厚、包块及压痛等。

(4)可行超声波检查、盆腔充气造影及腹腔镜检查,以确定是功能性痛经还是由器质性病变引起的痛经。月经血前列腺素测定可显示有异常增高。

(5)本病应注意与宫外孕、卵巢黄体破裂、卵巢囊肿扭转等急腹症以及急性盆腔炎、急性膀胱炎、泌尿系结石、阑尾炎、结肠炎、急性胃肠炎等疾病引起的小腹疼痛相鉴别。

【辨证论治】

痛经辨证首先当识别痛证的属性。根据疼痛发生的时间、性质、部位以及痛经的程度,结合月经期、量、色、质及兼证、舌脉,并根据素体情况等辨其寒、热、虚、实。一般痛在经前、经期,多属实证,痛在经后,多属虚证;疼痛剧烈拒按多属实证,隐隐作痛、喜揉喜按多属虚证;得热痛减多为寒,得热痛增多为热;痛甚

due to qi stagnation. Colic pain and cold pain are due to cold, while burning pain is due to heat. Pain in the sides of abdomen is due to liver disorder, while pain involving the loins is due to kidney disorder.

The basic therapeutic principle for treating dysmenorrhea is regulating qi and blood in the thoroughfare and conception vessels, including regulating qi, activating blood, dissipating cold, clearing away heat, supplementing asthenia and purging sthenia according to the syndromes. The treatment focuses either on the principal aspect by means of regulating blood to stop pain during menstruation or on the secondary aspect based on syndrome differentiation at other time.

(1) Syndrome of qi stagnation and blood stasis

Main symptoms: Unpressable lower abdominal pain or prolapsing pain 1-2 days before menstruation or during menstruation, profuse or scanty menstruation, dripping and unsmooth menorrhea, purplish and blacking color menses with blood clot or patches of putrid blood clot, alleviation after the removal of blood clot, distending pain in the chest, hypochondria and breasts, purplish tongue or with ecchymosis on the edge, deep and taut pulse.

Therapeutic methods: Soothing the liver to regulate qi and resolving stasis to stop pain.

Prescription and drugs: Modified Xuefu Zhuyu Tang composed of 10g of Danggui (*Radix Angelicae Sinensis*), 6g of Chuanxiong (*Rhizoma Chuanxiong*), 10g of Chishaoyao (*Radix Paeoniae Rubra*), 10g of Taoren (*Semen Persicae*), 10g of Honghua (*Flos Carthami*), 10g of Chuanniuxi (*Radix Cyathulae*), 10g of Xiangfu (*Rhizoma Cyperi*), 6g of Qingpi (*Pericarpium Citri Reticulatae Viride*), 10g of Zhike (*Fructus*

于胀,血块排出则疼痛减轻或刺痛者多为血瘀,胀甚于痛者多为气滞;绞痛、冷痛者属寒,灼痛者属热;痛在两侧少腹病多在肝,痛连腰际病多在肾。

痛经的治疗原则,以调理冲任气血为主。根据不同的证候,或行气,或活血,或散寒,或清热,或补虚,或泻实。治法分两步:月经期调血止痛以治标,平时辨证求因而治本。

一、气滞血瘀证

主要证候 每于经前一两日或经期小腹胀痛或坠痛,拒按,经量或多或少,淋漓不畅,经色紫黑有血块,或有大片腐肉样的血块排出后疼痛减轻,胸胁乳房胀痛,舌质紫暗,或边有瘀点,脉沉弦。

治 法 疏肝理气,化瘀止痛。

方 药 血府逐瘀汤加减:当归10 g,川芎6 g,赤芍药10 g,桃仁10 g,红花10 g,川牛膝10 g,香附10 g,青皮6 g,枳壳10 g,木香6 g,延胡索10 g,五灵脂10 g,甘草3 g。

Aurantii), 6g of Muxiang (*Radix Aucklaneliae*), 10g of Yanhusuo (*Rhizoma Corydalis*), 10g of Wulingzhi (*Faeces Trogopterorum*) and 3g of Gancao (*Radix Glycyrrhizae*).

Modification: For lower abdominal pain with cold sensation, 6g of Rougui (*Cortex Cinnamomi*) and 6g of Wuzhuyu (*Fructus Evodiae*) are added; for deep-red and profuse menorrhea, 10g of Mudanpi (*Cortex Moutan Radicis*) and 5g of Shensanqi (*Radix Notoginseng*) are added; for distending pain in the breast or even with mass, 6g of Chaihu (*Radix Bupleuri*) and 6g of Juhe (*Semen Citri Reticulatae*) are added; for nausea and vomiting, 5g of Sharen (*Fructus Amomi*) and 10g of Zisugeng (*Caulis Perillae*) are added; for membraniform dysmenorrhea, 10g of crude Shanzha (*Fructus Crataegi*) and 10g of Ezhu (*Rhizoma Curcumae*) are added.

(2) Syndrome of coagulation of cold dampness

Main symptoms: Unpressable lower abdominal cold pain before or during menstruation, alleviation of pain with warmth, scanty menorrhea with purplish color menses and clot or like juice of black soybean, cold sensation in the body and aversion to cold, loose stool, light purplish tongue with white and moist or white and greasy fur, deep and tense pulse.

Therapeutic methods: Warming meridians to disperse cold and draining dampness to eliminate stagnation.

Prescription and drugs: Modified Shaofu Zhuyu Tang composed of 6g of Rougui (*Cortex Cinnamomi*) (to be decocted later), 6g of Xiaohuixiang (*Fructus Foeniculi*), 6g of Paojiang (*baked Rhizoma Zingiberis*), 10g of Yanhusuo (*Rhizoma Corydalis*), 10g of Wulingzhi (*Faeces Trogopterorum*), 6g of Moyao (*Myrrha*), 10g of Danggui (*Radix Angelicae Sinensis*), 5g of Chuanxiong

加　减　若小腹疼痛伴有冷感者,加肉桂6 g,吴茱萸6 g;经色深红量多者,加牡丹皮10 g,参三七5 g;乳房胀痛甚则有块者,加柴胡6 g,橘核6 g;恶心呕吐,加砂仁5 g,紫苏梗10 g;膜样痛经,加生山楂10 g,莪术10 g。

二、寒湿凝滞证

主要证候　经前或经期小腹冷痛,按之痛甚,得热则舒,经行量少,色紫暗有块,或如黑豆汁,形寒畏冷,大便溏薄,舌淡紫,苔白润或白腻,脉沉紧。

治　法　温经散寒,利湿逐瘀。

方　药　少腹逐瘀汤加减:肉桂(后下)6 g,小茴香6 g,炮姜6 g,延胡索10 g,五灵脂10 g,没药6 g,当归10 g,川芎5 g,蒲黄(包煎)10 g,赤芍药10 g,苍术10 g。

(*Rhizoma Chuanxiong*), 10g of Puhuang (*Pollen Typhae*) (to be wrapped for decocting), 10g of Chishaoyao (*Radix Paeoniae Rubra*) and 10g of Cangzhu (*Rhizoma Atractylodis*).

Modification: For aversion to cold and cold limbs, 6g of sliced Fuzi (*Radix Aconiti Praeparata*) and 6g of Wuzhuyu (*Fructus Evodiae*) are added; for lower abdominal spasmodic pain, 20g of Baishaoyao (*Radix Paeoniae Alba*) and 5g of Gancao (*Radix Glycyrrhizae*) are added; for nausea and vomiting, 6g of Jiangbanxia (*Rhizoma Pinelliae*) and 6g of Muxiang (*Radix Aucklaneliae*) are added.

加 减 若畏寒肢冷,加附片6g,吴茱萸6g;小腹拘挛性疼痛,加白芍药20g,甘草5g;恶心呕吐加姜半夏6g,木香6g。

(3) Syndrome of qi and blood asthenia

Main symptoms: Dull pain or continuous pain or prolapsing sensation in the lower abdomen during or after menstruation, alleviation with pressure, profuse or scanty menses with ligh color and thin texture but without clot, pale complexion, dizziness, palpitation, lassitude, light-colored tongue with tooth print and thin fur as well as thin pulse.

Therapeutic methods: Strengthening the spleen and nourishing qi, invigorating blood and stopping bleeding.

Prescription and drugs: Modified Bazhen Tang composed of 12g of Dangshen (*Radix Codonopsis*), 12g of Baizhu (*Rhizoma Atractylodis Macrocephalae*), 10g of Fuling (*Poria*), 10g of Danggui (*Radix Angelicae Sinensis*), 10g of Baishaoyao (*Radix Paeoniae Alba*), 10g of Shudihuang (*Rhizoma Rehmanniae Praeparata*), 5g of stir-baked Gancao (*Radix Glycyrrhizae*), 10g of Huangqi (*Radix Astragali*) and 6g of Muxiang (*Radix Aucklaneliae*).

Modification: For aching in the loins, 10 g of Xu-

三、气血虚弱证

主要证候 经期或经净后小腹隐痛,绵绵不断,或有下坠感,按之痛减,经量多或少,色淡质稀无块,面色苍白,头昏心悸,神疲乏力,舌质淡,边有齿印,苔薄,脉细。

治 法 健脾益气,养血止痛。

方 药 八珍汤加减:党参12g,白术12g,茯苓10g,当归10g,白芍药10g,熟地黄10g,炙甘草5g,黄芪10g,木香6g。

加 减 若腰酸,加续断

duan (*Radix Dipsaci*) and 10g of Duzhong (*Cortex Eucommiae*) are added; for empty prolapsing sensation and pain in the lower abdomen, 6g of roasted Shengma (*Rhizoma Cimicifugae*) is added; for aversion to cold and cold limbs, 10g of Buguzhi (*Fructus Psoraleae*) is added; for anorexia and loose stool, 12g of stir-baked Maiya (*Fructus Hordei Germinatus*) and 10g of Liuqu (*Massa Medicata Fermentata*) are added; for profuse menorrhea, 10g of Ejiao (*Colla Corii Asini*) and 6g of charred Aiye (*Folium Artemisiae Argyi*) are added.

(4) Syndrome of liver and kidney asthenia

Main symptoms: Scanty menses with dull light color but without blood clot, dull pain in the lower abdomen after menstruation, aching sensation in the loins and knees, dizziness and tinnitus, light-red tongue with thin fur, deep and thin pulse.

Therapeutic methods: Nourishing blood and regulating the liver, replenishing the kidney and enriching essence.

Prescription and drugs: Modified Tiaogan Tang composed of 10g of Shanyao (*Rhizoma Dioscoreae*), 10g of Ejiao (*Colla Corii Asini*) (to be melted), 10g of Danggui (*Radix Angelicae Sinensis*), 10g of Baishaoyao (*Radix Paeoniae Alba*), 6g of Shanzhuyu (*Fructus Corni*), 10g of Bajitian (*Radix Morindae Officinalis*), 10g of Gouqizi (*Fructus Lycii*), 10g of Xiangfu (*Rhizoma Cyperi*), 10g of Shudihuang (*Rhizoma Rehmanniae Praeparata*), 10g of Shayuanzi (*Semen Astragali Complanati*) and 3g of Gancao (*Radix Glycyrrhizae*).

Modification: For severe aching in the loins, 10g of Xuduan is added; for dull pain in the sides of the lower abdomen, 10g of Yanhusuo and 10g of Juhe (*Semen Citri Reticulatae*) are added; for distending pain in the chest

10 g, 杜仲 10 g; 小腹空坠而痛, 加炙升麻 6 g; 畏寒肢冷, 加补骨脂 10 g; 纳差便溏加炒谷芽 12 g, 六曲 10 g; 经量过多, 加阿胶 10 g, 艾叶炭 6 g。

四、肝肾亏损证

主要证候 经来量少, 色暗淡, 无血块, 经后小腹隐痛, 腰膝酸软, 头晕耳鸣, 舌质淡红, 苔薄, 脉沉细。

治 法 养血调肝, 补肾填精。

方 药 调肝汤加减: 山药 10 g, 阿胶 (烊化) 10 g, 当归 10 g, 白芍药 10 g, 山茱萸 6 g, 巴戟天 10 g, 枸杞子 10 g, 香附 10 g, 熟地黄 10 g, 沙苑子 10 g, 甘草 3 g。

加 减 若腰酸甚, 加续断 10 g, 小腹两侧隐痛, 加川楝子 6 g, 延胡索 10 g, 橘核 10 g; 胸胁胀痛, 加青皮 6 g, 郁金

and hypochondria, 6g of Qingpi (*Pericarpium Citri Reticulatae Viride*) and 10g of Yujin (*Radix Curcumae*) are added; for frequent urination in the night, 10g of Yizhiren (*Fructus Alpiniae Oxyphyllae*) and 10g of Sangpiaoxiao (*Ootheca Mantidis*) are added.

[Other therapeutic methods]

(1) Chinese patent drugs

1) Tongjing Pill: 10g each time and three times a day, applicable to the treatment of cold coagulation and blood stasis.

2) Aifu Nuangong Pill: 10g each time and three times a day, applicable to the treatment of dysmenorrhea due to asthenia cold.

3) Yueyueshu Granulae: 1 bag each time and three times a day, applicable to the treatment of cold coagulation and blood stasis.

4) Yanhu Zhitong Tablets: 4 tablets each time and three times a day, applicable to the treatment of qi stagnation and blood stasis.

(2) Empirical and folk recipes

1) 30g of Yimucao (*Herba Leonuri*) is decocted with proper amount of brown sugar for oral taking, three times a day, applicable to the treatment of dysmenorrhea due to blood stasis.

2) 15g of Shengjiang (*Rhizoma Zingiberis Recens*) is decocted with 3 scallion stalks and proper amount of brown sugar, applicable to the treatment of dysmenorrhea due to cold dampness.

2.1.5　Amenorrhea

Amenorrhea is either primary or secondary. The former refers to non-occurrence of menstruation in women over 16 years old with the development of the second sex

10 g;夜尿频多,加益智仁10 g,桑螵蛸10 g。

【其他疗法】

1. 中成药

（1）痛经丸　每次服10 g,1 日 3 次,适用于寒凝血瘀证。

（2）艾附暖宫丸　每次服10 g,1 日 3 次,适用于虚寒性痛经。

（3）月月舒冲剂　每次服 1 包,1 日 3 次,适用于寒凝血瘀证。

（4）延胡止痛片　每次服 4 片,1 日 3 次,适用于气滞血瘀证。

2. 单验方

（1）益母草30 g,红糖适量,水煎服,1 日 3 剂,适用于血瘀证痛经。

（2）生姜15 g,葱白 3 根,红糖适量,水煎服,适用于寒湿痛经。

第五节　闭经

闭经有原发性和继发性之分。原发性闭经多指年龄超过 16 岁,第二性征已发育,

sign or women over 14 without the development of the second sex sign. The latter refers to stoppage of menstruation for 6 months or 3 cycles in women who had regular menstruation. Amenorrhea in adolescence, pregnancy and breast-feeding is physiological phenomenon.

Amenorrhea is usually caused by congenital defect, insufficiency of kidney qi, essence and blood; or by multiparity and excessive sexual life which impair the liver and kidney leading to deficiency of essence and blood and hypofunction of the thoroughfare and conception vessels; or by improper diet, overstrain and anxiety which damage spleen qi and leading to insufficiency of transformation; or by constitutional weakness, or serious disease and prolonged duration of illness, multiparity, loss of blood affecting fluid, deficiency of blood in the thoroughfare and conception vessels; or by impairment of the liver due to rage, stagnation of liver qi, unsmooth flow of qi which lead to stagnation of the thoroughfare and conception vessels; or by improper care during menstruation, or exogenous pathogenic factors attack, or internal impairment due to intake of uncooked and cold foods which result in cold coagulation in the thoroughfare and conception vessels; or by obesity, internal exuberance of phlegm-dampness, or failure of spleen yang to transport, leading to accumulation of dampness into phlegm in the thoroughfare and conception vessels as well as in the uterine collaterals.

[Key points for diagnosis]

(1) Non-occurrence of menarche after the age of 16

或年龄超过 14 岁,第二性征尚未发育,且无月经来潮者;继发性闭经则指以往曾建立正常月经、但此后因某种病理性原因而月经停止 6 个月,或按自身原来月经周期计算停经 3 个周期以上者。至于青春期前、妊娠期、哺乳期以及绝经后的无月经均属生理现象。中医古代医籍中称本病为"女子不月"、"经水断绝"、"血枯"等。

本病常由先天禀赋不足,肾气未盛,精血不充;或多产房劳、损及肝肾,以致精亏血少、冲任不盛;饮食劳倦,忧愁思虑,损伤脾气,化源不足;或素体虚弱,或大病久病、多产、失血伤津,冲任血少,血海空虚,以致经闭;或郁怒伤肝;肝气郁结,气机不利,以致冲任瘀滞、胞脉闭阻;或经期产后血室正开,调摄失慎,或外感寒邪,或内伤生冷,血为寒凝,冲任瘀阻;或素体肥胖,痰湿内盛,或脾阳失运、湿聚成痰,痰湿阻于冲任,胞脉闭塞等,病因所致。

【诊断要点】

(1) 年逾 16 岁月经尚未

or non-physiological stoppage of menstruation for 3 cycles.

(2) Careful examination is made of the general development, nutrition, mental state and development of the secondary sex characteristic in order to analyze the cause and nature of amenorrhea.

(3) Examination is made to see whether the external and internal genitals are normal and whether there is mass in the pelvis.

(4) Iodized oil roentgenograph is done to see whether there are abnormal development of the uterus, metrosynizesis and tuberculosis of endometrium.

(5) Diagnostic uterine curettage and pathological examination of endometrium are done to examine the functional states of the ovary and to see whether there are tuberculosis of endometrium and severe damage of endometrium.

(6) Sella turcica X-ray examination and CT scan are helpful for excluding pituitary tumor.

(7) Uteroscopy and peritoneoscopy are helpful for detecting organic pathological change of the uterus and pelvis.

(8) Chromosome nuclear analysis can be made in diagnosing primary amenorrhea.

(9) Test of hormones in the blood: FSH has obviously increased and estrin has decreased, suggesting hypofunction of the ovary; low FSH and LH values suggest hypofunction of the pituitary or hypothalamus; increase of LH, FSH and T values indicates amenorrhea due to polycystic ovary syndrome; increase of PRL value indicates amenorrhea due to hyperprolactin hematopathy.

(10) Cares should be taken to differentiate amenorrhea mentioned above from physiological amenorrhea due

初潮,或月经周期建立以后非生理性停经 3 个周期以上。

(2) 注意观察患者一般发育、营养、精神及第二性征发育等状态,有助于分析判断闭经的原因与性质。

(3) 注意检查患者内外生殖器官的发育状况,有无畸形或缺如,有无盆腔肿块。

(4) 通过子宫碘油造影,了解有无子宫畸形、宫腔粘连及子宫内膜结核。

(5) 诊断性刮宫及子宫内膜病理检查,有助于了解卵巢功能状态、有无子宫内膜结核及子宫内膜严重损伤。

(6) 蝶鞍 X 线摄片或 CT 检查有助于排除垂体肿瘤。

(7) 宫腔镜、腹腔镜检查可发现宫腔及盆腔器质性病变。

(8) 对原发性闭经患者可进行染色体核型分析。

(9) 血中激素水平测定:促卵泡激素(FSH)明显升高、雌激素(E)水平低下,提示卵巢功能减退;FSH 及 LH(促黄体生成激素)值低下,提示垂体或下丘脑功能低下;LH/FSH比值升高、T(睾酮)值升高,提示多囊卵巢综合征性闭经;PRL(泌乳素)值升高,提示高泌乳素血症性闭经。

(10) 本病应与妊娠、哺乳期、绝经期的生理性闭经相

to pregnancy, breastfeeding and menopause.

[Syndrome differentiation and treatment]

Non-occurrence of menarche after the normal age or development from scanty menorrhea to amenorrhea accompanied by other asthenia symptoms is of asthenia syndrome; while sudden occurrence of amenorrhea accompanied by other sthenia symptoms is of sthenia syndrome.

The treatment of amenorrhea is either nourishing for asthenia syndrome, such as nourishing the liver and kidney or regulating and nourishing qi and blood; or purging for sthenia syndrome, such as activating blood to resolve stasis, or regulating qi to remove stagnation, or expelling pathogenic factors to regulate menstruation. Both drastic purgation and drastic nourishing therapies are forbidden. The treatment of amenorrhea due to other diseases may concentrate on dealing with the diseases first.

(1) Syndrome of deficiency of the liver and kidney

Main symptoms: Non-occurrence of menarche after the normal age, or delayed menarche, delayed menstruation, scanty menorrhea, gradual amenorrhea, dizziness, tinnitus, aching and flaccid sensation in the loins and knees, dry mouth, feverish sensation over the palms, soles and chest, tidal fever and sweating, dark complexion or flushed cheeks, light-red tongue with scanty fur, and thin and taut pulse.

Therapeutic methods: Nourishing the liver and kidney, nourishing blood and regulating menstruation.

Prescription and drugs: Modified Guishen Wan composed of 10g of Shudihuang (*Rhizoma Rehmanniae Praeparata*), 10g of Danggui (*Radix Angelicae Sinensis*), 10g of Shanzhuyu (*Fructus Corni*), 10g of Gouqizi

鉴别。

【辨证论治】

闭经当分清虚实。一般而论,已逾正常女性初潮年龄而尚未行经,或月经逐渐稀发而停闭,伴有其他虚象的,多属虚证;如以往月经尚属正常而突然停闭,又伴其他实象的,则多是实证。

闭经的治疗原则,根据病证,虚者补而通之,或补益肝肾,或调养气血;实者泻而通之,或活血化瘀,或理气行滞,或除邪调经,切不可不分虚实,滥用攻破方药,亦不可一味峻补,反燥涩精血。至于因他病而致经闭者,又当或先治他病,病愈则月经可自调。

一、肝肾不足证

主要证候 月经超龄未至,或初潮延迟,月经后期、量少,渐至经闭,头晕耳鸣,腰酸膝软,口干咽燥,五心烦热、潮热汗出,面色晦黯或两颧潮红,舌质淡红少苔,脉细弦。

治 法 补益肝肾,养血调经。

方 药 归肾丸加减:熟地黄10 g,当归10 g,山茱萸10 g,枸杞子10 g,菟丝子12 g,潼蒺藜10 g,山药20 g,鸡血藤

(*Fructus Lycii*), 12g of Tusizi (*Semen Cuscutae*), 10g of Tongjili (*Semen Astragali Complanati*), 20g of Shanyao (*Rhizoma Dioscoreae*), 20g of Jixueteng (*Caulis Spatholobi*), 10g of Ejiao (*Colla Corii Asini*) (to be melted), 10g of Huainiuxi (*Radix Achyranthis Bidentatae*) and 10g of Zelan (*Herba Lycopi*).

Modification: For obvious tidal fever, 10g of Digupi (*Cortex Lycii*), 15g of roasted Biejia (*Carapax Trionycis*) and 10g of Baiwei (*Radix Cynanchi Atrati*) are added; for anorexia and loose stool, 10g of Fuling (*Poria*) and 10g of Baizhu (*Rhizoma Atractylodis Macrocephalae*) are added; for dry mouth, 10g of Maimendong (*Radix Ophiopogonis*) and 10g of Xuanshen (*Radix Scrophulariae*) are added; for dryness of the vagina, 10g of Lujiaojiao (*Colla Cornus Cervi*) and 10g of Ziheche (*Placenta Hominis*) (to be decocted first) are added; for severe aching sensation in the loins, 10g of Duzhong (*Cortex Eucommiae*) and 10g of Chuanxuduan (*Radix Dipsaci*) are added.

(2) Syndrome of asthenia of qi and blood

Main symptoms: Gradual development of menorrhea from delayed menorrhea, scanty menorrhea and light-colored menorrhea into amenorrhea, bright-white complexion or sallow complexion, lusterless hair or loss of hair, dizziness, blurred vision, palpitation, shortness of breath, no desire to speak, spiritual lassitude, anorexia, loose stool, light-colored lips and tongue as well as thin and weak pulse.

Therapeutic methods: Strengthening the spleen and nourishing qi, nourishing blood and regulating menstruation.

Prescription and drugs: Modified Bazhen Tang composed of 15g of Dangshen (*Radix Codonopsis Pilosu-*

20 g,阿胶（烊化）10 g,怀牛膝10 g,泽兰10 g。

加　减　若潮热明显者,加地骨皮10 g,炙鳖甲15 g,白薇10 g;纳差便溏加茯苓10 g,白术10 g;口干咽燥加麦门冬10 g,玄参10 g;阴道干涩,加鹿角胶10 g,紫河车（先煎）10 g;腰酸如折,加杜仲10 g,川续断10 g。

二、气血虚弱证

主要证候　月经由后期、量少、色淡而渐至经闭,面色㿠白或萎黄,毛发不泽或脱落,头昏眼花,心悸怔忡,气短懒言,神疲肢倦,纳少便溏,唇舌色淡,脉细弱。

治　法　健脾益气,养血调经。

方　药　八珍汤加味:党参15 g,黄芪10 g,白术10 g,

lae）, 10g of Huangqi （*Radix Astragali*）, 10g of Baizhu （*Rhizoma Atractylodis Macrocephalae*）, 10g of Fuling （*Poria*）, 10g of stir-baked Danggui （*Radix Angelicae Sinensis*）, 6g of Shudihuang （*Rhizoma Rehmanniae Praeparata*）, 10g of roasted Baishaoyao （*Radix Paeoniae Alba*）, 5g of Chuanxiong （*Rhizoma Chuanxiong*）, 20g of Shanyao （*Rhizoma Dioscoreae*）, 15g of Jixueteng （*Caulis Spatholobi*）, 10g of Zelan （*Herba Lycopi*）and 5g of roasted Gancao （*Radix Glycyrrhizae*）.

Modification：For disturbed sleep, 15g of Yejiaoteng （*Caulis Polygoni Multiflori*）and 10g of Suanzaoren （*Semen Ziziphi Spinosae*）are added; 10g of Gouji （*Rhizoma Cibotii*）and 10g of Duzhong （*Cortex Eucommiae*）are added; for anorexia, 6g of Muxiang （*Radix Aucklaneliae*）and 15g of Guya （*Fructus Oryzae Germinatus*）are added.

（3）Syndrome of qi stagnation and blood stasis

Main symptoms：Amenorrhea, mental depression, irritability, susceptibility to rage, distending fullness in the chest and hypochondria, pain or unpressable pain in the lower abdomen, purplish tongue or with ecchymosis and deep and unsmooth pulse.

Therapeutic methods：Promoting qi flow and activating blood, resolving stasis and promoting menstruation.

Prescription and drugs：Modified Xuefu Zhuyu Tang composed of 10g of Danggui （*Radix Angelicae Sinensis*）, 5g of Chuanxiong （*Rhizoma Chuanxiong*）, 10g of Chishaoyao （*Radix Paeoniae Rubra*）, 10g of Taoren （*Semen Persicae*）, 6g of Chaihu （*Radix Bupleuri*）, 10g of Honghua （*Flos Carthami*）, 10g of Zhike （*Fructus Aurantii*）, 12g of Xiangfu （*Rhizoma Cyperi*）, 10g of Chuanniuxi （*Radix Cyathulae*）and 15g of

茯苓10 g,炒当归10 g,熟地黄6 g,炒白芍药10 g,川芎5 g,山药20 g,鸡血藤15 g,泽兰10 g,炙甘草5 g。

加　减　若夜寐欠安者,加夜交藤15 g,酸枣仁10 g;腰酸,加狗脊10 g,杜仲10 g;纳差者,加木香6 g,谷芽15 g。

三、气滞血瘀证

主要证候　月经闭止不行,精神抑郁,烦躁易怒,胸胁胀满,小腹胀痛或拒按,舌紫暗,或有瘀点,脉沉涩。

治　法　行气活血,化瘀通经。

方　药　血府逐瘀汤加减:当归10 g,川芎5 g,赤芍药10 g,桃仁10 g,柴胡6 g,红花10 g,枳壳10 g,香附12 g,川牛膝10 g,泽兰15 g。

Zelan (*Herba Lycopi*).

Modification: For distending pain in the breast, 10g of Qingpi (*Pericarpium Citri Reticulatae Viride*) and 10g of Shanzha (*Fructus Crataegi*) are added; for dysphoria and dry mouth, 6g of Shanzhi (*Fructus Gardeniae*) and 10g of Zhimu (*Rhizoma Anemarrhenae*) are added; for lower abdominal cold pain, 6g of Rougui (*Cortex Cinnamomi*) and 6g of Wuzhuyu (*Fructus Evodiae*) are added.

(4) Syndrome of phlegm-dampness obstruction

Main symptoms: Amenorrhea, obesity, whitish complexion, fullness and oppression in the chest and hypochondria, spiritual lassitude, leukorrhagia, whitish greasy tongue fur and slippery pulse.

Therapeutic methods: Drying dampness and eliminating phlegm, activating blood and regulating menstruation.

Prescription and drugs: Modified Cangfu Daotan Wan composed of 12g of Cangzhu (*Rhizoma Atractylodis*), 10g of Fuling (*Poria*), 10g of Banxia (*Rhizoma Pinelliae*), 10g of Chenpi (*Pericarpium Citri Reticulatae*), 10g of Danxing (*Arisaema cum Bile*), 12g of Xiangfu (*Rhizoma Cyperi*), 10g of Danggui (*Radix Angelicae Sinensis*), 5g of Chuanxiong (*Rhizoma Chuanxiong*), 10g of Zhike (*Fructus Aurantii*), 12g of crude Shanzha (*Fructus Crataegi*), 10g of Zelan (*Herba Lycopi*) and 6g of Juanbai (*Herba Selaginellae*).

Modification: For chest distress, 10g of Houpo (*Cortex Magnoliae Officinalis*), 12g of Quangualou (*Fructus Trichosanthis*), 6g of Shichangpu (*Rhizoma Acori Graminei*) are added; for nausea and poor appetite, 6g of Sharen (*Fructus Amomi*) and 10g of Baizhu (*Rhizoma Atractylodis Macrocephalae*) are added; for

加 减 若乳房胀痛者，加青皮10 g，山楂10 g；心烦口干，加山栀6 g，知母10 g；小腹冷痛，加肉桂6 g，吴茱萸6 g。

四、痰湿阻滞证

主要证候 月经闭止不行，形体肥胖，面色白，胸胁满闷，呕恶痰多，神疲倦怠，带多色白，苔白腻，脉滑。

治 法 燥湿祛痰，活血调经。

方 药 苍附导痰丸加减：苍术12 g，茯苓10 g，半夏10 g，陈皮10 g，胆星10 g，香附12 g，当归10 g，川芎5 g，枳壳10 g，生山楂10 g，泽兰10 g，卷柏6 g。

加 减 若胸闷者，加厚朴10 g，全瓜蒌12 g，石菖蒲6 g；泛恶纳少者，加砂仁6 g，白术10 g；口腻加佩兰10 g，谷芽10 g；浮肿，加泽泻10 g，薏苡仁20 g。

greasy taste in the mouth, 10g of Peilan (*Herba Eupatorii*) and 10g of Guya (*Fructus Oryzae Germinatus*) are added; for edema, 10g of Zexie (*Rhizoma Alismatis*) and 20g of Yiyiren (*Semen Coicis*) are added.

[Other therapeutic methods]

(1) Chinese patent drugs

1) Danggui Pill(condensed pill): 8 pills each time and three times a day, applicable to the treatment of asthenia of qi and blood or qi stagnation and blood stasis.

2) Bazhen Yimu Pill: 6g each time and three times a day, applicable to the treatment of asthenia of qi and blood.

3) Qizhi Xiangfu Pill: 10g each time and three times a day, applicable to the treatment of phlegm-dampness syndrome.

4) Liuwei Dihuang Pill (condensed pill): 8 pills each time and three times a day, applicable to the treatment of deficiency of the liver and kidney.

5) Fangfeng Tongsheng Pill: 10g each time and three times a day, applicable to the treatment of phlegm-dampness syndrome.

(2) Empirical and folk recipes

1) 30 - 60g of Yimucao (*Herba Leonuri*) is decocted with proper amount of brown sugar, one dose a day.

2) 15g of Danggui (*Radix Angelicae Sinensis*), 30g of Yimucao (*Herba Leonuri*) and 15g of Huangqi (*Radix Astragali*) are decocted. The decoction, applicable to the treatment of amenorrhea of asthenia syndrome, is taken one dose a day.

3) 30g of Danshen (*Radix Salviae Miltiorrhizae*) is decocted with two eggs for 2 hours. The decoction, applicable to the treatment of amenorrhea of blood asthenia syndrome, is taken one dose a day.

【其他疗法】

1. 中成药

（1）当归丸（浓缩丸）每次服 8 粒,1 日 3 次,适用于气血虚或气滞血瘀证。

（2）八珍益母丸　每次服6 g,1 日 3 次,适用于气血虚弱证。

（3）七制香附丸　每次服10 g,1 日 3 次,适用于痰湿证。

（4）六味地黄丸（浓缩丸）　每次服 8 粒,1 日 3 次,适用于肝肾不足证。

（5）防风通圣丸　每次服10 g,1 日 3 次,适用于痰湿证。

2. 单验方

（1）益母草 30～60 g,红糖适量,水煎服,1 日 1 剂。

（2）当归15 g、益母草30 g、黄芪15 g,水煎服 1 日 1 剂,适用于虚证闭经。

（3）丹参30 g、鸡蛋 2 枚水煮 2 小时,食蛋饮汤,1 日 1 剂,适用于血虚证闭经。

2.1.6　Polycystic ovary syndrome

Polycystic ovary syndrome is marked by chronic anovulation, amenorrhea or scanty menorrhea, sterility, obesity, pilosity and bilateral cystic enlargement of ovary. It usually occurs among women ranging from 20 to 30 of age and is one of the commonly encountered gynecological diseases. It pertains to the conceptions of amenorrhea, irregular menstruation and sterility in TCM.

This disease is mainly caused by congenital weakness or early marriage, excessive sexual life and consumption of kidney qi; or by obesity or excessive intake of greasy and rich food or intemperance of food leading to impairment of the spleen and stomach and endogenous dampness; or by retention of blood after delivery, depression or impairment of the liver due to rage, stagnation of liver qi and qi stagnation and blood stasis; or by transformation of fire from prolonged stagnation leading to disharmony between qi and blood. All these factors may result in dysfunction of the viscera, disorder of qi and blood, obstruction of the meridians, accumulation of phlegm and dampness and abnormal accumulation in the thoroughfare vessel which lead to polycystic ovary syndrome.

[Key points for diagnosis]

(1) Irregular menorrhea appears first as scanty menorrhea and then turns into secondary amenorrhea, sterility, obesity and pilosity.

(2) Basal body temperature is unidirectional. Diagnostic curettage shows endometrial hyperplasia or exces-

第六节　多囊卵巢综合征

多囊卵巢综合征是以慢性无排卵、闭经或月经稀发、不孕、肥胖、多毛以及双侧卵巢呈多囊性增大为临床特征的综合症候群。发病年龄在20～30 岁,是妇科较为常见的疾病。根据其临床表现,属于中医学闭经、月经不调、不孕等范畴。

本病的主要病因可由禀赋薄弱或早婚房劳,肾气受损;素体肥胖或恣食膏粱厚味,或饮食失节,损伤脾胃,脾虚痰湿内生;经期产后余血未尽,抑郁或恼怒伤肝,肝气郁结,气滞血瘀;郁久化火气血失和。以上均可导致脏腑功能失常,气血失调,经络不畅,痰湿脂膜积聚,血海蓄溢失常而致本病。

【诊断要点】

(1) 月经不调,常先出现月经稀发或过少,渐可转为继发闭经、不孕、肥胖、多毛等症状。

(2) 基础体温呈单相,诊断性刮宫病理见子宫内膜呈

sive hyperplasia of endometrium and no secretory endo-metrium occurs; ultrasonic and abdominoscope examination indicates polycystic enlargement of ovary on both sides and intensified echo of thickened capsules. There are numerous cystic follicles 2 - 7mm in diameter under capsules.

(3) FSH value is low, serum LH/FSH is ≥3, E_1 and E_2≥1 higher than the normal cycle, and PRL is elevated.

(4) Clinically it should be differentiated from hyper-thecosis, granular-thecoma, hemopathy due to excessive prolactin, adrenal-ovary tumor and Cushing's syndrome.

[Syndrome differentiation and treatment]

Polycystic ovary syndrome is marked by asthenia of the principal aspect and sthenia of the secondary aspect. Kidney asthenia is the principal aspect, while phlegm-dampness, liver depression transforming into fire, qi stagnation and blood stasis are the secondary aspect. Both aspects interact on each other. The viscera involved are the liver, spleen and kidney. The location of the disease is in the thoroughfare and conception vessels. Clinically this syndrome is divided into kidney asthenia, phlegm-damp-ness, liver depression transforming into fire and qi stag-nation with blood stasis.

The treatment mainly concentrates on nourishing the kidney followed by strengthening the spleen to regulate qi and resolve phlegm, soothing the liver to relieve depres-sion and reduce fire as well as activating blood to resolve stasis and regulating menstruation. The treatment and se-lection of herbs are based on the differentiation of syn-dromes according to the pathological conditions in question.

增生期或增生过长,无分泌期改变;超声及腹腔镜检查双侧卵巢多囊性增大,被膜增厚回声强。被膜下可见数目较多、直径 2~7 mm。

(3) 激素测定 FSH 值偏低,血清 LH/FSH ≥ 3, E_1/E_2≥1高于正常周期,PRL 也可升高。

(4) 临床上注意与卵巢卵泡膜增多症、颗粒-卵巢泡膜细胞瘤、高催乳素血症、产生雄激素的肾上腺-卵巢瘤、库欣氏综合征等疾病相鉴别。

【辨证论治】

多囊卵巢综合征是本虚标实证,肾虚为本,痰湿、肝郁化火、气滞血瘀为标,两者互为因果,涉及的脏腑是肝脾肾,病位在冲任,临证可分肾虚、痰湿、肝郁化火、气滞血瘀四种。

治疗以补肾治其本,健脾理气化痰,疏解肝郁泻火,活血化瘀调经治其标,标本同治。同时还应根据月经周期的不同时间和患者的体质情况辨证论治,选方用药。

（1）Kidney asthenia syndrome

Main symptoms：Delayed menstruation with scanty and light-colored menses, gradual amenorrhea, occasional irregular menstruation, failure to be pregnant long after marriage, dizziness and tinnitus, aching and weak sensation in the loins and knees, dispiritedness, or cold sensation in the body and cold limbs, clear and profuse urine, loose stool, sexual frigidity, or obesity and pilosity, light-colored tongue with whitish thin fur and deep-thin pulse.

Therapeutic methods：Nourishing the kidney to replenish essence, regulating and nourishing the thoroughfare and conception vessels.

Prescription and drugs：Modified Yougui Wan composed of 10g of Shudihuang（*Rhizoma Rehmanniae Praeparata*）, 20g of Shanyao（*Rhizoma Dioscoreae*）, 10g of Shanzhuyu（*Fructus Corni*）, 10g of Gouqizi（*Fructus Lycii*）, 10g of Lujiaojiao（*Colla Cornus Cervi*）, 12g of Tusizi（*Semen Cuscutae*）, 10g of Duzhong（*Cortex Eucommiae*）, 10g of Danggui（*Radix Angelicae Sinensis*）, 6g of Rougui（*Cortex Cinnamomi*）and 6g of prepared Fuzi（*Radix Aconiti Praeparata*）.

Modification：For scanty menstruation, delayed menstruation or amenorrhea, 12g of Zelan（*Herba Lycopi*）, 12g of Chuanniuxi（*Radix Cyathulae*）and 20g of Jixueteng（*Caulis Spatholobi*）are added; for patients in puberty or with maldevelopment of the uterus, 10g of Ziheche（*Placenta Hominis*）（to be decocted first）, 10g of Heshouwu（*Radix Polygoni Multiflori*）, 10g of Roucongrong（*Herba Cistanches*）and 10g of Yinyanghuo（*Herba Epimedii*）are added.

（2）Phlegm-dampness syndrome

Main symptoms：Scanty menorrhea, delayed men-

一、肾虚证

主要证候　月经后期，量少，色淡，渐至闭经，偶有先后无定期，婚久不孕，头晕耳鸣，腰膝酸软，精神不振，或形寒肢冷，小便清长，大便不实，性欲淡漠，或形体肥胖多毛，舌质淡，苔薄白，脉沉细。

治　法　补肾填精，调补冲任。

方　药　右归丸加减：熟地黄10 g，山药20 g，山茱萸10 g，枸杞子10 g，鹿角胶10 g，菟丝子12 g，杜仲10 g，当归10 g，肉桂6 g，制附子6 g。

加　减　若月经量少、错后或闭经者，加泽兰12 g，川牛膝12 g，鸡血藤20 g；青春期患者或伴子宫发育不良者，可加紫河车（先煎）10 g，何首乌10 g，肉苁蓉10 g，淫羊藿10 g。

二、痰湿证

主要证候　月经量少，经

struation or even amenorrhea, failure to be pregnant long after marriage, or leukorrhagia, dizziness and heavy sensation in the head, chest oppression, nausea, lassitude of limbs, or profuse sputum in the throat, loose stool, obesity, pilosity, whitish greasy tongue fur and slippery pulse.

Therapeutic methods: Resolving phlegm and eliminating dampness, regulating qi and menstruation.

Prescription and drugs: Cangfu Daotan Tang composed of 10g of Cangzhu (*Rhizoma Atractylodis*), 10g of Xiangfu (*Rhizoma Cyperi*), 12g of Fuling (*Poria*), 10g of Fabanxia (*Rhizoma Pinelliae*), 10g of Chenpi (*Pericarpium Citri Reticulatae*) and 3g of Gancao (*Radix Glycyrrhizae*), 10g of Danxing (*Arisaema cum Bile*), 10g of Zhike (*Fructus Aurantii*), 10g of Liuqu (*Massa Medicata Fermentata*) and 3 slices of Shengjiang (*Rhizoma Zingiberis Recens*).

Modification: For obesity and pilosity, 10g of Shancigu (*Bulubus Iphigeniae*), 10g of Xiakucao (*Spica Prunellae*), 15g of Zaojiaoci (*Spina Gleditsiae*) and 10g of Shichangpu (*Rhizoma Acori Graminei*) are added for resolving phlegm and activating collaterals; for mass in the lower abdomen, 15g of Kunbu (*Thallus Laminariae seu Eckloniae*), 15g of Haizao (*Sargassum*), 10g of Xiakucao (*Spica Prunellae*) and 12g of Ezhu (*Rhizoma Curcumae*) are added for softening hardness and dissipating abdominal mass.

(3) Syndrome of liver depression transforming into fire

Main symptoms: Amenorrhea, or scanty menorrhea, or irregular menstruation, failure to be pregnant long after marriage, muscular building, thick hair, acne on the face, distending pain in the chest, hypochondria and breasts, or lactorrhea, dry mouth with preference for

行延后甚或闭经,婚久不孕,或带下量多,头晕头重,胸闷泛恶,四肢倦怠,或喉间多痰,大便不实,形体肥胖,多毛,苔白腻,脉滑。

治 法 化痰除湿,理气调经。

方 药 苍附导痰汤:苍术10 g,香附10 g,茯苓12 g,法半夏 10 g,陈皮10 g,甘草3 g,胆星10 g,枳壳10 g,六曲10 g,生姜3 片。

加 减 若形体肥胖,多毛明显者,酌加山慈菇10 g,夏枯草10 g,皂角刺15 g,石菖蒲10 g,以化痰活络;若小腹结块形成者,加昆布 15 g,海藻15 g,夏枯草10 g,莪术12 g,以软坚散结消癥。

三、肝郁化火证

主要证候 闭经、或月经稀发、量少,或先后无定期,婚久不孕,形体壮实,毛发浓密,面部痤疮,经前乳房胸胁胀痛,或有溢乳,口干喜冷饮,大

drinking water, constipation, yellowish thin tongue fur and taut and rapid pulse.

Therapeutic methods: Soothing the liver to relieve depression and clearing away heat to reduce fire.

Prescription and drugs: Modified Danzhi Xiaoyao San composed of 10g of Mudanpi (*Cortex Moutan Radicis*), 10g of Zhizi (*Fructus Gardeniae*), 10g of Danggui (*Radix Angelicae Sinensis*), 15g of Baishaoyao (*Radix Paeoniae Alba*), 6g of Chaihu (*Radix Bupleuri*), 10g of Baizhu (*Rhizoma Atractylodis Macrocephalae*), 5g of roasted Gancao (*Radix Glycyrrhizae*) and 10g of Chuanniuxi (*Radix Cyathulae*).

Modification: For obvious constipation, proper amount of Dahuang (*Radix et Rhizoma Rhei*) is added for clearing away heat and reducing fire to promote defecation; for lactorrhea, 60g of stir-baked Maiya (*Fructus Hordei Germinatus*) and 10g of Kudingcha (*Folium Ilicis*) are added; for distension and fullness in the chest, hypochondria and breasts, 15g of Yujin (*Radix Curcumae*), 15g of Wangbuliuxing (*Semen Vaccariae*) and 10g of Lulutong (*Fructus Liquidambaris*) are added for soothing the liver, dredging collaterals and dissipating nodules.

(4) Syndrome of qi stagnation and blood stasis

Main symptoms: Delayed menstruation, or scanty and unsmooth menorrhea, unpressable abdominal pain during menstruation acompanied by blood clot, alleviation of abdominal pain after removal of blood clot, or even amenorrhea; occasional scanty menorrhea, sterility after marriage, mental depression, distending fullness in the chest and hypochondria, purplish tongue or with ecchymosis on the edge and tip, deep and taut pulse.

Therapeutic methods: Regulating qi and activating

便秘结,苔薄黄,脉弦数。

治　法　疏肝解郁,清热泻火。

方　药　丹栀逍遥散加减:牡丹皮10 g,栀子10 g,当归10 g,白芍药15 g,柴胡6 g,白术10 g,炙甘草5 g,川牛膝10 g。

加　减　若大便秘结明显者,加大黄适量清热泻火通便;若溢乳者,酌加炒麦芽60 g,苦丁茶10 g;若乳房胸胁胀满甚者,酌加郁金15 g,王不留行15 g,路路通10 g,疏肝通络散结。

四、气滞血瘀证

主要证候　月经延后,或量少不畅,经行腹痛拒按,伴有血块,块出疼减,甚者闭经不行。偶或月经量多,婚后不孕,精神抑郁,胸胁胀满,舌质黯紫,或边尖瘀点,脉沉弦。

治　法　理气活血,化瘀

blood, resolving stasis and regulating menstruation.

Prescription and drugs: Modified Gexia Zhuyu Tang composed of 10g of Danggui (*Radix Angelicae Sinensis*), 5g of Chuanxiong (*Rhizoma Chuanxiong*), 10g of Chishaoyao (*Radix Paeoniae Rubra*), 10g of Taoren (*Semen Persicae*), 6g of Honghua (*Flos Carthami*), 10g of Zhike (*Fructus Aurantii*), 10g of Yanhusuo (*Rhizoma Corydalis*), 10g of Wulingzhi (*Faeces Trogopterorum*), 10g of Mudanpi (*Cortex Moutan Radicis*), 10g of Baishaoyao (*Radix Paeoniae Alba*), 10g of Xiangfu (*Rhizoma Cyperi*) and 5g of Gancao (*Radix Glycyrrhizae*).

Modification: For chest distension, breast distension, lower abdominal distending pain, dysphoria and susceptibility to rage before menstruation, 10g of Qingpi (*Pericarpium Citri Reticulatae Viride*), 9g of Muxiang (*Radix Aucklaneliae*) and 6g of Chaihu (*Radix Bupleuri*) are added for soothing the liver to relieve stagnation and activating qi to stop pain; for mass in the abdomen, 10g of Sanleng (*Rhizoma Sparganii*), 10g of Ezhu (*Rhizoma Curcumae*), 10g of Moyao (*Myrrha*) and 10g of Lulutong (*Fructus Liquidambaris*) are added for activating blood, resolving stasis and dissipating abdominal mass.

[Other therapeutic methods]

(1) Chinese patent drugs

1) Yougui Pill: 1 pill each time and three times a day, applicable to the treatment of kidney asthenia syndrome.

2) Qizhi Xiangfu Pill: For resolving phlegm and drying dampness, 6g each time, applicable to the treatment of phlegm-dampness syndrome.

3) Xiaoyao Pill: 10g each time and three times a day, applicable to the treatment of liver depression syn-

调经。

方　药　膈下逐瘀汤加减：当归10 g，川芎5 g，赤芍药10 g，桃仁10 g，红花6 g，枳壳10 g，延胡索10 g，五灵脂10 g，牡丹皮10 g，白芍药10 g，香附10 g，甘草5 g。

加　减　经前胸胁、乳房、小腹胀痛，心烦易怒者，酌加青皮10 g，木香9 g，柴胡6 g，舒肝解郁，行气止痛。若腹中包块久不消散，加三棱10 g，莪术10 g，没药10 g，路路通10 g，活血化瘀消癥。

【其他疗法】

1. 中成药

（1）右归丸　每次1丸，1日3次，适用于肾虚型。

（2）七制香附丸　化痰燥湿。每次6 g，适用于痰湿证。

（3）逍遥丸　每次服10 g，1日3次，适用于肝

drome.

4) Dahuang Zhechong Pill: 1 pill each time and twice or 3 times a day with boiled water or ginger decoction, applicable to the treatment of blood stasis syndrome.

(2) Empirical and folk recipes

1) Huanang Tang composed of 30 g of Dongguaren (*Semen Benincasae*), 30g of Xiakucao (*Spica Prunellae*), 30g of Juhe (*Semen Citri Reticulatae*), 20 g of Zhebeimu (*Bulbus Fritillariae Thunbergii*), 10g of Taoren (*Semen Persicae*), 10g of Mudanpi (*Cortex Moutan Radicis*), 10g of Chishaoyao (*Radix Paeoniae Rubra*), 10g of Bianxu (*Herba Polygoni Avicularis*), 10g of Sangzhi (*Ramulus Mori*). These herbs are decocted in water and the decoction is orally taken one dose a day. One menstrual cycle is a course of treatment. This treatment is applicable to dampness-heat syndrome.

2) Yiren Shanzha Yimucao Tang composed of 30g of Yiyiren (*Semen Coicis*), 15g of Shanzha (*Fructus Crataegi*), 30g of Yimucao (*Herba Leonuri*) and 20g of stir-baked Baibiandou (*Semen Lablab Album*). These ingredients are cooked into porridge for treating phlegm-dampness syndrome.

2.1.7 Premenstrual syndrome

Premenstrual syndrome refers to physiological and mental changes before menstruation, such as irritability, susceptibility to rage, nervousness, edema, diarrhea, headache and distending pain in the breasts without obvious organic changes in examination. This syndrome usually occurs 7 - 14 days before menstruation and disappears after menstruation. The incidence is 30%- 40%.

郁证。

（4）大黄䗪虫丸　每次1丸，1日2～3次。温开水或姜水送下，适用于血瘀证。

2. 单验方

（1）化囊汤　冬瓜仁30 g，夏枯草30 g，橘核30 g，浙贝母20 g，桃仁10 g，牡丹皮10 g，赤芍药10 g，萹蓄10 g，桑枝10 g，水煎服，每日1次，1个周期为1个疗程，适用于湿热证。

（2）苡仁山楂益母草汤　薏苡仁30 g，山楂15 g，益母草30 g，炒白扁豆20 g，煮粥常食用，适用于痰湿证。

第七节　经前期综合征

经前期综合征是指妇女在月经期前反复出现生理、精神以及行为方面的改变，如烦躁易怒、精神紧张、浮肿、腹泻、头痛、乳房胀痛等症状，严重者可影响生活和工作，但经检查一般并无明显器质性改变。本病多发生于经前7～14

This syndrome is usually caused by emotional factors and dysfunction of the viscera, susceptibility to depression, liver depression and qi stagnation leading to transformation of fire and disturbing cardiac spirit; or by invasion of liver qi into the spleen and stomach, disharmony between the spleen and stomach, accumulation and retention of phlegm-dampness as well as obstruction of breast collaterals; or by constitutional yin asthenia, relative hyperactivity of liver qi, upward adverse flow of qi and disharmony of the lucid orifices; or by constitutional asthenia of the spleen and kidney, insufficiency of kidney yang, decline of fire in mingmen (gate of life), lack of warmth for the spleen, dysfunction of the spleen in transformation and transportation, retention of dampness, retention of fluid in the skin and migrating into the stomach and intestines. It is clear that this syndrome is mainly caused by dysfunction of the liver and is related to the heart, spleen and kidney.

According to the clinical symptoms, this syndrome pertains to the conceptions of headache during menstruation, fever during menstruation, body pain during menstruation, edema during menstruation, diarrhea during menstruation, dizziness during menstruation, abnormal emotional changes during menstruation and distending pain in breasts during menstruation in TCM, generally known as symptoms before and after menstruation.

[Key points for diagnosis]

(1) Before or during menstruation there are regular mental tension, depression, anxiety, irritability, insomnia, headache, vertigo, distending pain in chest, hypochondria and breasts, fever, edema, diarrhea and oral ulceration, or even psychosis in a few extremely serious ca-

天,月经期后自行消失。发病率为30%～40%。

本病的发生与情志因素及脏腑功能失调有关,若素性抑郁,肝郁气滞,久而化火,上扰心神;肝气横犯克伐脾胃,脾胃失和,痰湿蕴阻,乳络失畅;素体阴虚,肝气偏旺,气逆于上,清窍失和;素体脾肾亏虚,肾阳不足,命门火衰,脾失温煦,运化不健,水湿停聚,泛溢于肌肤,下注于胃肠而发病。可见本病关键尤以肝的功能失调为主要原因,与心、脾、肾等脏密切相关。

根据本病的临床症状,可分属于中医学的"经行头痛"、"经行发热"、"经行身痛"、"经行浮肿"、"经行泄泻"、"经行眩晕"、"经行情志异常"、"经行乳房胀痛"等范畴,总称为"经行前后诸征"。

【诊断要点】

(1) 在经前或经期周期性出现精神紧张、抑郁忧虑、烦躁失眠、头痛眩晕、胸胁乳房胀痛、发热、浮肿、泄泻、口腔溃疡等症状,极少数症状严重

ses.

(2) The basal body temperature appears bi-directionally and no organic changes are found in examination; the breasts are normal or have nodules with tenderness; estrin has increased, pregnendione is low; the ratio between estrin and progestogen has increased; in a few cases lactin has elevated.

(3) This syndrome should be differentiated from other organic diseases, such as neurosis, schizophrenia, regular psychosis, disorders of the heart, kidney, intestine and stomach as well as breast tumor.

[Syndrome differentiation and treatment]

This syndrome is clinically divided into asthenia and sthenia types. The asthenia type is marked by kidney asthenia and spleen asthenia. The sthenia syndrome is marked by qi stagnation. The viscera involved are the liver, the spleen and the kidney. Usually two viscera or three viscera are involved at the same time or simultaneous disease of qi and blood. Since clinical symptoms are complicated, clinical syndrome differentiation should be done in light of the time, location and nature of the symptoms as well as the conditions of the tongue and pulse.

(1) Syndrome of liver depression and qi stagnation

Main symptoms: Hypochondriac distension and oppression, distending pain in the breast, depression, frequent sighing, irritability, susceptibility to rage, lower abdominal pain, whitish thin tongue fur and thin and taut pulse before menstruation.

Therapeutic methods: Soothing the liver to regulate qi and activating blood to dredge collaterals.

Prescription and drugs: Modified Xiaoyao San com-

者可类似精神病患者。

（2）基础体温多呈双相型曲线，妇科检查无器质性改变；乳房检查可正常或有触痛性结节；性激素测定可有雌激素水平升高，孕酮偏低，雌/孕激素比值增高，少数病例可有泌乳素增高。

（3）本病应与其他功能性或器质性疾病鉴别。如与神经官能症，精神分裂症，周期性精神病，心、肾疾病，肠胃道疾病，乳房肿瘤等病相鉴别。

【辨证论治】

本病在临床上分为虚、实两大类。虚证以肾虚、脾虚多见；实证则以气滞多见。涉及的脏腑以肝、脾、肾功能失调为主，常表现为两脏或三脏同时发病或气血同病。由于本病临床症状复杂多样，临证时要对不同症状，根据发生的时间、部位、性质，结合舌脉及全身表现以进行辨证。

一、肝郁气滞证

主要证候 经前两胁胀闷，乳房胀痛，性情抑郁，叹息时舒，烦躁易怒，小腹胀痛，舌苔薄白，脉细弦。

治 法 疏肝理气，活血通络。

方 药 逍遥散加减：

posed of 6g of Chaihu (*Radix Bupleuri*), 12g of
Baishaoyao (*Radix Paeoniae Alba*), 12g of Danggui
(*Radix Angelicae Sinensis*), 10g of Xiangfu (*Rhizoma
Cyperi*), 6g of Qingpi (*Pericarpium Citri Reticulatae
Viride*), 6g of Chenpi (*Pericarpium Citri Reticula-
tae*), 10g of Yujin (*Radix Curcumae*), 10g of Sigualuo
(*Retinervus Luffae Fructus*), 10g of Danshen (*Radix
Salviae Miltiorrhizae*) and 3g of crude Gancao (*Radix
Glycyrrhizae*).

Modification: For untouchable distending pain in
the breasts, 10g of Lulutong (*Fructus Liquidambaris*)
and 10g of Chishaoyao (*Radix Paeoniae Rubra*) are added; for mass in breasts, 10g of Juhe (*Semen Citri Reticulatae*), 10g of Wangbuliuxing (*Semen Vaccariae*) and
10g of Xiakucao (*Spica Prunellae*) are added; for bitter
taste in the mouth and constipation, 6g of Shanzhi (*Fructus Gardeniae*) and 6g of Chuanlianzi (*Fructus Toosendan*); for dizziness and headache, 15g of Gouteng (*Ramulus Uncariae cum Uncis*) and 12g of Baijili (*Fructus
Tribuli*) are added; for restless sleep in the night, 20g of
Qinglongchi (*Dens Draconis*) and 10g of Hehuanpi (*Cortex Albiziae*) are added.

(2) Syndrome of yin asthenia and liver hyperac-
tivity

Main symptoms: Dizziness and headache, restlessness, occasional tidal fever, feverish sensation over
palms, soles and chest, irritating sensation in the eyes,
tinnitus, dry mouth and throat, aching sensation in the
loins and spine, red tongue and thin and rapid pulse during
menstruation or before and after menstruation.

Therapeutic methods: Nourishing yin and blood,
suppressing liver yang.

Prescription and drugs: Qiju Dihuang Wan com-

柴胡 6 g，白芍药 12 g，当归
12 g，香附 10 g，青皮 6 g，陈皮
6 g，郁金 10 g，丝瓜络 10 g，丹
参 10 g，生甘草 3 g。

加　减　若乳房胀痛不
能触衣者，加路路通 10 g，赤芍
药 10 g；乳房有块者，加橘核
10 g，王不留行 10 g，夏枯草
10 g；口苦便秘者，加山栀 6 g，
川楝子 6 g；头晕头痛者，加钩
藤 15 g，白蒺藜 12 g；夜寐欠安
者，加青龙齿 20 g，合欢皮
10 g。

二、阴虚肝旺证

主要证候　经期或月经
前后眩晕头痛，烦躁不安，时
有潮热，五心烦热，目涩耳鸣，
咽干口燥，腰脊酸楚，舌质偏
红，脉细数。

治　法　滋阴养血，平潜
肝阳。

方　药　杞菊地黄丸：

posed of 10g of Gouqizi (*Fructus Lycii*), 10g of Juhua (*Flos Chrysanthemi*), 20g of Shanyao (*Rhizoma Dioscoreae*), 10g of Shudihuang (*Rhizoma Rehmanniae Praeparata*), 10g of Mudanpi (*Cortex Moutan Radicis*), 10g of Fuling (*Poria*), 10g of Shanzhuyu (*Fructus Corni*), 10g of Danggui (*Radix Angelicae Sinensis*), 10g of Baishaoyao (*Radix Paeoniae Alba*), 15g of Gouteng (*Ramulus Uncariae cum Uncis*) (to be decocted later), 10g of Baijili (*Fructus Tribuli*) and crude Gancao (*Radix Glycyrrhizae*).

Modification: For dry mouth and oral erosion, 5g of Huanglian (*Rhizoma Coptidis*) and 5g of Dengxincao (*Medulla Junci*) are added; for loose stool, 10g of Baizhu (*Rhizoma Atractylodis Macrocephalae*) and 10g of roasted Muxiang (*Radix Aucklaneliae*) are added; for insomnia, 10g of Suanzaoren (*Semen Ziziphi Spinosae*) and 15 g of Yejiaoteng (*Caulis Polygoni Multiflori*) are added; for pain in the limbs, 20 g of Jixueteng (*Caulis Spatholobi*) and 10g of Duhuo (*Radix Angelicae Pubescentis*) are added.

(3) Syndrome of spleen and kidney asthenia

Main symptoms: Facial dropsy, edema of limbs, loose stool, even diarrhea, anorexia, epigastric distension, aching and weak sensation in the loins and knees, lassitude, dizziness, nausea, aversion to cold and cold limbs, whitish and slippery tongue fur as well as deep and weak pulse.

Therapeutic methods: Warming and invigorating kidney yang, strengthening the spleen and resolving dampness.

Prescription and drugs: Modified Jiangu Tang composed of 15g of Dangshen (*Radix Codonopsis Pilosulae*), 10g of Baizhu (*Rhizoma Atractylodis Macrocephalae*), 10g of Fuling (*Poria*), 12g of Shanyao (*Rhizoma Di-*

枸杞子10 g,菊花10 g,山药20 g,熟地黄10 g,牡丹皮10 g,茯苓10 g,山茱萸10 g,当归10 g,白芍药10 g,钩藤(后下)15 g,白蒺藜10 g,生甘草。

加 减 若口干口糜者,加黄连5 g,灯心草5 g;大便溏薄,加白术10 g,煨木香10 g;失眠,加酸枣仁10 g,夜交藤15 g;肢体疼痛,加鸡血藤20 g,独活10 g。

三、脾肾两虚证

主要证候 经期或经行前后,面浮肢肿,大便不实,甚则泄泻,纳少脘胀,腰膝酸软,身倦乏力,头晕呕恶,畏寒肢冷,舌苔白滑,脉沉弱。

治 法 温补肾阳,健脾化湿。

方 药 健固汤加减。党参15 g,白术10 g,茯苓10 g,山药12 g,薏苡仁 20 g,巴戟天10 g,补骨脂10 g,陈皮6 g,炮

oscoreae）, 20g of Yiyiren（*Semen Coicis*）, 10g of Baji-tian（*Radix Morindae Officinalis*）, 10 g of Buguzhi（*Fructus Psoraleae*）, 6g of Chenpi（*Pericarpium Citri Reticulatae*）, 5g of Paojiang（processed *Rhizoma Zingiberis*）, 5g of stir-baked Gancao（*Radix Glycyrrhizae*）and 10g of Muxiang（*Radix Aucklaneliae*）.

Modification: For nausea, 10g of Banxia（*Rhizoma Pinelliae*）and 5g of Sharen（*Fructus Amomi*）are added; for morning diarrhea, 12g of Yizhiren（*Fructus Alpiniae Oxyphyllae*）and 10g of Roudoukou（*Semen Myristicae*）are added; for frequent urination in the night, 10g of Duzhong（*Cortex Eucommiae*）and 10g of Xuduan（*Radix Dipsaci*）are added; for poor appetite, 10g of Guya（*Fructus Oryzae Germinatus*）and 10g of Shanzha（*Fructus Crataegi*）are added.

[**Other therapeutic methods**]

(1) Chinese patent drugs

1) Yueju Pill: 10g each time and three times a day, applicable to the treatment of liver depression and qi stagnation.

2) Xiaoyao Pill: 10g each time and three times a day, applicable to the treatment of blood asthenia and liver depression.

3) Shenling Baizhu Pill: 6g each time and twice a day, applicable to the treatment of spleen asthenia.

4) Qiju Dihuang Liquid: 1 bottle each time and three times a day, applicable to the treatment of yin asthenia and liver hyperactivity.

(2) Empirical and folk recipes

1) 15g of Chenpi（*Pericarpium Citri Reticulatae*）and 15g of Lujiaoshuang（*Cornu Cervi Deglatinatum*）are decocted with wine for oral taking. This decoction is applicable to the treatment of distending pain in the

姜5 g,炙甘草5 g,木香10 g。

加　减　若泛恶欲吐者,加半夏10 g,砂仁5 g;鸡鸣泄泻,加益智仁 12 g,肉豆蔻10 g;夜间尿频,加杜仲10 g,续断10 g;食欲不振,加谷芽10 g,山楂10 g。

【其他疗法】

1. 中成药

（1）越鞠丸　每次服10 g,1日3次,适用于肝郁气滞证。

（2）逍遥丸　每次服10 g,1日3次,适用于血虚肝郁证。

（3）参苓白术丸　每次服6 g,1日2次,适用于脾虚证。

（4）杞菊地黄口服液每次1支,1日3次,适用于阴虚肝旺证。

2. 单验方

（1）陈皮15 g,鹿角霜15 g,黄酒、水各半煎服,适用于经前乳房胀痛。

breasts.

2) 30g of Yiyiren (*Semen Coicis*), 15g of Fuling (*Poria*) and 10 Chinese dates are decocted for oral taking. This decoction is taken one dose a day in summer, applicable to the treatment of edema before menstruation.

2.1.8　Perimenopausal syndrome

About 1/3 of the women in perimenopausal period do not have subjective symptoms because of neural and endocrine auto-regulation. In about 2/3 of the women there appear a series of symptoms due to deficiency of sexual hormone known as perimenopausal syndrome, usually occurring in women aging from 45 to 55. The incidence is about 85%. About 25% cases are severe. There is difference in the onset due to individual difference. In serious cases, treatment is necessary. This syndrome can also be caused by operation or actinotherapy or chemotherapy.

This syndrome is usually caused by decline of kidney qi, near exhaustion of reproductive substance (tiangui), deficiency of the thoroughfare and conception vessels and insufficiency of essence and blood before and after menopause; or by asthenia of kidney yang and malnutrition of meridians and vessels; or by frequent asthenia of blood; or by multiparity and excessive sexual life, or serious disease and prolonged illness and severe asthenia of kidney yin that lead to failure of yang to keep in latency as well as asthenia of yin and hyperactivity of yang; or by deficiency of kidney yin that fails to nourish the heart and liver, leading to hyperactivity of heart and liver fire; or by fre-

（2）薏苡仁 30 g，茯苓 15 g，大枣 10 枚，水煎服，入夏后每日 1 剂，适用于经前浮肿。

第八节　围绝经期综合征

围绝经期妇女约 1/3 能通过神经内分泌的自我调节达到新的平衡而无自觉症状，2/3 妇女则可出现一系列性激素减少所致的症状，称为围绝经期综合征。一般发生于 45~55 岁之间，其发生率为 85%，较重者占 25% 左右；发病程度个体差异较大，严重者需要治疗。非围绝经期妇女因手术或放射、化疗等人工的方法致绝经后，也可引起本病。

本病的病因主要是妇女年届绝经前后，肾气渐衰，天癸将竭，冲任亏虚，精血不足，而出现肾阴不足，阳失潜藏；或肾阳虚衰，经脉失于温养等阴阳平衡失调状况；加之素体阴血亏虚；或多产房劳，或大病久病失养，肾阴亏虚益甚，阴虚则阳失潜藏，而致阴虚阳亢；肾阴不足，不能涵养心肝，易致心肝火旺；或素体阳虚，过用寒凉，损及肾阳。故本病

quent asthenia of yang and excessive intake of cold foods consuming kidney yang. This syndrome is marked by kidney asthenia, disturbance of the heart, liver and spleen as well as disorder of yin, yang, qi and blood.

There is no such a term of perimenopausal period in TCM literature. But the symptoms are included in recurrence of menstruation in old women, hysteria and lily disease, collectively known as symptoms before and after menopause.

[Key points for diagnosis]

(1) Flushed cheeks, tidal fever, sweating, aversion to cold after sweating, palpitation and chest oppression, dizziness and tinnitus, headache and insomnia, or pain in the waist, back and joints, dry and itching skin as well as emotional changes like depression, anxiety, susceptibility to irritability and even emotional disorders in climacterium or after removal of ovary followed by disorder of menstruation or menopause.

(2) FSH and LH have obviously increased, but E_2 has decreased.

(3) This syndrome should be differentiated from angina pectoris, primary hypertension, perimenopausal psychosis, benign and malignant tumor of genitalia, urethrocystitis and hyperplasic arthritis.

[Syndrome differentiation and treatment]

Kidney asthenia is the root cause of this syndrome which is usually of asthenia. Even if the syndrome is of sthenia, it is often mingled with asthenia. The viscera involved are the heart, spleen and kidney. Syndrome differ-

以肾虚致病为基础,心、肝、脾诸脏功能紊乱,阴阳气血失调为病发之现状。中医古籍中无此病名记载,但其症状散见于"老年经断复来"、"脏躁"、"百合病"等病证之中,中医学称之为"绝经前后诸证"或"经断前后诸证"。

【诊断要点】

(1) 妇女在更年期或卵巢切除术后,伴随出现月经紊乱,或绝经,而出现潮红、潮热汗出、汗后有畏冷感、心悸胸闷、眩晕耳鸣、头痛失眠,或有腰背关节疼痛、皮肤干燥瘙痒以及精神情绪的改变,如抑郁忧愁、多思善虑,或易于激动、焦虑急躁,甚至喜怒无常等。

(2) 血清促卵泡生成激素(FSH)明显升高,促黄体生成激素(LH)亦升高,雌二醇(E_2)明显下降。

(3) 本病应与心绞痛、原发性高血压、精神神经系统的围绝经期精神病及生殖系统的良性或恶性肿瘤、尿道膀胱炎,以及增生性关节炎等疾病相鉴别。

【辨证论治】

本病以肾虚为本,虚多实少,即便有实证,亦多为虚中夹实,纯实证不多见。累及的脏腑主要是心、肝、脾、肾。临

entiation should be done in light of the clinical manifestations, menstruation and the conditions of the tongue and pulse so as to make clear whether it is due to asthenia of kidney yin or kidney yang or disharmony between the heart and kidney or asthenia of both the heart and spleen or liver depression.

证时应根据临床表现、月经情况、舌脉的变化，辨证其属肝肾阴虚、肾阳虚、心脾两虚，或是肝郁证等。

(1) Yin asthenia syndrome of the liver and kidney

Main symptoms: Dizziness and tinnitus, flushed cheeks and high fever, occasional sweating, feverish sensation over the palms, soles and chest, insomnia and dreaminess, aching and weak sensation in the loins and knees, dryness and pruritus of skin, dry mouth and retention of feces, scanty yellowish urine, or scanty menstruation with red menses, or disturbance of menstrual disorder, alternate sudden profuse uterine bleeding and dripping uterine bleeding, red tongue with scanty fur and thin pulse.

Therapeutic methods: Nourishing the liver and kidney, fostering yin and suppressing yang.

Prescription and drugs: Modified Zuogui Wan composed of 10g of Shengdihuang (*Radix Rehmanniae*), 10g of Shudihuang (*Radix Rehmanniae Praeparata*), 10g of Gouqizi (*Fructus Lycii*), 10g of Shanzhuyu (*Fructus Corni*), 20 g of Shanyao (*Rhizoma Dioscoreae*), 10g of Fuling (*Poria*), 10g of Mudanpi (*Cortex Moutan Radicis*), 10g of Guiban (*Plastrum Testudinis*), 15g of Longgu (*Os Draconis*), 15g of Nüzhenzi (*Fructus Ligustri Lucidi*) and 15g of Mohanlian (*Herba Ecliptae*).

Modification: For insomnia, 15g of Yejiaoteng (*Caulis Polygoni Multiflori*) and 12g of Suanzaoren (*Semen Ziziphi Spinosae*) are added; for severe headache, 15g of Gouteng (*Ramulus Uncariae cum Uncis*), 10g of Tianma (*Rhizoma Gastrodiae*) and 10g of Shi-

一、肝肾阴虚证

主要证候　绝经前后，眩晕耳鸣，潮红烘热，时有汗出，五心烦热，失眠多梦，腰膝酸软，皮肤干燥瘙痒，口干便结，尿少色黄，或月经先期量少，色红，或周期紊乱，崩漏交替，舌红苔少，脉细致。

治　法　滋补肝肾，育阴潜阳。

方　药　左归丸加减：生地黄、熟地黄各10 g，枸杞子10 g，山茱萸10 g，山药20 g，茯苓10 g，牡丹皮10 g，龟版10 g，龙骨15 g，女贞子15 g，墨旱莲15 g。

加　减　若彻夜难眠者，加夜交藤15 g，酸枣仁12 g；头痛甚者，加钩藤15 g，天麻10 g，石决明10 g；口干者，加玄参10 g，麦门冬10 g；多汗，

jueming (*Concha Haliotidis*) are added; for dry mouth, 10g of Xuanshen (*Radix Scrophulariae*) and 10g of Maimendong (*Radix Ophiopogonis*) are added; for profuse sweating, 6g of Wuweizi (*Fructus Schisandrae*) and 30g of Fuxiaomai (*Fructus Tritici Levis*) are added; for pruritus of skin, 6g of Chantui (*Periostracum Cicadae*) and 10g of Baixianpi (*Cortex Dictamni*) are added; for constipation, 10g of Baiziren (*Semen Platycladi*) and 6g of Huomaren (*Fructus Cannabis*) are added.

(2) Yang-deficiency syndrome

Main symptoms: Before and after menopause, grayish complexion, dispiritedness, puffy face, edema of limbs, chilly body and aversion to cold, anorexia and abdominal distension, loose stool, frequent and profuse urine, irregular menstruation, or sudden profuse uterine bleeding, whitish and thin leukorrhea, bulgy tongue with tooth print and whitish thin coating as well as deep and thin pulse.

Therapeutic methods: Warming the kidney and supporting yang, strengthening the spleen and assisting transportation.

Prescription and drugs: Modified Yougui Wan composed of 10g of Lujiaojiao (*Colla Cornus Cervi*), 15g of Dangshen (*Radix Codonopsis Pilosulae*), 10g of Baizhu (*Rhizoma Atractylodis Macrocephalae*), 10g of Buguzhi (*Fructus Psoraleae*), 10g of Xianmao (*Rhizoma Curculiginis*), 10g of Yinyanghuo (*Herba Epimedii*), 15g of Shanyao (*Rhizoma Dioscoreae*), 10g of Shanzhuyu (*Fructus Corni*), 10g of Duzhong (*Cortex Eucommiae*) and 10g of Tusizi (*Semen Cuscutae*).

Modification: For morning diarrhea, 10g of Muxiang (*Radix Aucklaneliae*) and 10g of Roudoukou (*Semen Myristicae*) are added; for frequent urination and

加五味子6 g,浮小麦30 g;皮肤瘙痒甚者,加蝉蜕6 g,白鲜皮10 g;便秘者,加柏子仁10 g,火麻仁6 g。

二、肾阳虚证

主要证候 绝经前后,面色晦黯,精神委靡,面浮肢肿,形寒畏冷,纳差腹胀,大便溏薄,小便频多,月经紊乱,或崩中漏下,带多色白清稀,舌淡胖边有齿印,苔薄白,脉沉细。

治 法 温肾扶阳,健脾助运。

方 药 右归丸加减:鹿角胶10 g,党参15 g,白术10 g,补骨脂10 g,仙茅10 g,淫羊藿10 g,山药15 g,山茱萸10 g,杜仲10 g,菟丝子10 g。

加 减 若晨起腹泻加煨木香10 g,肉豆蔻10 g;尿频失禁加益智仁10 g,金樱子

incontinence of urine, 10g of Yizhiren (*Fructus Alpiniae Oxyphyllae*) and 10g of Jinyingzi (*Fructus Rosae Laevigatae*) are added; for epigastric distension, 12g of Fuling (*Poria*) and 5g of Sharen (*Fructus Amomi*) are added; for swelling of limbs, 10g of Huangqi (*Radix Astragali*), 10g of Fulingpi (*Epidermis Poriae*) and 10g of Fangji (*Radix Stephaniae Tetrandrae*) are added; for chest oppression, 6g of Shichangpu (*Rhizoma Acori Graminei*) and 10g of Yujin (*Radix Curcumae*) are added.

(3) Liver depression syndrome

Main symptoms: Mental depression, anxiety, sentimentality, irritability, chest oppression, susceptibility to sighing, distending pain in hypochondria, feverish sweating, disturbance of menstruation, profuse menorrhea in the late stage with dark red color, red tongue with thin and white or thin and yellow fur as well as taut pulse before and after menopause.

Therapeutic methods: Soothing the liver to relieve depression and regulating qi to nourish yin.

Prescription and drugs: Modified Xiaoyao San composed of 10g of Baishaoyao (*Radix Paeoniae Alba*), 10g of Danggui (*Radix Angelicae Sinensis*), 5g of Chaihu (*Radix Bupleuri*), 10g of Shengdihuang (*Radix Rehmanniae*), 10g of Fuling (*Poria*), 10g of Yujin (*Radix Curcumae*), 15g of Shanyao (*Rhizoma Dioscoreae*), 6g of Chenpi (*Pericarpium Citri Reticulatae*) and 5g of Gancao (*Radix Glycyrrhizae*).

Modification: For transformation of heat from liver depression with restless fever, bitter taste in the mouth and dry throat, 6g of Zhizi (*Fructus Gardeniae*) and 10g of Mudanpi (*Cortex Moutan Radicis*) are added; for anorexia and loose stool, 10g of Baizhu (*Rhizoma Atractylodis Macrocephalae*) and 15g of Taizishen (*Radix*

10 g;脘腹作胀加茯苓12 g,砂仁5 g;四肢肿胀加黄芪10 g,茯苓皮10 g,防己10 g;胸闷者加石菖蒲6 g,郁金10 g。

三、肝郁证

主要证候　绝经前后,精神抑郁,多愁善感,烦躁易怒,胸闷叹息,两胁胀痛,烘热汗出,月经紊乱,后期量少,色暗红,舌红,苔薄白或薄黄,脉弦。

治　法　疏肝解郁,理气益阴。

方　药　逍遥散加减:白芍药10 g,当归10 g,柴胡5 g,生地黄10 g,茯苓10 g,郁金10 g,山药15 g,陈皮6 g,甘草5 g。

加　减　若肝郁化热见烦热、口苦咽干者,加栀子6 g,牡丹皮10 g;纳少便溏者,加白术10 g,太子参15 g;夜寐欠宁者,加青龙齿(先煎)20 g,酸枣仁10 g。

Pseudostellariae) are added; for restless sleep in the night, 20g of Qinglongchi (*Dens Draconis*) (to be decocted first) and 10g of Suanzaoren (*Semen Ziziphi Spinosae*) are added.

(4) Syndrome of simultaneous asthenia of heart and spleen

Main symptoms: Feverish sweating, palpitation and shortness of breath, amnesia and insomnia, sallow complexion, facial dropsy, lassitude, epigastric and abdominal distension, anorexia and loose stool, disturbance of menstruation, or sudden profuse vaginal bleeding or dripping vaginal bleeding with light color and thin texture, light-colored tongue with whitish thin fur and thin and weak pulse before and after menopause.

Therapeutic methods: Strengthening the spleen and nourishing qi, nourishing the heart and tranquilizing mind.

Prescription and drugs: Modified Guipi Tang composed of 10g of Huangqi (*Radix Astragali*), 10g of Dangshen (*Radix Codonopsis Pilosulae*), 10g of Baizhu (*Rhizoma Atractylodis Macrocephalae*), 10g of Danggui (*Radix Angelicae Sinensis*), 10g of Fushen (*Sclerotium Poriae Circum Radicem Pini*), 6g of Yuanzhi (*Radix Polygalae*), 10g of Suanzaoren (*Semen Ziziphi Spinosae*), 10g of Chenpi (*Pericarpium Citri Reticulatae*), 10g of Muxiang (*Radix Aucklaneliae*), 5g of Gancao (*Radix Glycyrrhizae*) and 5 Chinese dates.

Modification: For incessant vaginal bleeding, 20g of calcined Longgu (*Os Draconis*) and 20g of calcined Muli (*Caro Ostreae*) are added; for aching in the loins and lassitude as well as aversion to cold and cold limbs, 10g of Buguzhi (*Fructus Psoraleae*) and 10g of Duzhong (*Cortex Eucommiae*) are added; for facial dropsy and

四、心脾两虚证

主要证候　绝经前后,烘热汗出,心悸气短,健忘失眠,面色萎黄,面目虚浮,倦怠乏力,脘腹作胀,纳少便溏,月经紊乱,或崩或漏,色淡质稀,舌质淡,苔薄白,脉细弱。

治　法　健脾益气,养心安神。

方　药　归脾汤加减:黄芪10 g,党参10 g,白术10 g,当归10 g,茯神10 g,远志6 g,酸枣仁10 g,陈皮10 g,木香10 g,甘草5 g,大枣5枚。

加　减　若阴道流血不止,加煅龙骨20 g,煅牡蛎20 g;腰酸乏力、畏寒肢冷加补骨脂10 g,杜仲10 g;面浮足肿加薏苡仁20 g,玉米须10 g。

foot edema, 20g of Yiyiren (*Semen Coicis*) and 10g of Yumixu (*Stigma Maydis*) are added.

[Other therapeutic methods]

(1) Chinese patent drugs

1) Liuwei Dihuang Pill: 6g each time and three times a day, applicable to the treatment of yin asthenia syndrome.

2) Qiju Dihuang Pill: 6g each time and three times a day, applicable to the treatment of yin asthenia and yang sthenia syndrome.

3) Danzhi Xiaoyao Pill: 6 –9g each time and three times a day, applicable to the treatment of stagnant heat in the liver meridian.

4) Jingui Shenqi Pill: 6g each time and three times a day, applicable to the treatment of yang asthenia syndrome.

(2) Empirical and folk recipes

1) Zaohe Decoction: 30g of Suanzaoren (*Semen Ziziphi Spinosae*) is decocted in water. After removal of the residue, 50g of fresh Baihe (*Bulbus Lilii*) is decocted in the decoction. The decoction is taken orally and the cooked Baihe (*Bulbus Lilii*) is eaten in the morning and evening.

2) Huaixiaomai Decoction: 30g of Huaixiaomai (*Fructus Tritici Levis*) and 6g of Gancao (*Radix Glycyrrhizae*) are decocted in water. After the removal of the residue, 5 Chinese dates and 5 dried longan pulps are decocted in the decoction with mild fire for oral taking.

【其他疗法】

1. 中成药

（1）六味地黄丸　每次6 g，1 日 3 次，适用于阴虚证。

（2）杞菊地黄丸　每次6 g,1 日 3 次,适用于阴虚阳旺证。

（3）丹栀逍遥丸　每次6～9 g,1 日 3 次,适用于肝经郁热证。

（4）金匮肾气丸　每次6 g,1 日 3 次,适用于阳虚证。

2. 单验方

（1）枣合饮　酸枣仁30 g,水煎后去渣,用药液煎煮鲜百合50 g,熟后饮汤食百合,早晚分服。

（2）淮小麦饮　淮小麦30 g,甘草6 g,加水煎汤,去渣留汁,加大枣 5 枚、桂圆肉 5 枚,文火煎煮饮用。

2.2 Endometriosis and adenomyosis

2.2.1 Endometriosis

Endometriosis means that the endometrium with growing function appears outside the uterus. Such a problem usually occurs among women aging 20 - 50. The incidence peak ranges from 30 to 40. According to the clinical manifestations, this problem pertains to the conceptions of dysmenorrhea, sterility, abdominal mass and irregular menstruation in TCM.

Endometriosis is usually caused by mental depression, unsmooth flow of qi, retention of blood stasis; or by invasion of pathogenic cold in the uterus during menstruation and after delivery; or by improper sexual intercourse and consumption of kidney qi; or by weakness of visceral qi and unsmooth flow of qi and blood; or by flow of blood into the thoroughfare and conception vessels as well as uterine collaterals during menstruation and delivery; or by operational wound and impairment of the thoroughfare and conception vessels leading to abnormal flow of blood and blood stasis. Prolonged retention of blood stasis may transform into heat or lead to abdominal mass.

[Key points for diagnosis]

(1) Secondary dysmenorrhea is often found and about

第二章　子宫内膜异位症和子宫腺肌病

第一节　子宫内膜异位症

具有生长功能的子宫内膜组织出现在子宫腔被覆粘膜以外的身体其他部位时，即称为子宫内膜异位症。本病是妇科的一种常见疾病，好发于20～50岁的妇女，发病高峰在30～40岁。根据本病的临床症状可归纳为"痛经"、"不孕"、"癥瘕"、"月经失调"等范畴。

本病的发生多因情志抑郁、气机不畅、瘀血阻滞；或经行、产后血室正开，寒邪侵袭，血遇寒凝；或房事不节，肾气受损；或脏气虚弱，气血运行不畅而瘀阻；或经产时余血流注于子宫冲任脉络之外；或手术创伤，冲任之脉受损，血不循经，离经外溢而致瘀血阻滞。瘀血留滞日久可以化热，亦可变生癥瘕等病。

【诊断要点】

（1）育龄期女性有继发性

40% accompanied with primary or secondary sterility among woman of childbearing age.

(2) Abdominal pain, which appears 1 – 2 days before menstruation, becomes most serious on the first day of menstruation and gradually gets relieved after menstruation. The location of pain is usually in the lower abdomen and lumbosacral region, radiating to vagina, perineum, anus or medial side of leg. Focus in the retrouterine excavation and uterosacral ligament may lead to coital pain, distending and prolapsing sensation in anus that are worsened during menstruation. It may be accompanied by prolonged menstrual duration and increased menorrhea. Rupture of cyst in endometriosis may result in acute abdominal pain and intra-abdominal bleeding.

(3) The basal body temperature usually appears in bi-directional curve. Gynecological examination finds fixed retroversion of uterus. Painful hard nodules can be felt on the postuterine wall and uterosacral ligament. Fixed and painful cystic mass can be felt beside the uterus. Occasionally purplish nodules can be found in vaginal fornix and cervix.

(4) Type B ultrasonic examination suggests thick liquid in unilateral or bilateral ovary or enlargement of the uterus.

(5) Peritoneoscopy may find endometriosis focus or bluish-purplish or brownish sticky cystic enlargement of ovary in the retrouterine excavation and sacral ligament. Biopsy of doubtful focus is necessary for accurate diagnosis.

(6) Endometriosis should be differentiated from primary dysmenorrhea, hysteromyoma, benign and malig-

痛经,约40%的患者伴有原发或继发性不孕症。

(2) 腹痛于经前1～2天开始,以经期第1天为最剧,月经干净后逐渐缓解。其部位多在下腹及腰骶部疼痛,并向阴道、会阴、肛门或大腿内侧放射。子宫直肠陷凹及子宫骶骨韧带有病灶时可伴有性交疼痛、肛门坠胀感,并在经期加剧。也可伴有月经量增多及经期延长。卵巢内膜异位囊肿(巧克力囊肿)破裂时,可引起急性腹痛及腹腔内出血。

(3) 基础体温多呈双相型曲线。妇科检查:子宫位置后倾、固定,于子宫后壁及子宫骶骨韧带可扪及硬性触痛性结节,子宫旁可扪及囊性肿块,常较固定,并有触痛,偶见阴道穹窿及宫颈处有紫蓝色结节。

(4) B超检查可提示一侧或两侧卵巢部位有较粘稠的液性暗区或子宫增大。

(5) 腹腔镜检查可在子宫直肠陷窝、骶骨韧带等处发现子宫内膜异位病灶,或卵巢囊性增大,表面呈紫蓝色或有褐黄色粘连。对可疑病灶进行活检可明确诊断。

(6) 本病应与原发性痛经、子宫肌瘤、卵巢良性及恶

nant uterine tumor, chronic pelvitis, and pelvic tuberculosis, etc.

[Syndrome differentiation and treatment]

The main syndrome of endometriosis is blood stasis syndrome. This disease is usually sthenia at the primary stage and gradually turns into a syndrome of asthenia mingled with sthenia. Simple asthenia syndrome is seldom seen. Apart from blood stasis syndrome, other symptoms are often accompanied. Syndrome differentiation should be done in light of the time, nature and location of the symptoms; changes of menstrual cycle, quantity, color and texture; and other general symptoms in order to decide whether the syndrome is due to kidney asthenia and blood asthenia, or cold coagulation and blood stasis, or qi stagnation and blood stasis, or heat stagnation and blood stasis.

(1) Syndrome of kidney asthenia and blood stasis

Main symptoms: Abdominal pain during or after menstruation, scanty or profuse menorrhea, unsmooth menorrhea, blackish menses, or menorrhea with blood clot, aching and weak sensation in the loins and knees, blackish complexion, or accompanied by sterility, grayish tongue or tongue with ecchymosis on the tongue edge and thin and taut pulse.

Therapeutic methods: Replenishing the kidney and activating blood, resolving stasis and regulating menstruation.

Prescription and drugs: Modified Hupo San composed of 3g of Hupo powder (*Succinum*) (to be taken separately), 12g of Danggui (*Radix Angelicae Sinensis*), 12g of Chishaoyao (*Radix Paeoniae Rubra*), 10g of Danshen (*Radix Salviae Miltiorrhizae*), 6g of Chuanxiong (*Rhizoma Chuanxiong*), 10g of Puhuang (*Pollen*

性肿瘤、慢性盆腔炎、盆腔结核等病相鉴别。

【辨证论治】

本病临床主证是血瘀证，且贯穿疾病的整个过程。疾病初期以实证为主，病久伤正，因实致虚而表现为虚实夹杂证，纯虚证极少见。除血瘀主证外均兼有其他症状，临床可根据病症发生的时间、性质、部位和月经的期、量、色、质的变化及舌脉与其他全身证状，辨证有属肾虚血瘀、寒凝血瘀、气滞血瘀、热郁血瘀的不同，分别论治。

一、肾虚血瘀证

主要证候 经行或经后腹痛，经量或多或少，经行不畅，经色紫黯，或有血块，腰酸腿软，面色黧黑，或伴不孕，舌质偏暗，或舌边有瘀点，脉细弦。

治 法 补肾活血，化瘀调经。

方 药 琥珀散加减：琥珀粉（吞）3 g，当归12 g，赤芍药12 g，丹参10 g，川芎6 g，蒲黄（包煎）10 g，炒五灵脂10 g，菟丝子10 g，淫羊藿10 g，肉桂6 g，莪术10 g，红花10 g。

Typhae) (to be wrapped for decocting), 10g of stir-baked Wulingzhi (*Faeces Trogopterorum*), 10g of Tusizi (*Semen Cuscutae*), 10g of Yinyanghuo (*Herba Epimedii*), 6g of Rougui (*Cortex Cinnamomi*), 10g of Ezhu (*Rhizoma Curcumae*) and 10g of Honghua (*Flos Carthami*).

Modification: For severe abdominal pain, 6g of prepared Ruxiang (*Olibanum*), 6g of prepared Moyao (*Myrrha*), 5g of stir-baked Chuanlianzi (*Fructus Toosendan*) and 10 g of Yanhusuo (*Rhizoma Corydalis*) are added; for profuse menorrhea with blood clot, 3g of Shensanqi (*Radix Notoginseng*) (to be taken separately) is added; for scanty and unsmooth menstruation, 10g of Chuanniuxi (*Radix Cyathulae*) and 10g of Zelanye (*Folium Lycopi*) are added; for lumbago, 10g of Duzhong (*Cortex Eucommiae*) and 10g of Sangjisheng (*Ramulus Taxilli*) are added; for prolapsing and distending sensation in the anus, 12g of Zhike (*Fructus Aurantii*) and 12 g of Baijiangcao (*Herba Patriniae*) are added; for cyst in endometriosis, 10g of Huangyaozi (*Rhizoma Dioscoreae Bulbiferae*), 15g of Baijiangcao (*Herba Patriniae*) and 6g of Liujinu (*Herba Artemisiae Anomalae*) are added.

(2) Syndrome of cold coagulation and blood stagnation

Main symptoms: Unpressable cold pain in lower abdomen, aggravation before or after menstruation, alleviation with warmth, even nausea, vomiting, scanty menorrhea, unsmooth menorrhea, difficulty in getting pregnant, pale complexion, aversion to cold, cold limbs, light-white or light-purplish tongue or tongue with ecchymosis on the tongue edge, deep and tense or deep, thin and unsmooth pulse.

加　减　若小腹痛甚,加制乳香6 g,制没药6 g,炒川楝子5 g,延胡索10 g;经量多,夹有血块者,加参三七(研粉另吞)3 g;经行量少不畅,加川牛膝10 g,泽兰叶10 g;腰痛,加杜仲10 g,桑寄生10 g;肛门坠胀加枳壳12 g,败酱草12 g;卵巢有异位囊肿者,加黄药子10 g,败酱草15 g,刘寄奴6 g。

二、寒凝血滞证

主要证候　小腹冷痛拒按,经前或经行加剧,得热痛减,甚则恶心呕吐,经行量少,排出不畅,不易受孕,面色苍白,形寒怕冷,四肢不温,舌淡白或淡紫,或边有瘀点,脉沉紧或沉细涩。

Therapeutic methods: Warming meridians to disperse cold, and resolving stasis to dredge collaterals.

Prescription and drugs: Modified Wenjing Tang composed of 10g of Dangshen (*Radix Codonopsis Pilosulae*), 10g of Danggui (*Radix Angelicae Sinensis*), 5g of Chuanxiong (*Rhizoma Chuanxiong*), 15g of Danshen (*Radix Salviae Miltiorrhizae*), 10g of Niuxi (*Radix Achyranthis Bidentatae*), 6g of Rougui (*Cortex Cinnamomi*), 6g of Xiaohuixiang (*Fructus Foeniculi*), 6g of Ganjiang (*Rhizoma Zingiberis*), 10g of Ezhu (*Rhizoma Curcumae*), 12g of Wuyao (*Radix Linderae*), 6g of Aiye (*Folium Artemisiae Argyi*) and 10g of Zishiying (*Fluoritum*).

Modification: For aversion to cold and cold limbs, 8g of Fuzi (*Radix Aconiti Praeparata*) and 6g of Rougui (*Cortex Cinnamomi*) are added; for lower abdominal distending pain, 12g of Xiangfu (*Rhizoma Cyperi*) and 10g of Zhike (*Fructus Aurantii*) are added; for scanty and unsmooth menorrhea, 10g of Liujinu (*Herba Artemisiae Anomalae*) and 10g of Chongweizi (*Semen Leonuri*) are added.

(3) Syndrome of qi stagnation and blood stasis

Main symptoms: Unpressable lower abdominal distending pain, aggravation during or after menstruation, relative profuse menorrhea, purplish red menses, mingled with blood clot, alleviation of abdominal pain after removal of blood clot, or relative scanty menorrhea, unsmooth menorrhea, distending pain in the breasts before menstruation, chest oppression and restlessness, or mental depression, prolapsing and distending sensation in the anus, purplish and blackish tongue or tongue with ecchymosis on the edge, taut or taut and thin pulse.

Therapeutic methods: Soothing the liver and regu-

治　法　温经散寒,化瘀通络。

方　药　温经汤加减:党参10 g,当归10 g,川芎5 g,丹参15 g,牛膝10 g,肉桂6 g,小茴香6 g,干姜6 g,莪术10 g,乌药12 g,艾叶6 g,紫石英10 g。

加　减　若形寒怕冷、四肢不温者,加附子8 g,肉桂6 g;小腹胀痛,加香附12 g,枳壳10 g;经行量少不畅者,加刘寄奴10 g,茺蔚子10 g。

三、气滞血瘀证

主要证候　小腹胀痛拒按,经行或经后加剧,经量偏多,色紫红,夹有血块,血块排出后腹痛减轻,或经量偏少,排出不畅,经前乳房胀痛,胸闷烦躁,或精神抑郁不舒,肛门坠胀,舌紫黯,或边有瘀斑,脉弦或弦细。

治　法　疏肝理气,化瘀

lating qi, resolving stasis and dredging collaterals.

Prescription and drugs: Modified Xiaoyao San combined with Xuefu Zhuyu Tang composed of 10g of Danggui (*Radix Angelicae Sinensis*), 6g of Chuanxiong (*Rhizoma Chuanxiong*), 10g of Chishaoyao (*Radix Paeoniae Rubra*), 6g of Chaihu (*Radix Bupleuri*), 12g of Xiangfu (*Rhizoma Cyperi*), 10g of stir-baked Chuan-lianzi (*Fructus Toosendan*), 10g of Taoren (*Semen Persicae*), 10g of Honghua (*Flos Carthami*), 10g of Zhike (*Fructus Aurantii*), 10g of Niuxi (*Radix Achyranthis Bidentatae*), 12g of Danshen (*Radix Salviae Miltiorrhizae*) and 10g of Yujin (*Radix Curcumae*).

Modification: For severe lower abdominal pain, 6g of Ruxiang (*Olibanum*) and 6g prepared Moyao (*Myrrha*) and 4g of Xuejie (*Resina Draconis*) (to be ground into powder and taken separately) are added; for distending pain and mass in the breasts, 6g of Qingpi (*Pericarpium Citri Reticulatae Viride*) and 10 g of Ju-he (*Semen Citri Reticulatae*) are added; for profuse menorrhea, 3g of Sanqi powder (*Radix Notoginseng*) (to be taken separately) and 10g of charred Guanzhong (*Rhizoma Dryopteris Gassirhizomae*) are added; for irritability and susceptibility to rage, 10g of Mudanpi (*Cortex Moutan Radicis*) and 6g of Zhizi (*Fructus Gardeniae*) are added; for stagnant mass in the lower abdomen, 6g of Zhechong (*Eupolyphaga seu Steleophaga*) are added.

(4) Syndrome of heat stagnation and blood stasis

Main symptoms: Lower abdominal pain, aggravation during menstruation, fever or even high fever during menstruation and gradual improvement after menstruation, profuse menorrhea at the beginning with red color and thick texture or with blood clot, bitter taste in the mouth and dry throat, retention of dry feces, yellowish

通络。

方 药 逍遥散合血府逐瘀汤加减：当归10g，川芎6g，赤芍药10g，柴胡6g，香附12g，炒川楝子10g，桃仁10g，红花10g，枳壳10g，牛膝10g，丹参12g，郁金10g。

加 减 若小腹痛甚加制乳香6g，制没药6g，血竭（研末另吞）4g；乳房胀痛有块者，加青皮6g，橘核10g；经量过多，加参三七粉（另吞）3g，贯众炭10g；烦躁易怒，加牡丹皮10g，栀子6g；下腹有瘀块，加䗪虫6g。

四、热郁血瘀证

主要证候 下腹疼痛，经行加剧，经期发热，甚或高热，经净后渐至正常，月经先期量多，色红，质稠，或有血块，口苦咽干，大便干结，小便色黄次频，带下色黄，性交疼痛，舌

urine and frequent urination, yellowish leukorrhea, coital pain, red tongue with thin and yellow fur, thin and rapid pulse or thin and taut pulse.

Therapeutic methods: Activating blood and resolving stasis, clearing away heat and dissipating nodules.

Prescription and drugs: Modified Qingjing Siwu Tang composed of 10g of Danggui (*Radix Angelicae Sinensis*), 6g of Chuanxiong (*Rhizoma Chuanxiong*), 10g of Shengdihuang (*Radix Rehmanniae*), 10g of Chishaoyao (*Radix Paeoniae Rubra*), 10g of Mudanpi (*Cortex Moutan Radicis*), 12g of Hongteng (*Caulis Sargentodoxae*), 12g of Baijiangcao (*Herba Patriniae*), 10g of stir-baked Chuanlianzi (*Fructus Toosendan*), 10g of Taoren (*Semen Persicae*), 12g of Wulingzhi (*Faeces Trogopterorum*), 10g of Xiakucao (*Spica Prunellae*) and 10g of Shanzha (*Fructus Crataegi*).

Modification: For dysphoria and susceptibility to rage, 6g of Zhizi (*Fructus Gardeniae*) and 10g of Huangqin (*Radix Scutellariae*) are added; for low fever, 10g of Digupi (*Cortex Lycii Radicis*) and 6g of Qinghao (*Herba Artemisiae Annuae*) are added; for profuse menorrhea, 12g of crude Diyu (*Radix Sanguisorbae*) and 10g of charred Guanzhong (*Rhizoma Dryopteris Gassirhizomae*) are added; for constipation, 6g of Dahuang (*Radix et Rhizoma Rhei*) and 10g of Zhishi (*Fructus Aurantii Immaturus*) are added; for yellowish leukorrhagia, 10g of Chungenpi (*Cortex Toonae Sinensis*) and 6 g of Huangbai (*Cortex Phellodendri*) are added.

[Other therapeutic methods]

(1) Chinese patent drugs

1) Danggui Pill: 8 pills each time and three times a day; applicable to the treatment of the syndrome of qi stagnation and blood stasis.

质红,苔薄黄,脉细数或细弦数。

治　法　活血化瘀,清热散结。

方　药　清经四物汤加减:当归10g,川芎6g,生地黄10g,赤芍药10g,牡丹皮10g,红藤12g,败酱草12g,炒川楝子10g,桃仁10g,五灵脂12g,夏枯草10g,山楂10g。

加　减　若心烦易怒,加栀子6g,黄芩10g;伴有低热,加地骨皮10g,青蒿6g;经量过多,加生地榆12g,贯众炭10g;大便秘结,加大黄6g,枳实10g;带多色黄,加椿根皮10g,黄柏6g。

【其他疗法】

1. 中成药

（1）当归丸　每服8粒,1日3次,适用于气滞血瘀证。

2) Tongjing Pill: 6g each time and three times a day, applicable to the treatment of the syndrome of cold coagulation and blood stasis.

(2) Empirical and folk recipes

1) Dilong (*Pheretima*), Wugong (*Scolopendra*), Zhechong (*Eupolyphaga seu Steleophaga*), Rougui (*Cortex Cinnamomi*) and Chenxiang (*Lignum Aquilariae Resinatum*) of the same amount are ground into powder. 3g is taken each time and three times a day, applicable to the treatment of blood stasis syndrome.

2) 3g of Sanqi (*Radix Notoginseng*), 20g of Danshen (*Radix Salviae Miltiorrhizae*) and 2 eggs are decocted together in 300ml water. When the eggs are well cooked, the shells are removed and the rest is put into the decoction to boil for some time. After the removal of the residue, the decoction and egg are taken. Such a decoction begins 2 days before menstruation, which is taken once a day for 5 days. This decoction is applicable to the treatment of blood stasis syndrome.

(3) External therapy

1) Enema: 30g of Sanleng (*Rhizoma Sparganii*), 30g of Ezhu (*Rhizoma Curcumae*), 20g of Sumu (*Lignum Sappan*), 15g of Honghua (*Flos Carthami*), 30g of Loufengfang (*Nidus Polistis*), 15g of Pugongying (*Herba Taraxaci*) and 20g of Hongteng (*Caulis Sargentodoxae*) are decocted in water into 100 - 150ml of decoction for enema, once a day and 20 - 30 minutes each time for retaining the decotion and 10 days making up one course of treatment. Or the cotton cushion is rinsed in the decoction and applied to the lower abdomen with iontophoresis apparatus, once a day, 20 - 30 minutes each time and 10 times making up one course of treatment. This treatment can be used to treat, excluding the syndrome of cold coagulation and blood stasis, the other three types of

（2）痛经丸　每服6 g,1日3次,适用于寒凝血瘀证。

2. 单验方

（1）地龙、蜈蚣、䗪虫、肉桂、沉香等分,研细末,每服3 g,1日3次,适用于血瘀证。

（2）三七3 g,丹参20 g,加鸡蛋2枚,水300 ml同煮,蛋熟后去壳再煮片刻,去药渣,食蛋饮汤。于月经前2天开始每天服1次,连服5天,适用于血瘀证。

3. 外治法

（1）灌肠法　三棱30 g,莪术30 g,苏木20 g,红花15 g,露蜂房30 g,蒲公英15 g,红藤20 g煎至100～150 ml,进行保留灌肠,每日1次,每次保留药液20～30分钟,10天为1个疗程。亦可将上液用棉垫浸透敷于下腹,用离子透入仪进行中药离子透入,每日1次,每次20～30分钟,10次为1个疗程。除寒凝血瘀证外,其他三种证型均可采用。

syndrome.

2) Insertion of drugs into the vagina: Zhongrushi (*Stalactitum*), Ruxiang (*Olibanum*), Moyao (*Myrrha*), Sanleng (*Rhizoma Sparganii*) and Ezhu (*Rhizoma Curcumae*) of the same amount are ground into fine powder, sifted and sterilized. Each time 5 - 10g is inserted into posterior fornix and stuffed with a cotton ball with a remaining thread. The inserted powder is removed after 24 hours. One month makes up one course of treatment. This treatment, applicable to the treatment of nodules and mass in the posterior fornix after endometriosis, can be used continuously for 2 - 4 courses.

2.2.2 Adenomyosis

Adenomyosis refers to invasion of endometrium into myometrium, usually seen among pluripara at the age of 30 - 50. Half of the cases are complicated by hysteromyoma. In some cases, endometriosis appears at the same time. After menopause, the symptoms gradually get improved and the focus becomes shrunk and eventually disappears. According to the clinical manifestations, adenomyosis pertains to the conceptions of dysmenorrhea, abdominal mass and irregular menstruation in TCM.

This disease is mainly caused by retention of blood stasis in the thoroughfare and conception vessels as well as the uterus. Blood stasis is caused by emotional depression, inhibited flow of liver qi, obstructed activity of qi, unsmooth circuation of blood and qi stagnation; abdominal mass results from stagnation of qi and blood due to excessive intake of uncooked and cold foods or attack by exogenous pathogenic cold which coagulates blood. Constitutional asthenia of spleen qi and hypofunction in transpor-

（2）阴道纳药法　钟乳石、乳香、没药、三棱、莪术各等份，压成细末过筛，消毒备用，每次取药末 5～10 g，纳药入阴道后穹窿，以有尾棉球填塞，24 小时取出，1 个月为 1 个疗程，连用 2～4 个疗程，适用于本病后穹隆有结节和包块者。

第二节　子宫腺肌病

子宫内膜侵入子宫肌层，称为子宫腺肌病。其发病多见于 30～50 岁经产妇，半数的病例合并子宫肌瘤，部分与子宫内膜异位症并存，绝经后症状缓解，病灶萎缩消失。子宫腺肌病根据临床表现，属中医学"痛经"、"癥瘕"、"月经不调"等范畴。

本病主要是瘀血阻滞冲任、胞宫所致。平素情志抑郁，肝气不舒，气机不利，血行不畅，气滞而血瘀；或经前、经期恣食生冷，或感受寒凉，血遇寒则凝，气血瘀滞，日久结块，形成癥瘕；或素体脾虚气弱，运血无力，血行迟滞，日久成瘀。

ting blood will slow the flow of blood and gradually lead to stasis. Retention of blood stasis in the thoroughfare and conception vessels as well as uterus blocks uterine collaterals and causes dysmenorrhea.

[Key points for diagnosis]

(1) Progressive secondary dysmenorrhea is the typical symptom. But in some cases there is no dysmenorrhea.

(2) The commonly seen symptoms are changes of menstruation marked by profuse menorrhea and prolonged menstruation.

(3) Pelvic examination indicates even enlargement of the uterus, hard texture with tenderness, obvious tenderness of the uterus before menstruation, shrinkage after menstruation, difference in size, number and location with the complication of hysteromyoma.

(4) Type B ultrasonic examination indicates even spherical enlargement of the uterus and low echo of multiple follicle-like in the muscular wall of the uterus.

(5) Iodized oil roentgenograph of the uterus suggests enlargement of the uterine cavity, appearance of diverticulum-like spherical prominence with the iodized oil flowing into the muscular layer.

(6) Pathological examination shows thickening and hardness of the uterine wall, especially the posterior wall, thick myofiber zone and small cysts in the superior wall of the section, occasional appearance of old blood.

[Syndrome differentiation and treatment]

The main clinical manifestation is blood stasis syndrome, pertaining to sthenia syndrome. But it may develop into a syndrome mingled with both asthenia and sthenia due to profuse menorrhea, menostaxis and excessive loss of blood. Syndrome differentiation should be done based

【诊断要点】

(1) 继发性痛经进行性加重是典型的症状,但部分病例可无痛经。

(2) 月经的改变,以月经量增多、经期延长为常见。

(3) 盆腔检查,子宫呈均匀性增大,质硬有压痛,月经前子宫触痛明显,月经后可缩小,合并子宫肌瘤时,则依肌瘤的大小、数目、部位而异。

(4) B超检查,子宫均匀性增大呈球形,肌壁有多发小囊样低回声反射。

(5) 子宫碘油造影显示,子宫腔增大,碘油溢入肌层形成憩室样球形隆起。

(6) 病理检查,子宫壁增厚而硬,后壁更明显,切面上肌壁间夹杂有粗厚的肌纤维带和小囊腔,其中偶见陈旧血液。

【辨证论治】

本病临床表现为血瘀证,为实证。但因月经量多,经期延长,日久失血较多,致虚实夹杂证。因此临床辨证时要根据疼痛的性质、部位、程度、

on the nature, location, degree and duration of pain; in light of the quantity, color and texture of menses; based on the conditions of the tongue and pulse as well as general manifestations so as to decide whether the syndrome is of sthenia or a mixture of both sthenia and asthenia.

Dysmenorrhea usually occurs before and during menstruation. Lower abdominal cold pain or colic may be due to cold coagulation and blood stasis if it gets improved with warmth. Lower abdominal distending pain complicated by distending pain in the breasts is due to cold coagulation and blood stasis. Prolapsing pain in the lower abdomen with scanty and light-colored menses as well as lassitude is due to qi asthenia and blood stasis.

The treatment usually concentrates on resolving abdominal mass. If it is due to cold coagulation and blood stasis, the treatment should be warming the meridians to disperse cold; if it is due to qi stagnation and blood stasis, the treatment should be promoting qi flow and activating blood; if it is due to qi asthenia and blood stasis, the treatment should be nourishing qi and activating blood.

(1) Syndrome of cold coagulation and blood stasis

Main symptoms: Lower abdominal cold pain or colic worsened by pressure, or lower abdominal mass, profuse or scanty menses with purplish color and blood clot, alleviation of abdominal pain after removal of blood clot, cold limbs, purplish and blackish tongue with ecchymosis and whitish and slippery fur, deep and taut or deep and tense pulse before menstruation.

Therapeutic methods: Warming meridians and dispersing cold, resolving stasis and eliminating mass.

Prescription and drugs: Modified Shaofu Zhuyu Tang composed of 10g of stir-baked Xiaohuixiang (*Fructus Foeniculi*), 10g of Ganjiang (*Rhizoma Zingiberis*),

持续时间及月经量、色、质的变化和舌脉及全身表现辨虚实孰多孰少,辨其为实证,还是虚实夹杂之证。

痛经多发生于经前、经期。小腹冷痛或绞痛,得热稍减者,为寒凝血瘀;小腹胀痛并伴胸胁乳房胀痛者,属气滞血瘀;小腹疼痛下坠,月经量少色淡,倦怠乏力者,为气虚血瘀。

治疗总以化瘀消癥为主,其中寒凝血瘀者,宜温经散寒;气滞血瘀者,又当行气活血;气虚血瘀者,则应以益气活血为法。

一、寒凝血瘀证

主要症状 经期经前小腹冷痛或绞痛,按之痛甚,痛势剧烈,或下腹结块,月经量多或少,色紫黯,有血块,块下痛减,四肢厥冷,舌质紫黯,有瘀斑、瘀点,苔白滑,脉沉弦或沉紧。

治 则 温经散寒,化瘀消癥。

方 药 少腹逐瘀汤加减:炒小茴香10 g,干姜10 g,桂枝6 g,赤芍药12 g,当归

6g of Guizhi (*Ramulus Cinnamomi*), 12g of Chishaoyao (*Radix Paeoniae Rubra*), 10g of Danggui (*Radix Angelicae Sinensis*), 6g of Chuanxiong (*Rhizoma Chuanxiong*), 10 g of Sanleng (*Rhizoma Sparganii*), 10g of Ezhu (*Rhizoma Curcumae*), 10g of Wuyao (*Radix Linderae*), 12g of Kunbu (*Thallus Laminariae seu Eckloniae*) and 5g of crude Gancao (*Radix Glycyrrhizae*).

Modification: For profuse menorrhea, Sanleng (*Rhizoma Sparganii*) and Ezhu (*Rhizoma Curcumae*) are deleted while 15g of Xianhecao (*Herba Agrimoniae*), 15g of Yimucao and 6g of Paojiangtan (*Charred Rhizoma Zingiberis*) are added for reinforcing the effect for warming yang, resolving stasis and stopping bleeding.

(2) Syndrome of qi stagnation and blood stasis

Main symptoms: Unbearable lower abdominal pain before and during menstruation, or lower abdominal mass, profuse menses with deep-red color and blood clot, slight alleviation of pain after removal of blood clot, premenstrual dysphoria and susceptibility to rage, distending pain in chest, hypochondria and breasts, blackish tongue or tongue with ecchymosis and taut pulse.

Therapeutic methods: Promoting qi flow and activating blood, resolving stasis and dissipating nodules.

Prescription and drugs: Modified Xuefu Zhuyu Tang composed of 8g of Chaihu (*Radix Bupleuri*), 10g of prepared Xiangfu (*Rhizoma Cyperi*), 10g of Chuanniuxi (*Radix Cyathulae*), 12g of Zhike (*Fructus Aurantii*), 10g of Taoren (*Semen Persicae*), 10g of Honghua (*Flos Carthami*), 6g of Chuanxiong (*Rhizoma Chuanxiong*), 10g of Yanhusuo (*Rhizoma Corydalis*), 10g of Sanleng (*Rhizoma Sparganii*), 10g of Ezhu (*Rhizoma Curcumae*), 12g of Wulingzhi (*Faeces Trogopterorum*) and 12g of Kunbu (*Thallus Laminariae seu Eckloniae*).

10 g,川芎6 g,三棱10 g,莪术10 g,乌药10 g,昆布12 g,生甘草5 g。

加　减　若经量多者,去三棱、莪术,加仙鹤草15 g,益母草15 g,炮姜炭6 g,以增温阳化瘀止血之功。

二、气滞血瘀证

主要症状　经前经期小腹胀痛难忍,拒按,或下腹结块,月经量多,色黯红有血块,块下痛稍减,经前心烦易怒,胸胁乳房胀痛,舌质紫黯或有瘀斑瘀点,脉弦。

治　则　行气活血,消瘀散结。

方　药　血府逐瘀汤加减:柴胡8 g,制香附10 g,川牛膝10 g,枳壳12 g,桃仁10 g,红花10 g,川芎6 g,延胡索10 g,三棱10 g,莪术10 g,五灵脂12 g,昆布12 g。

Modification: For premenstrual abdominal pain, 10g of prepared Moyao (*Myrrha*) and 20g of Jixueteng (*Caulis Spatholobi*) are added for promoting qi flow, activating blood and stopping pain; for profuse menorrhea, Sanleng (*Rhizoma Sparganii*) and Ezhu (*Rhizoma Curcumae*) are deleted while 30g of Yimucao (*Herba Leonuri*), 30 g of Qiancaotan (Charred *Radix Rubiae*) (*infused into decoction*) and 3g of Sanqi powder (*Radix Notoginseng*) are added for resolving stasis and stopping bleeding.

(3) Syndrome of qi asthenia and blood stasis

Main symptoms: Unbearable and prolapsing pain in the lower abdomen, profuse or delayed menstruation with light color and thin texture menses, or lower abdominal mass, lassitude, anorexia, grayish tongue or tongue with ecchymosis, thin and unsmooth pulse.

Therapeutic methods: Nourishing qi and activating blood, resolving stasis and dissipating abdominal mass.

Prescription and drugs: Modified Sijunzi Tang combined with Siwu Tang composed of 15g of Dangshen (*Radix Codonopsis Pilosulae*), 12g of Baizhu (*Rhizoma Atractylodis Macrocephalae*), 10g of Fuling (*Poria*), 12g of Chishaoyao (*Radix Paeoniae Rubra*), 6g of Chuanxiong (*Rhizoma Chuanxiong*), 10g of stir-baked Danggui (*Radix Angelicae Sinensis*), 12g of Sanleng (*Rhizoma Sparganii*), 12g of Ezhu (*Rhizoma Curcumae*), 10g of prepared Xiangfu (*Rhizoma Cyperi*) and 6g of processed Gancao (*Radix Glycyrrhizae*).

Modification: For the onset of abdominal pain, 10g of Yanhusuo (*Rhizoma Corydalis*), 10g of prepared Moyao (*Myrrha*) and 3g of Xuejie powder (*Resina Draconis*) (infused into decoction) are added; for prolonged or profuse menstruation, Sanleng (*Rhizoma Sparganii*)

加　减　若经前经期腹痛已作，加制没药10 g，鸡血藤20 g，以行气活血止痛。

若经行量多者，经期去三棱、莪术活血逐瘀之品，加益母草30 g，茜草炭30 g，三七粉（冲）3 g以化瘀止血。

三、气虚血瘀证

主要症状　经行小腹坠痛，疼痛难忍，月经量多或经期延长，色淡质稀，或下腹结块，倦怠乏力，纳少，舌质淡黯或有瘀斑瘀点，脉细涩。

治　则　益气活血，化瘀消癥。

方　药　四君子汤合四物汤加减。党参15 g，白术12 g，茯苓10 g，赤芍药12 g，川芎6 g，炒当归10 g，三棱12 g，莪术12 g，制香附10 g，炙甘草6 g。

加　减　若腹痛发作时，加延胡索10 g，制没药10 g，血竭粉3 g（冲）；若经期延长或经行量多者，经期去破血逐瘀之三棱、莪术，加益母草15 g， and Ezhu (*Rhizoma Curcumae*) are deleted during menstruation while 15g of Yimucao (*Herba Leonuri*), 15g of Wuzeigu (*Os Sepiae*), 15g of Xianhecao (*Herba Agrimoniae*) and 3g of Sanqi powder (*Radix Notoginseng*) (infused into decoction) are added for reinforcing the effect for resolving stasis and stopping bleeding.

[Other therapeutic methods]

(1) Chinese patent drugs

1) Yanhu Zhitong Tablet: 4 tablets each time and three times a day, applicable to the treatment of qi stagnation and blood stasis syndrome.

2) Aifu Nuangong Pill: 10g each time and three times a day, applicable to the treatment of cold coagulation and blood stasis syndrome.

3) Fuke Huisheng Bolus: 1 bolus each time and twice a day, applicable to the treatment of qi asthenia and blood stasis syndrome.

(2) Empirical and folk recipes

1) 45g of Yimucao (*Herba Leonuri*) and 15g of Yanhusuo (*Rhizoma Corydalis*) are decocted together with 2 eggs in 600ml of water. When the eggs are well cooked, the shells are removed and the rest is put into the decoction to boil for a while. After the removal of the residue, the decoction and eggs are taken. This treatment begins 2 days before menstruation. The decoction and eggs are taken once a day for 5 days, applicable to the treatment of qi stagnation and blood stasis syndrome.

2) 30g of Lizhihe (*Semen Litchi*) and 30g of Huixiang (*Fructus Foeniculi*) are stir-baked black and ground into fine powder. Each time 3g is taken with warm wine and twice a day. This treatment begins 3 days before menstruation, applicable to the treatment of cold coagulation and blood stasis type.

3) 30g of Dangshen (*Radix Codonopsis Pilosulae*),

乌贼骨15 g,仙鹤草15 g,三七粉（冲）3 g,以增化瘀止血之功。

【其他疗法】

1. 中成药

（1）延胡止痛片　每次服 4 片,1 日 3 次,适用于气滞血瘀证。

（2）艾附暖宫丸　每次服10 g,1 日 3 次,适用于寒凝血瘀证。

（3）妇科回生丹　每次服 1 丸,每日 2 次,适用于气虚血瘀型。

2. 单验方

（1）益母草45 g,延胡索15 g,鸡蛋 2 枚,上药加水600 ml同煮,蛋熟后去壳再煮片刻,去药渣,吃蛋饮汤。于月经前 2 天开始每天服 1 次,连服 5 天,适用于气滞血瘀证。

（2）荔枝核30 g,茴香30 g,将上 2 味炒黑,研极细末,每服3 g,温酒送下,经前 3 天开始服,每天 2 次,服至经净,适用于本病寒凝血瘀证。

（3）党参30 g,黄芪10 g,

10g of Huangqi (*Radix Astragali*) and 30g of Danshen (*Radix Salviae Miltiorrhizae*) are decocted in 500ml of water. After boiling, the herbs continue to be decocted with mild fire for 30 minutes. 30 g of brown sugar is added into the decoction. The decoction is taken as tea for 10 days. This treatment begins 3 days before menstruation, applicable to the treatment of qi asthenia and blood stasis syndrome.

(3) Enema with Chinese medicinal herbs

15g of Danshen (*Radix Salviae Miltiorrhizae*), 15g of Chishaoyao (*Radix Paeoniae Rubra*), 10g of Taoren (*Semen Persicae*), 15g of Sanleng (*Rhizoma Sparganii*), 15g of Ezhu (*Rhizoma Curcumae*), 15g of Haizao (*Sargassum*), 10g of Zhechong (*Eupolyphaga seu Steleophaga*), 10g of Yanhusuo (*Rhizoma Corydalis*), 10g of Chuanlianzi (*Fructus Toosendan*), 15g of Lizhihe (*Semen Litchi*) and 10g of Muxiang are decocted into 100ml for enema, once a night. This therapy is effective for promoting qi flow to activate blood and expelling stasis to stop pain. For cold coagulation and blood stasis syndrome, 3g of Xixin (*Herba Asari*) and 10g of Guizhi (*Ramulus Cinnamomi*) are added for warming meridians and dredging collaterals.

丹参30 g,将上药加水 500 ml,煮沸后用微火煎 30 分钟取汁,加入30 g红糖当茶饮,于经前 3 天开始,可连服 10 天,适用于气虚血瘀证。

3. 中药灌肠

丹参15 g,赤芍药15 g,桃仁10 g,三棱15 g,莪术15 g,海藻15 g,䗪虫10 g,延胡索10 g,川楝子10 g,荔枝核15 g,木香10 g,浓煎 100 ml,保留灌肠,每晚 1 次。行气活血,祛瘀止痛;若寒凝血瘀者,加细辛3 g,桂枝10 g,以温经通络。

2.3 Sterility

第三章
不孕症

Sterility is a commonly encountered gynecological disease. About 10% of the couples at the age of 25 - 35 suffer from sterility. This percentage is increasing year by year. In the human reproduction procedure, a number of factors may affect pregnancy and lead to sterility. This chapter only discusses female sterility.

不孕症是妇科临床常见疾病,在正常适龄夫妇中约有10%左右伴发不孕症,且有逐年上升趋势。其发病年龄多集中在 25~35 岁。在人类生殖活动过程中,由综合性的、多方面的因素影响了受孕的任何一个环节,都可导致不孕症。本节所论述的不孕症,主要是指不孕原因在女方,亦谓之女性不孕症。

2.3.1 Primary sterility

第一节   原发性
不孕症

Couples of proper age with normal sexual life without using contraception for two years without pregnancy is called sterility. No experience of pregnancy after marriage is known as primary sterility.

育龄夫妇有正常性生活、同居 2 年以上,未采取避孕措施而不能受孕者,称为不孕症。婚后从未受孕者,称为原发性不孕。

The kidney governs reproduction, stores essence and functions as the prenatal base of life. Only when kidney qi is superabundant, essence and blood are sufficient, the thoroughfare and conception vessels are full as well as menstruation is regular can sexual intercourse result in pregnancy. Any factors that affect any links in this procedure may cause sterility. So sterility is closely related to the kidney. Since the kidney is the dominant one

肾主生殖而藏精气,当肾气盛,精血充沛,天癸至,月事以时下,两精相搏,则可受孕。反之,由于某些因素影响了上述任何一个环节,都会导致不孕。因此,不孕与肾的关系最为密切。肾虚可导致肝、脾、心等脏腑功能失调,出现肝肾

among the fiver zang and six fu organs, asthenia of the kidney may lead to dysfunction of the liver, spleen and heart. The dysfunction of these viscera further leads to insufficiency of the liver and kidney, asthenia of both the spleen and kidney as well as disharmony between the heart and kidney that result in disturbance of qi and blood in the thoroughfare and conception vessels and failure of the uterus to conceive fetus.

[Key points for diagnosis]

(1) Couples of proper age with regular sexual life and without contraception for two years without pregnancy is called sterility. Examination concentrates on the type of build, the secondary sex characteristic and pubes, etc. Gynecological examination is done to see whether there are organic changes.

(2) Assay of ovarian function: BBT tests ovulation. For instance, uni-directional BBT indicates no ovulation; bidirectional BBT, temperature difference $\leqslant 0.3℃$, or continuous high fever for $1-2$ days, or gradual increase of body temperature indicate ovulation with hypofunction of yellow body of ovary. Smear examination of the exfoliated cells in the vagina: If the smear examination indicates simple action of estrin or hypofunction of estrin, it suggests no ovulation. Examination of cervical mucus: cervical marks-estimation is for monitoring of ovulation.

(3) Diagnostic curettage and histological examination of endometrium before menstruation or 6 hours within menstruation: This examination is helpful for understanding both the morbid changes in the cervix and uterus and the functions of yellow body of ovary. Hyperplasic endometrium indicates no ovulation while secretory endometrium suggests ovulation; early secretory endometrium

不足、脾肾两虚、心肾不交等证,并影响冲任气血紊乱,则胞宫难以摄精成孕。

【诊断要点】

(1) 婚后 2 年以上,夫妇同居,性生活规律,未避孕而不受孕,体格检查着重于患者体型、第二性征发育、阴毛分布等;妇科检查判断有无性器发育异常等。

(2) 卵巢功能测定:基础体温(BBT)可检测排卵情况,如 BBT 为单相型的则无排卵,如 BBT 为双相型,但温差小于或等于 0.3℃,或高温相持续时间小于 1~2 天,或体温上升缓慢,则提示为有排卵而黄体功能不足。阴道脱落细胞涂片检查:如表现单纯雌激素作用或雌激素功能低下则提示无排卵功能。宫颈粘液检查:以宫颈评分监测排卵。

(3) 经前或行经 6 小时内诊断性刮宫及子宫内膜组织学检查,既可了解宫颈及宫腔的病变又可了解黄体功能状态,若为增生期内膜则视为无排卵,若为分泌期内膜提示有排卵;若为分泌早期或分泌不

or insufficiency of secretion suggests ovulation with hypo-function of yellow body of ovary.

(4) Hormone level test is done to analyze whether ovary, pituitary gland and hypothalamus have affected ovulation.

(5) Type B ultrasonic examination is helpful for detecting development of ovum and understanding whether there are organic changes of the uterus and ovary.

(6) Hysterosalpingography is helpful for detecting the pathological changes of the uterus and the conditions of the oviduct.

(7) Abdominoscopy and uterioscopy are helpful for direct observation of the pelvis and the uterus.

(8) PCT tests the ability of semen in penetrating cervical mucus and in survival.

(9) Immune examination of serum and cervical mucus.

(10) Sterility should be differentiated from some congenital defects of genitalia.

[Syndrome differentiation and treatment]

Primary sterility, either asthenia or sthneia, should be differentiated according to the age of menarche, menstruation, the secondary sex characteristic and constitution. Primary sterility of asthenia nature is marked by late occurrence of menarche, delayed menstruation, scanty menorrhea with light or grayish color and thin texture and scanty leukorrhea. Primary sterility of asthenia nature is marked by scanty menorrhea with grayish color and multiple blood clots, unpressable distending pain in lower abdomen. The root cause lies in the kidney, but the liver, spleen and qi and blood must be taken into consideration.

足表示虽有排卵但黄体功能欠佳。

（4）激素水平测定：用以分析卵巢、垂体及下丘脑功能有无异常而影响排卵。

（5）B超检查可了解子宫、卵巢有无器质性病变及监测卵泡发育与排卵。

（6）子宫输卵管造影术可了解宫腔病变及输卵管通畅程度。

（7）腹腔镜、宫腔镜检查则可直观了解盆腔脏器及宫腔。

（8）性交后试验（PCT）以测试精子穿透宫颈粘液的能力与存活情况。

（9）血清及宫颈粘液免疫学检查。

（10）某些严重的先天性器官缺如及畸形或纯属男方原因者，应注意加以鉴别。

【辨证论治】

原发性不孕症应根据初潮年龄、月经带下的情况以及第二性征发育、体质状况等辨别虚实。初潮年龄较晚，行经落后，量少，色淡或暗，质薄，带下甚少，属虚；量少，色暗，多血块，小腹胀痛拒按，属实。其根本在于肾，但肝、脾、气血的影响也是非常重要的。临证应当注意辨别。

(1) Syndrome of kidney qi asthenia

Main symptoms: No pregnancy long after marriage, late occurrence of menarche, delayed menstruation, scanty menorrhea with light or grayish color, even amenorrhea, blackish complexion, aching in the loins and flaccidity of legs, sexual frigidity, leukorrhagia with thin texture, clear and profuse urine, loose stool, scanty pubes, small uterus, light-colored tongue with whitish fur, deep and thin pulse or deep and slow pulse.

Therapeutic methods: Warming the kidney and replenishing essence, nourishing the thoroughfare and conception vessels.

Prescription and drugs: Modified Yulinzhu composed of 15g of Dangshen (*Radix Codonopsis Pilosulae*), 10g Fuling (*Poria*), 15g of Shanyao (*Rhizoma Dioscoreae*), 10g of Shudihuang (*Rhizoma Rehmanniae Praeparata*), 10g of Shanzhuyu (*Fructus Corni*), 10g of Danggui (*Radix Angelicae Sinensis*), 6g of Chuanxiong (*Rhizoma Chuanxiong*), 10g of Xuduan (*Radix Dipsaci*), 10g of Tusizi (*Semen Cuscutae*), 10g of Duzhong (*Cortex Eucommiae*), 10g of Lujiaojiao (*Colla Cornus Cervi*) and 10g of Ziheche (*Placenta Hominis*).

Modification: For severe lumbago and lower abdominal cold, 6g of Xiaohuixiang (*Fructus Foeniculi*), 10g of Zishiying (*Fluoritum*) and 10g Yinyanghuo (*Herba Epimedii*) are added; for thin and profuse leukorrhea, 10g of Jinyingzi (*Fructus Rosae Laevigatae*) and 10g of Qianshi (*Semen Euryales*) are added; for loose stool, 6g of Paojiang (*baked Rhizoma Zingiberis*), 6g of toasted Muxiang (*Radix Aucklaneliae*) and 10g of stir-baked Baibiandou (*Semen Lablab Album*) are added; for frequent urination, 10g of Yizhiren (*Fructus Alpiniae Oxyphyllae*) and 10g of Sangpiaoxiao (*Ootheca Mantidis*)

一、肾气亏损证

主要证候 婚后久不孕，月经初潮较晚，经期错后而至，量少色淡或暗，甚至经闭，面色晦黯黧黑，腰酸腿软，性欲淡漠，带下量多、清稀，小便清长，大便溏薄，妇科检查阴毛稀疏，子宫偏小，舌淡苔白，脉沉细或沉迟。

治 法 温肾填精，补益冲任。

方 药 毓麟珠加减：党参15 g，茯苓10 g，山药15 g，熟地黄10 g，山茱萸10 g，当归10 g，川芎6 g，续断10 g，菟丝子10 g，杜仲10 g，鹿角胶（霜）15 g，紫河车10 g。

加 减 若腰酸如折，小腹清冷，加小茴香6 g，紫石英10 g，淫羊藿10 g；带下清稀量多，加金樱子10 g，芡实10 g；大便溏薄，加炮姜6 g，煨木香6 g，炒白扁豆10 g；小便频多，加益智仁10 g，桑螵蛸10 g；形体消瘦，五心烦热，加牡丹皮10 g，龟版（先煎）10 g，白薇6 g，知母10 g。

are added; for emaciation and feverish sensation over palms, soles and chest, 10g of Mudanpi (*Cortex Moutan Radicis*), 10g of Guiban (*Plastrum Testudinis*) (to be decocted first), 6g of Baiwei (*Radix Cynanchi Atrati*) and 10g of Zhimu (*Rhizoma Anemarrhenae*) are added.

(2) Syndrome of liver and kidney deficiency

Main symptoms: No pregnancy long after marriage, delayed menstruation, scanty, light-colored or grayish menorrhea, even amenorrhea, emaciation, feverish sensation over palms, soles and chest, dizziness, tinnitus, palpitation, insomnia, aching in the loins and flaccidity of legs, red tongue with scanty fur, taut pulse or thin and taut pulse.

Therapeutic methods: Nourishing the liver and kidney, replenishing essence and nourishing yin.

Prescription and drugs: Modified Erzhi Dihuang Tang composed of 15g of Nüzhenzi (*Fructus Ligustri Lucidi*), 15g of Hanliancao (*Herba Ecliptae*), 15g of Shanyao (*Rhizoma Dioscoreae*), 10g of Shudihuang (*Rhizoma Rehmanniae Praeparata*), 10g of Shanzhuyu (*Fructus Corni*), 10g of Danggui (*Radix Angelicae Sinensis*), 10g of Baishaoyao (*Radix Paeoniae Alba*), 10g of Fuling (*Poria*), 10g of Xuduan (*Radix Dipsaci*), 10g of Gouqizi (*Fructus Lycii*), 10g of Ziheche (*Placenta Hominis*) and 5g of Gancao (*Radix Glycyrrhizae*).

Modification: For palpitation, 10g of Suanzaoren (*Semen Ziziphi Spinosae*) and 10g of Hehuanpi (*Cortex Albiziae*) are added; for restless sleep in the night, 10g of Heshouwu (*Radix Polygoni Multiflori*) and 10g of Fushen (*Sclerotium Poriae Circum Radicem Pini*) are added; for afternoon low fever, 15g of Guiban (*Plastrum Testudinis*) and 15g of Biejia (*Carapax Trionycis*) are added.

二、肝肾不足证

主要证候 婚后久不怀孕,经期错后而至,量少色淡或暗,甚至经闭,形体消瘦,五心烦躁,头晕耳鸣,心悸失眠,腰酸腿软,舌质红,苔少,脉弦或细弦。

治 法 补益肝肾,填精养阴。

方 药 二至地黄汤加减:女贞子15 g,旱莲草15 g,山药15 g,熟地黄10 g,山茱萸10 g,当归10 g,白芍药10 g,茯苓10 g,续断10 g,枸杞子10 g,紫河车10 g,甘草5 g。

加 减 心悸怔忡加酸枣仁10 g,合欢皮10 g;夜寐欠安加何首乌10 g,茯神10 g;午后低热加龟版15 g,鳖甲15 g。

(3) Syndrome of qi and blood asthenia

Main symptoms: No pregnancy long after marriage, scanty menorrhea with light color, or amenorrhea, sallow complexion, lusterless skin, physical weakness, spiritual lassitude, dizziness, shortness of breath and palpitation, accompanied by maldevelopment of the uterus, light-colored tongue with white fur, thin and weak pulse.

Therapeutic methods: Nourishing qi and blood, strengthening and invigorating the uterine collaterals.

Prescription and drugs: Modified Bazhen Tang composed of 15g of Huangqi (*Radix Astragali*), 12g of Dangshen (*Radix Codonopsis Pilosulae*), 10g of Baizhu (*Rhizoma Atractylodis Macrocephalae*), 10g of Fuling (*Poria*), 20g of Shanyao (*Rhizoma Dioscoreae*), 10g of Danggui (*Radix Angelicae Sinensis*), 6g of Chuanxiong (*Rhizoma Chuanxiong*), 10g of Baishaoyao (*Radix Paeoniae Alba*), 10g of Shudihuang (*Rhizoma Rehmanniae Praeparata*), 12g of Nüzhenzi (*Fructus Ligustri Lucidi*), 12g of Ejiao (*Colla Corii Asini*) and 10g of Xiangfu (*Rhizoma Cyperi*).

Modification: For severe aching in the loins, 10g of Chuanduan (*Radix Dipsaci*), 10g of Ziheche (*Placenta Hominis*) and 12g of Tusizi (*Semen Cuscutae*) are added; for palpitation, 10g of Suanzaoren (*Semen Ziziphi Spinosae*) and 10g of Yuanzhi (*Radix Polygalae*) are added; for restless sleep in the night, 10g of Heshouwu (*Radix Polygoni Multiflori*) and 12g of Yejiaoteng (*Caulis Polygoni Multiflori*) are added; for aversion to cold, 8g of Fuzi (*Radix Aconiti Praeparata*) and 10g of Buguzhi (*Fructus Psoraleae*) are added.

(4) Syndrome of liver and heart qi stagnation

Main symptoms: No pregnancy long after marriage,

三、气血虚弱证

主要证候 婚后多年不孕,月经量少色淡,或闭经,面色萎黄,肌肤不泽,形体虚弱,神疲乏力,头晕目眩,心悸气短,可伴子宫发育不良,舌淡苔白,脉细弱。

治 法 补益气血,固养胞脉。

方 药 八珍汤加减:黄芪15g,党参12g,白术10g,茯苓10g,山药20g,当归10g,川芎6g,白芍药10g,熟地黄10g,女贞子12g,阿胶12g,香附10g。

加 减 若腰酸甚者,加川断10g,紫河车10g,菟丝子12g;心悸怔忡加酸枣仁10g,远志10g;夜寐欠安加何首乌10g,夜交藤12g;畏寒肢冷加附子8g,补骨脂10g。

四、心肝气郁证

主要证候 婚后多年不

mental upsets, depression, irritability, irregular menstruation, scanty menorrhea with blackish color, or unsmooth menorrhea, or abdominal pain during menstruaton, distending pain in the breasts before menstruation, discomfort in the chest and hypochondria, insomnia and dreaminess, deep-red tongue with thin and white fur, taut pulse or thin pulse.

Therapeutic methods: Soothing the liver to relieve depression and regulating qi and blood.

Prescription and drugs: Modified Kaiyu Zhongyu Tang composed of 12g of Danggui (*Radix Angelicae Sinensis*), 12g of Chishaoyao(*Radix Paeoniae Rubra*), 12g of Baishaoyao (*Radix Paeoniae Alba*), 10g of Baizhu (*Rhizoma Atractylodis Macrocephalae*), 10g of Fuling (*Poria*), 10g of Xiangfu (*Rhizoma Cyperi*), 6g of Qingpi (*Pericarpium Citri Reticulatae Viride*), 6g of Chaihu (*Radix Bupleuri*), 10g of Yujin (*Radix Curcumae*), 6g of Chuanlianzi (*Fructus Toosendan*), 10g of Yanhusuo (*Rhizoma Corydalis*), 10g of Danshen (*Radix Salviae Miltiorrhizae*) and 10g of Niuxi (*Radix Achyranthis Bidentatae*) are added.

Modification: For unsmooth menorrhea, 12g of Honghua (*Flos Carthami*), 15g of Yimucao (*Herba Leonuri*), 12g of Shanzha (*Fructus Crataegi*) and 10g of Zelan (*Herba Lycopi*) are added; for distending pain and nodules in the breasts, 10g of Juye (*Folium Citri Tangerinae*), 10g of Juhe (*Semen Citri Reticulatae*), 12g of Quangualou (*Fructus Trichosanthis*) and 10g of Lulutong (*Fructus Liquidambaris*) are added; for restlessness and susceptibility to rage, 6g of Zhizi (*Fructus Gardeniae*), 10g of Mudanpi (*Cortex Moutan Radicis*) and 15g of Gouteng (*Ramulus Uncariae cum Uncis*) are added; for dizziness and tinnitus, 12g of Nüzhenzi (*Fructus Ligustri Lucidi*) and 12g of Sangshenzi (*Fructus Mori*) are added.

孕,精神不安,抑郁烦躁,月经先后不定期,量少色黯,或经行不畅,或经期腹痛,经前乳房胀痛,胸胁不舒,失眠多梦,舌质黯红,苔薄白,脉弦或细弦。

治 法 疏肝解郁,调和气血。

方 药 开郁种玉汤加减:当归12 g,赤芍药12 g,白芍药 1 2g,白术 10 g,茯苓 10 g,香附10 g,青皮6 g,柴胡6 g,郁金10 g,川楝子6 g,延胡索10 g,丹参10 g,牛膝10 g。

加 减 若经行不畅加红花12 g,益母草15 g,山楂 12 g,泽兰10 g;乳房胀痛结块加橘叶10 g,橘核10 g,全瓜蒌12 g,路路通10 g;烦躁易怒加栀子 6 g,牡丹皮10 g,钩藤15 g;头晕耳鸣加女贞子12 g,桑椹子12 g。

[Other therapeutic methods]

(1) Chinese patent drugs

1) **Ankun Zanyu Pill**: 1 pill each time and twice a day, applicable to the treatment of kidney qi asthenia syndrome in sterility.

2) **Dingkun Bolus**: 1 bolus each time during menstruation and twice a day, applicable to the treatment of kidney qi asthenia syndrome in sterility.

3) **Aifu Nuangong Pill**: 5g each time and twice a day, applicable to the treatment of cold syndrome in sterility.

4) **Shenrong Lutai Paste**: 1 spoon each time and twice a day, applicable to the treatment of kidney yang asthenia syndrome in sterility.

(2) Empirical and folk recipes

1) Mu'er Tang composed of 30g of Baimu'er (*Tremella Fuciformis*) and 8g of Lujiaojiao (*Colla Cornus Cervi*). Baimu'er (*Tremella Fuciformis*) is washed and cooked in proper amount of water. Then 15g of Bingtang (*crystal sugar*) and Lujiaojiao (*Colla Cornus Cervi*) are added into the decoction. This decoction is applicable to the treatment of kidney yin asthenia syndrome.

2) 500g of black-boned chicken, 60g of Danggui (*Radix Angelicae Sinensis*) and 7 slices of ginger are decocted in water with proper amount of salt. The decoction is taken orally in seven days, applicable to the treatment of blood asthenia syndrome.

3) 100g of Ziheche (*Placenta Hominis*) is ground into powder that is put into capsules for oral taking, applicable to the treatment of kidney asthenia syndrome.

2.3.2 Secondary sterility

Failure to be pregnant without contraceptions in two

【其他疗法】

1. 中成药

（1）安坤赞育丸　每次服1丸,1日2次,适用于本病肾气亏损证。

（2）定坤丹　于经间后每次服1丸,1日2次,适用于本病肾气亏损证。

（3）艾附暖宫丸　每次服5g,1日2次,适用于本病寒证。

（4）参茸鹿胎膏　每次服1匙,1日2次,适用于肾阳虚不孕证。

2. 单验方

（1）木耳汤　白木耳30g,鹿角胶8g,冰糖15g;白木耳洗净,加水适量,煎熬后,加入鹿角胶和冰糖拌均匀,熬至烊化,适用于肾阴虚证。

（2）乌骨鸡500g,当归60g,生姜七片,盐适量煎汤,分七天服,用于血虚证。

（3）紫河车100g打粉,装入胶囊,分次服,适用于肾虚证。

第二节　继发性不孕症

曾有过妊娠（包括分娩与

years after last pregnancy (including delivery and abortion) is called secondary sterility. Secondary sterility is usually due to improper care during menstruation and after delivery, or intemperance in sexual life and invasion of pathogenic factors into the uterus that lead to downward migration of blood stasis or damp-heat to block the uterine collaterals as well as the thoroughfare and conception vessels; or due to emotional upsets, stagnation of liver qi, disharmony between qi and blood as well as obstruction of the thoroughfare and conception vessels; or due to obesity, excessive intake of greasy and rich foods that lead to endogenous phlegm-dampness obstructing the thoroughfare and conception vessels. The conception of sterility in TCM is similar to sterility caused by salpingitis, endometriosis and immune disorder in Western medicine.

[Key points for diagnosis]

(1) Failure to be pregnant without contraceptions in two years after last pregnancy accompanied by irregular menstruation, premenstrual distension or distending pain in the breasts, dysmenorrhea, aching, prolapsing and distending pain in the loins and abdomen, abnormal changes of leukorrhea, mass in the abdomen, occasional low fever, sexual frigidity, dyspareunia, or anxiety, insomnia and depression.

(2) Hysterosalpingography is helpful for detecting morbid changes in the uterus and the conditions of oviduct; abdominoscopy and uteroscopy are helpful for direct observation of the organs in the pelvis and uterus, such as inflammation and mass in the reproductive system.

(3) Diagnostic curettage and histological examination of endometrium before menstruation or 6 hours within menstruation: This examination is helpful for understanding both the morbid changes in the cervix and uterus and

流产)史,以后未采取避孕措施而连续 2 年不再受孕者,称为继发性不孕。继发性不孕的发生常因经期、产后摄生不慎,或房事不节,邪入胞宫,与血相搏结,以致瘀血或湿热下注,胞脉受阻,任脉不通,两精不能抟合而不孕。或因七情内伤,肝气郁结,疏泄失常,气血不和,冲任瘀滞而致不孕。或因素体肥胖,恣食膏粱厚味,以致痰湿内生,冲任胞脉闭塞,而致不能摄精成孕。相当于西医输卵管炎症造成的梗阻性不孕、子宫内膜异位症的不孕、免疫性不孕等。

【诊断要点】

(1) 婚后曾有过妊娠,以后未避孕连续 2 年未再受孕,常伴有月经失调及经前乳胀或胀痛,痛经,腰腹酸胀坠痛,带下异常,腹部有包块,时有低热,性欲淡漠,性交障碍,性交痛,或有焦虑、失眠、忧郁等精神异常表现。

(2) 子宫输卵管造影术可了解宫腔病变及输卵管通畅程度;腹腔镜、宫腔镜检查则可直观盆腔脏器及宫腔内有无生殖系统炎症、肿块等。

(3) 经前或行经 6 小时内诊断性刮宫及子宫内膜组织学检查,既可了解宫颈及宫腔的病变,又可了解黄体功能状

the functions of yellow body of ovary. Hyperplasic endometrium indicates no ovulation while secretory endometrium suggests ovulation; early secretory endometrium or insufficiency of secretion suggests ovulation with hypofunction of yellow body of ovary.

(4) Type B ultrasonic examination is helpful for detecting development of ovum and understanding whether there are organic changes of the uterus and ovary.

(5) Hormone level test is done to analyze whether ovary, pituitary gland and hypothalamus have affected ovulation.

(6) PCT tests the ability of semen in penetrating cervical mucus and in survival.

(7) Immune examination of serum and cervical mucus is done to determine whether sterility is immune sterility or not.

[Syndrome differentiation and treatment]

The examination of secondary sterility may be done in light of pregnancy and abortion or history of other disease that may cause sterility, usually marked by asthenia of the root aspect and sthenia of the branch aspect or mixture of asthenia and sthenia. Clinically various factors have to be taken into consideration in differentiating syndromes in light of the differentiation of diseases.

(1) Syndrome of qi stagnation and blood stasis

Main symptoms: Experience of pregnancy after marriage, sterility due to abortion, premature delivery and gynecological operation, delayed menstruation, scanty and unsmooth menorrhea with purplish and blackish color or with blood clot, often accompanied by dysmenorrhea, unpressable pain in the lower abdomen, purplish and blackish tongue or with ecchymoses, taut and unsmooth

态。若为增生期内膜则视为无排卵,若为分泌期内膜提示有排卵;若为分泌早期或分泌不足表示虽有排卵但黄体功能欠佳。

(4) B超检查可了解子宫、卵巢有无器质性病变及监测卵泡发育与排卵。

(5) 性激素水平测定:以分析卵巢、垂体及下丘脑功能有无异常而影响排卵。

(6) 性交后试验(PCT)以测试精子穿透宫颈粘液的能力与存活情况。

(7) 血清及宫颈粘液免疫学检查以确定是否为免疫性不孕。

【辨证论治】

继发性不孕症可追溯其妊娠或流产史,或有可致不孕的其他病史。常有本虚标实,或虚实夹杂之证,临证须根据相关因素仔细辨析。

一、气滞血瘀证

主要证候 婚后曾受孕,因流产、早产及妇科手术后多年不孕,月经后期,量少不畅,经血紫黑,或有血块,常伴痛经,小腹胀痛拒按,舌紫黯,或有瘀点,脉弦涩。

pulse.

Therapeutic methods: Activating blood, resolving stasis and dredging uterine collaterals.

Prescription and drugs: Modified Shaofu Zhuyu Tang composed of 12g of Danggui (*Radix Angelicae Sinensis*), 10g of Chishaoyao (*Radix Paeoniae Rubra*), 6g of Chuanxiong (*Rhizoma Chuanxiong*), 10g of Taoren (*Semen Persicae*), 10g of Honghua (*Flos Carthami*), 10 g of Chuanniuxi (*Radix Cyathulae*), 12g of Wulingzhi (*Faeces Trogopterorum*), 10g of Xiangfu (*Rhizoma Cyperi*), 10g of Wuyao (*Radix Linderae*), 10g of Zhike (*Fructus Aurantii*), 15g of Danshen (*Radix Salviae Miltiorrhizae*) and 12g of Yanhusuo (*Rhizoma Corydalis*).

Modification: For severe abdominal pain, 6g of Moyao (*Myrrha*), 6g of prepared Ruxiang (*Olibanum*) and 9g of Gegen (*Radix Puerariae*) are added; for lower abdominal cold pain, 10g of Aiye (*Folium Artemisiae Argyi*), 6g of Rougui (*Cortex Cinnamomi*) and 10g of Xiaohuixiang (*Fructus Foeniculi*) are added; for abdominal pain with low fever, 15g of Baijiangcao (*Herba Patriniae*), 10g of Mudanpi (*Cortex Moutan Radicis*), 10g of Pugongying (*Herba Taraxaci*) and 10g of Digupi (*Cortex Lycii*) are added; for serious blood stasis with strong physique, Poxiao Dangbao Tang can be used.

(2) Syndrome of interior retention of phlegm-dampness

Main symptoms: Sterility for years due to abortion, obesity, bright-white complexion, profuse and sticky leukorrhea, scanty and delayed menorrhea, or even amenorrhea, chest oppression and nausea, lassitude and fatigue, sexual frigidity, light-colored bulgy tongue with whitish greasy fur and slippery pulse.

治 法 活血化瘀,疏通胞脉。

方 药 少腹逐瘀汤加减:当归12 g,赤芍药10 g,川芎 6 g,桃仁10 g,红花10 g,川牛膝10 g,五灵脂12 g,香附10 g,乌药10 g,枳壳10 g,丹参15 g,延胡索12 g。

加 减 若腹痛甚加制没药6 g,制乳香6 g,葛根9 g;小腹冷痛加艾叶10 g,肉桂6 g,小茴香10 g;时有腹痛低热者,加败酱草15 g,牡丹皮10 g,蒲公英 10 g,地骨皮10 g;如血瘀较重,身体健壮者,可用朴硝荡胞汤治之。

二、痰湿内阻证

主要证候 婚后曾因流产而后多年不孕,形体肥胖,面色㿠白,头晕心悸,白带量多、质稠粘,月经后期量少,甚或闭经,胸闷泛恶,倦怠乏力,性欲淡漠,舌淡胖,苔白腻,

Therapeutic methods: Drying dampness and resolving phlegm, strengthening the spleen and regulating qi.

Prescription and drugs: Modified Qigong Wan composed of 10g of Banxia (*Rhizoma Pinelliae*), 10g of Cangzhu (*Rhizoma Atractylodis*), 10g of Baizhu (*Rhizoma Atractyloidis Macrocephalae*), 10g of Fuling (*Poria*), 10g of Chenpi (*Pericarpium Citri Reticulatae*), 10g of Shenqu (*Massa Medicata Fermentata*), 9g of Shichangpu (*Rhizoma Acori Graminei*), 6g of Houpo (*Cortex Magnoliae Officinalis*), 10g of Xiangfu (*Rhizoma Cyperi*), 6g of Chuanxiong (*Rhizoma Chuanxiong*), 10g of Yuanzhi (*Radix Polygalae*) and 15g of Haizao (*Sargassum*).

Modification: For dizziness and headache, 6g of Qianghuo (*Rhizoma seu Radix Notopterygii*) and 12g of Baijili (*Fructus Tribuli*) are added; for lumbago and tinnitus, 10g of Duzhong (*Cortex Eucommiae*), 10g of Buguzhi (*Fructus Psoraleae*) and 10g of Tusizi (*Semen Cuscutae*) are added; for chest oppression and anorexia, 15g of Yiyiren (*Semen Coicis*) and 10g of Peilan (*Herba Eupatorii*) are added; for delayed and scanty menorrhea, 10g of Taoren (*Semen Persicae*) and 10g of Honghua (*Flos Carthami*) are added.

(3) Syndrome of downward migration of damp-heat

Main symptoms: Sterility for years due to gynecological operation, profuse and sticky leukorrhea with white or yellow color and foul smell, lower abdominal pain, irregular menstruation, red tongue with yellow and greasy fur as well as taut and rapid pulse.

Therapeutic methods: Clearing away heat and eliminating dampness and regulating the thoroughfare and

脉滑。

治 法 燥湿化痰,健脾理气。

方 药 启宫丸加减:半夏10 g,苍术10 g,白术10 g,茯苓10 g,陈皮10 g,神曲10 g,石菖蒲9 g,厚朴6 g,香附10 g,川芎6 g,远志10 g,海藻15 g。

加 减 若头晕头痛,加羌活6 g,白蒺藜10 g;腰痛耳鸣,加杜仲10 g,补骨脂10 g,菟丝子10 g;胸闷、纳呆加薏苡仁15 g,佩兰10 g;月经错后量少加桃仁10 g,红花10 g。

三、湿热下注证

主要证候 妇科手术后多年不孕,带下量多,质地稠粘,色白或黄,时有臭味,少腹疼痛,月经失调,舌红,苔黄腻,脉弦数。

治 法 清化湿热,调畅冲任。

conception vessels.

Prescription and drugs: Modified Simiao Wan combined with Hongteng Baijiang San composed of 10g of Huangbai (*Cortex Phellodendri*), 10g of Cangzhu (*Rhizoma Atractylodis*), 10g of Niuxi (*Radix Achyranthis*), 15g of Yiyiren (*Semen Coicis*), 15g of Hongteng (*Caulis Sargentodoxae*), 12g of Baijiangcao (*Herba Patriniae*), 10g of Fuling (*Poria*), 10g of Xiangfu (*Rhizoma Cyperi*), 10g of Yanhusuo (*Rhizoma Corydalis*), 12g of Lulutong (*Fructus Liquidambaris*), 15g of Tianxianteng (*Herba Aristolochiae*) and 10g of Zhike (*Fructus Aurantii*).

Modification: For lower abdominal distending pain, 6g of Moyao (*Myrrha*) and 6g of prepared Ruxiang (*Olibanum*) are added; for yellow and greasy tongue fur and bitter taste in the mouth, 6g of Danxing (*Arisaema cum Bile*) and 10g of Gualoupi (*Pericarpium Trichosanthis*) are added; for profuse leukorrhea, 10 g of Fuling (*Poria*), 10g of Zexie (*Rhizoma Alismatis*) and 15g of Chungenpi (*Cortex Toonae Sinensis*) are added; for predominant heat in damp-heat, Longdan Xiegan Tang can be used.

[**Other therapeutic methods**]

(1) Chinese patent drugs

1) Danggui Pill: 15g each time and twice a day, applicable to the treatment of qi stagnation and blood stasis syndrome.

2) Yimu Bazhen Pill: 10g each time and three times a day, applicable to the treatment of qi stagnation and blood stasis syndrome.

3) Fuke Qianjin Tablet: 10g each time and twice a day, applicable to the treatment of damp-heat syndrome.

(2) External therapy

1) Enema: Tongguan Tang composed of Danggui

方　药　四妙丸合红藤败酱散加减：黄柏10 g,苍术10 g,牛膝10 g,薏苡仁15 g,红藤15 g,败酱草12 g,茯苓10 g,香附10 g,延胡索10 g,路路通12 g,天仙藤15 g,枳壳10 g。

加　减　小腹胀痛,加制没药6 g,制乳香6 g;苔黄腻、口苦,加胆星6 g,瓜蒌皮10 g;带下过多,加土茯苓10 g,泽泻10 g,椿根皮15 g;湿热偏于热者,用龙胆泻肝汤治之。

【其他疗法】

1. 中成药

（1）当归丸　每次服15 g,1 日 2 次,适用于气滞血瘀证。

（2）益母八珍丸　每次服10 g,1 日 3 次,适用于气滞血瘀证。

（3）妇科千金片　每次服10 g,1 日 2 次,适用于湿热证。

2. 外治法

（1）灌肠法　通管汤

(*Radix Angelicae Sinensis*), Chishaoyao (*Radix Paeoniae Rubra*), Honghua (*Flos Carthami*), Pugongying (*Herba Taraxaci*), Zaojiaoci (*Spina Gleditsiae*), Baijiangcao (*Herba Patriniae*), Hongteng (*Caulis Sargentodoxae*), Taoren (*Semen Persicae*), Chuanxiong (*Rhizoma Chuanxiong*), Chaihu (*Radix Bupleuri*), Xiangfu (*Rhizoma Cyperi*) and Lulutong (*Fructus Liquidambaris*) (15g for each). These herbs are decocted in 300ml of water into 100ml of decoction for enema. This treatment is given once a day and 10 times make up one course of treatment, applicable to the treatment of sterility due to inflammation of appendage and obstruction of oviduct. It should be suspended during menstruation.

2) Oviduct Infusion: 4ml of Danshen (*Radix Salviae Miltiorrhizae*) injection added with 0.9% of normal saline of 40 - 60ml is infused into the oviduct to treat sterility due to the obstruction of oviduct.

3) Hot compression: 20g of Danshen (*Radix Salviae Miltiorrhizae*), 15g of Zaojiaoci (*Spina Gleditsiae*), 30g of Tougucao (*Herba Speranskiae*), 20g of Rougui (*Cortex Cinnamomi*), 20g of Honghua (*Flos Carthami*), 10g of Chuanwu (*Radix Aconiti*), 10g of Weilingxian (*Radix Clematidis*), 6g of Moyao (*Myrrha*), 6g of Ruxiang (*Olibanum*), 20g of Chishaoyao (*Radix Paeoniae Rubra*) and 20g of Danggui (*Radix Angeliae Sinensis*) are ground into fine powder. The powder, after being steamed with a little alcohol, is applied to both sides of the abdomen. This compression is applied once a day and 40 minutes each time. 10 days make up one course of treatment.

（当归、赤芍药、红花、蒲公英、皂角刺、败酱草、红藤、桃仁、川芎、柴胡、香附、路路通各15 g，加 300 ml 水，煎成100 ml），保留灌肠，每日 1 次，10 次为 1 个疗程。经期停用。可治疗因附件炎症、输卵管阻塞所致不孕症。

（2）输卵管注入法　丹参注射液 4 ml 加入 0.9%生理盐水 40～60 ml 中，行子宫输卵管通液术，治疗输卵管阻塞而致的不孕症。

（3）热敷法　丹参20 g，皂角刺15 g，透骨草30 g，肉桂20 g，红花20 g，川乌10 g，威灵仙10 g，没药6 g，乳香6 g，赤芍药 20 g，当归 20 g 研成细末，滴少许白酒蒸后热敷于下腹两侧，每日 1 次，热敷约 40 分钟，10 天为 1 个疗程。

2.4　Edeitis

2.4.1　Bartholinitis and Bartholin's cyst

Bartholinitis is caused by invasion of pathogen into the greater vestibular gland. In acute bartholinitis, the greater and smaller lips of pudendum on the same side become tumescent and painful. This problem is known as pudendal pain or pudendal swelling in TCM. Under infection, swelling of the gland duct causes adhesion and obstruction which lead to abscess of the greater vestibular gland. After the abatement of acute inflammation, pus is absorbed and develops into cyst known as pudendal cocoon in TCM.

Bartholinitis is usually caused by improper sexual activity, pudendal infection and retention of damp-heat during menstruaton and after delivery and operation as well as disharmony between qi and blood; or by frequent asthenia of the spleen, dysfunction of the spleen in transformation and transportation, or by transformation of heat from liver depression and downward migration of damp toxin.

[Key points for diagnosis]

(1) At the acute stage, one side of the pudendum is swelling and painful, making it difficult to walk. Suppuration leads to aggravation of local pain accompanied by general symptoms such as fever. Under interior pressure, abscess may rupture automatically, resulting in abatement of inflammation. If the rupture is not big enough to drain

第四章　生殖器官炎症

第一节　前庭大腺炎及囊肿

前庭大腺因病原体侵入而引发的炎症为前庭大腺炎。急性前庭大腺炎时,该侧大小阴唇发赤肿胀、疼痛,中医称为"阴痛"、"阴肿"。在感染状态下,腺管肿胀,以致粘连堵塞,可形成前庭大腺脓肿。在急性炎症消退后,脓液逐渐吸收而形成囊肿,中医称为"阴茧"。

本病多有不洁性交史,经期、产后、手术后等外阴部感染湿热,湿热之邪稽留,气血失和,蕴而为患;或素体脾虚,运化失司,或肝郁化热,湿毒下注。

【诊断要点】

(1) 急性期,外阴一侧肿痛,甚至难以行走。化脓时局部疼痛加剧,并伴有发热等全身症状。当脓肿内压力增大,可自行破溃,炎症渐消退而愈;倘破口过小,引流不畅,炎

pus, the inflammation will linger for a period of time and relapse may be caused accordingly. At the chronic stage, there are no subjective symptoms except slight discomfort in the external genitals.

(2) In acute bartholinitis, one side of the lip of the pudendum becomes reddish, tumescent, feverish with obvious tenderness. When abscess is developed, local fluid wave can be felt. If it becomes putrid, pus may come out from the rupture. At the chronic stage with the formation of cyst, local round cystic mass-like substance can be detected. Routine smear examination should be done with the suppurating secreta.

(3) Detailed inquiry of the medical history and smear examination of the secreta are helpful for excluding bacterial inflammation of the greater vestibular gland.

[Syndrome differentiation and treatment]

The main manifestations of this disease are swelling and pain in the vagina, or suppuration and rupture, accompanied by chills and fever. Relapse consumes healthy qi and makes the disease difficult to heal. Clinically the differentiation of syndrome should be done in light of the nature and degree of the pathological conditions as well as the accompanied symptoms. Usually sudden onset with chills and fever suggests heat and sthenia syndrome. Incomplete treatment and lingering of the disease or slow onset often lead to asthenia syndrome or syndrome with the mixture of asthenia and sthenia.

(1) Damp-heat syndrome

Main symptoms: At the acute stage, adhesion and obstruction of greater vestibular gland without infection may lead to retention cyst of the greater vestibular gland like cocoon. Infection leads to local redness, swelling, hot sensation, pain and pruritus, the prolonged duration

症可持续不消,并会反复急性发作;慢性炎期,除外阴稍有不适外,无明显自觉症状。

（2）急性炎症时可见一侧阴唇下端红肿、发热、触痛明显,形成脓肿时局部有波动感,如已败溃则可见脓液自破口流出。慢性期形成囊肿时,局部可查见圆形囊性之块物。对脓性分泌物应常规行涂片检查。

（3）详细询问病史及分泌物涂片检查有助于排除淋菌性前庭大腺炎。

【辨证论治】

本病的主要表现症状是阴户肿胀,疼痛,或成脓破溃,可伴见寒战发热等症状。病情反复发作,可致正气渐虚,使病情缠绵不愈。一般情况下,凡起病急,伴寒战高热者,多属热、属实;若未能彻底治疗,而病状缠绵,或起病较缓者,往往属虚,或虚实夹杂,临床当仔细审证论治。

一、湿热证

主要证候　急性期,前庭大腺管粘连堵塞而腺体未发生感染时,则可形成前庭大腺潴留性囊肿,状如蚕茧,感染后局部红、肿、热、痛,阴痒,稍

of which results in suppuration with yellowish greasy tongue fur and rapid pulse.

Therapeutic methods: Clearing away heat and relieving toxin, draining dampness and relieving pain.

Prescription and drugs: Modified Longdan Xiegan Tang composed of 9g of Longdancao (*Radix Gentianae*), 9g of stir-baked Huangbai (*Cortex Phellodendri*), 10g of Huangqin (*Radix Scutellariae*), 6g of Shanzhi (*Fructus Gardeniae*), 10g of Zexie (*Rhizoma Alismatis*), 5g of Mutong (*Caulis Akebiae*), 6g of Chaihu (*Radix Bupleuri*), 10g of Danggui (*Radix Angelicae Sinensis*), 10g of Chishaoyao (*Radix Paeoniae Rubra*), 10g of Cheqianzi (*Semen Plantaginis*) (to be wrapped for decocting), 12g of Zihuadiding (*Herba Violae*) and 5g of Gancao (*Radix Glycyrrhizae*).

Modification: For obvious pudendal redness, swelling, hotness and pain, 15 g of Jinyinhua (*Flos Lonicerae*), 15g of Pugongying (*Herba Taraxaci*) and 15g of Banbianlian (*Herba Lobeliae Chinesis*) are added for clearing away heat and relieving toxin; for severe pudendal distension, swelling and pain, 6g of processed Ruxiang (*Olibanum*), 6g of processed Moyao (*Myrrha*), 10g of Baizhi (*Radix Angelicae*) and 15g of Zaojiaoci (*Spina Gleditsiae*) are added; for severe pudendal pruritus due to relative predominant damp-heat, 20g of Yiyiren (*Semen Coicis*) and 10g of Difuzi (*Fructus Kochiae*) are added.

(2) Syndrome of blood stasis

Main symptoms: At the chronic stage, the symptoms are thickening and roughness of the local skin with cyanotic color, pudendal pruritus, or accompanied by cocoon-like mass in the pudendum, purplish tongue with slight yellow and greasy fur, and thin pulse.

久则化脓,苔黄腻,脉数。

治　法　清热解毒,利湿止痛。

方　药　龙胆泻肝汤加减:龙胆草9 g,炒黄柏9 g,黄芩10 g,山栀6 g,泽泻10 g,木通5 g,柴胡6 g,当归10 g,赤芍药10 g,车前子(包煎)10 g,紫花地丁12 g,甘草5 g。

加　减　外阴红、肿、热、痛明显者,加入金银花15 g,蒲公英15 g,半边莲15 g等清热解毒之品;外阴肿胀疼痛剧烈者,加入制乳香6 g,制没药6 g,白芷10 g,皂角刺15 g等药;阴痒颇剧,湿热偏甚者,加入薏苡仁20 g,地肤子10 g等。

二、血瘀证

主要证候　慢性期,局部皮肤肥厚、粗糙,呈紫褐色,外阴瘙痒,或伴有阴茧状,舌质边紫,苔微黄腻,脉细。

Therapeutic methods: Activating blood and resolving stasis, clearing away damp-heat.

Prescription and drugs: Modified Xuefu Zhuyu Tang composed of 10g of Taoren (*Semen Persicae*), 10g of Honghua (*Flos Carthami*), 10g of Danggui (*Radix Angelicae Sinensis*), 10g of Chishaoyao (*Radix Paeoniae Rubra*), 10g of Chuanniuxi (*Radix Cyathulae*), 10g of stir-baked Zhike (*Fructus Aurantii*), 6g of Chaihu (*Radix Bupleuri*), 6g of Jiegeng (*Radix Platycodi*), 10g of Shudihuang (*Radix Rehmanniae Praeparata*), 9g of stir-baked Huangbai (*Cortex Phellodendri*) and 20g of Yiyiren (*Semen Coicis*).

Modification: For severe pudendal pruritus, 10g of Cangzhu (*Rhizoma Atractylodis*), 6g of Jingjie (*Herba Schizonepetae*) and 10g of Difuzi (*Fructus Kochiae*) are added; for prolonged duration of disease with greater pudendal cocoon, 6g of Zhechong (*Eupolyphaga seu Steleophaga*), 6g of roasted Guizhi (*Ramulus Cinnamomi*), 15g of Shijianchuan (*Herba Salviae Chinensis*), 10g of Mudanpi (*Cortex Moutan Radicis*) and 10g of Wulingzhi (*Faeces Trogopterorum*) are added.

[**Other therapeutic methods**]
External therapy

1) **External application of Pugongying (*Herba Taraxaci*)**: 60g of Pugongying (*Herba Taraxaci*) is washed, pounded and mixed up with a little honey. The mixture is applied to the affected part once a day, applicable to the treatment of acute bartholinitis with abscess.

2) **Lotion**: 15g of Yejuhua (*Flos Chrysanthemi Indici*), 30 g of Zihuadiding (*Herba Violae*), 15g of Longdancao (*Radix Gentianae*), 15g of Pugongying (*Herba Taraxaci*) and 15g of Huangbai (*Cortex Phellodendri*) are decocted. The decoction is used to fumigate and wash the affected part, twice a day. This treatment is applica-

治　法　活血化痰,清利湿热。

方　药　血府逐瘀汤加减:桃仁10 g,红花10 g,当归10 g,赤芍药10 g,川牛膝10 g,炒枳壳10 g,柴胡6 g,桔梗6 g,熟地黄10 g,炒黄柏9 g,薏苡仁20 g。

加　减　阴痒甚者加入制苍术10 g,荆芥6 g,地肤子10 g;病程长、阴茧较大者,加入䗪虫、炙桂枝各6 g,石见穿15 g,牡丹皮10 g,五灵脂10 g。

【其他疗法】
外治法

(1) 蒲公英外敷方　鲜蒲公英60 g,将蒲公英洗净捣烂,加少许蜜糖调匀敷于患处,每日换药1次,适用于急性前庭大腺炎有脓肿者。

(2) 外用搽剂　野菊花15 g,紫花地丁30 g,龙胆草15 g,蒲公英15 g,黄柏15 g,煎汤趁热先薰后洗,每日2次,适用于急、慢性前庭大腺炎或有湿疹者。

ble to the treatment of acute and chronic bartholinitis or with eczema.

2.4.2 Cervicitis

Cervicitis is either acute or chronic. Clinically acute infection usually lead to cervicitis, a commonly encountered gynecological disease among half of the married women. Cervicitis is responsible for cervical cancer to a certain extent. It is usually caused by improper care during menstruation and after delivery, giving rise to invasion of damp toxin into the thoroughfare and conception vessels and affecting the belt vessel; or by constitutional weakness, dysfunction of the spleen in transformation, interior retention of dampness and impairment of the thoroughfare and conception vessels; or by transformation of heat from accumulation of pathogenic dampness, putrefaction due to accumulation of damp-heat and downward migration into the lower energizer.

[Key points for diagnosis]

(1) The clinical manifestations of this disease are profuse leukorrhea with milk-like and sticky texture or with pus-like and light yellow color, or bloody leukorrhea, or bleeding after sexual intercourse, pudendal pruritus and pain; even lumbosacral pain, prolapsing pain in the lower abdomen, dysmenorrhea and dyspareunia; or frequent urination, stabbing pain in urination and difficulty in urination. Bacterial infection is usually accompanied by fever. In serious cases sterility can be caused.

(2) In acute cervicitis, gynecological examination may find cervical congestion, edema, even exfoliation and necrosis as well as discharge of excessive pyogenic mucus. Erosion of cervix is either granular or mastoid. The erosion is graded into mild, medium and serious degrees.

第二节　子宫颈炎

子宫颈炎是女性生殖器官炎症中最常见的一种,约占已婚妇女的半数以上;可分为急性和慢性两类,临床上急性感染常转化为慢性宫颈炎,而且和宫颈癌的发生有一定关系。本病多因经期产后,血室正开,调护不当,摄生不洁,湿毒秽浊之邪乘虚内侵,直伤冲任,致带脉失约;或素体虚弱,脾运失健,湿浊内停,伤及任带二脉;或湿邪蕴久化热,湿热壅蒸郁腐,流注下焦所致。

【诊断要点】

(1) 本病临床表现以白带增多,呈乳白色黏液状或淡黄色脓性,或有血性白带,或性交后出血,外阴痒痛;甚则腰骶部疼痛、下腹坠痛及痛经、性交痛;还可有尿频、尿刺痛、排尿困难。若淋菌感染者常伴有发热。本病严重者可引起不孕。

(2) 妇科检查:急性子宫颈炎时可见宫颈充血、水肿,甚至表皮剥脱、坏死,大量脓性黏液排出。子宫颈糜烂呈颗粒型和乳突型,糜烂面积分

Sometimes cervical polyp, Naboth's cysts and cervical hypertrophy can be found.

(3) Routine blood test in acute cervicitis finds increase of white cells. Smear of secreta from the vagina finds a large number of pus cells. Gram's stain finds bacteria. Pathogenic bacteria are visible in the culture of the secreta.

(4) This disease should be differentiated from cervical cancer. Cervical smear can be used to detect cancer cells. Or vaginoscopy is used to examine the cervix. Biopsy may be used to examine the skeptic part. Besides, cervicitis should be differentiated from trichomoniasis, mycotic, tuberculous, amebic and bilharzial cervicitis, old cervical laceration and severe eversion of the cervix.

[Syndrome differentiation and treatment]

(1) Syndrome of accumulation of damp-heat

Main symptoms: Erosion and congestion of cervix, profuse leukorrhea with yellow or yellow and white color, or multi-colored sticky and pus-like leukorrhea with stinky odor, accompanied by pudendal pruritus, prolapsing pain in the lower abdomen, reddish tongue with yellowish greasy or whitish greasy fur and taut pulse.

Therapeutic methods: Clearing away heat and draining dampness.

Prescription and drugs: Modified Yihuang Tang composed of 10g of Huangbai (*Cortex Phellodendri*), 10g of Cheqianzi (*Semen Plantaginis*), 12g of Cangzhu (*Rhizoma Atractylodis*), 10g of Baizhu (*Rhizoma Atractylodis Macrocephalae*), 20g of Yiyiren (*Semen Coicis*), 10g of Huainiuxi (*Radix Achyranthis Bidentatae*), 10g of Zexie (*Rhizoma Alismatis*), 15g of Chun-

为轻、中、重三度。还可见宫颈息肉、宫颈腺体囊肿及宫颈肥大。

(3) 急性子宫颈炎血常规化验可见白细胞增高。阴道分泌物涂片可见大量脓细胞，革兰染色可发现细菌；分泌物培养可见致病菌。

(4) 本病应与子宫颈癌相鉴别。宫颈刮片检查找癌细胞，或行阴道镜检查，可疑部位活检以明确诊断。此外，还应与滴虫性、真菌性、结核性、阿米巴性、血吸虫性宫颈炎以及陈旧性子宫颈裂伤及重度子宫颈外翻鉴别。

【辨证论治】

一、湿热蕴结证

主要证候　宫颈糜烂、充血，带下量多，色黄或黄白相间，或赤白带下，质稠粘，呈脓样，有腥臭味，伴阴部瘙痒，小腹坠痛，舌质偏红，苔黄腻或白腻，脉弦。

治　法　清热利湿。

方　药　易黄汤加减：黄柏10 g，车前子10 g，苍术12 g，白术10 g，薏苡仁20 g，怀牛膝10 g，泽泻10 g，椿根皮15 g，牡丹皮10 g，败酱草10 g，小蓟10 g，白果15 g。

genpi (*Cortex Toonae Sinensis*), 10g of Mudanpi (*Cortex Moutan radicis*), 10g of Baijiangcao (*Herba Patriniae*), 10g of Xiaoji (*Herba Cephalanoploris*) and 15g of Baiguo (*Semen Ginkgo*).

Modification: For prolapsing and distending sensation in the lower abdomen, 10g of Zhike (*Fructus Aurantii*) and 6g of Chaihu (*Radix Bupleuri*) are added; for multi-colored leukorrhea, 10g of roasted Huaihua (*Flos Sophorae*) and 10g of Diyutan (Charred *Radix Sanguisorbae*) are added; for leukorrhea with stinky odor, 15g of Hongteng (*Caulis Sargentodoxae*) and 10g of Yuxingcao (*Herba Houttuyniae*) are added; for severe lumbago, 10g of Sangjisheng (*Ramulus Taxilli*) and 10g of Xuduan (*Radix Dipsaci*) are added.

(2) Syndrome of exuberance of heat toxin

Main symptoms: Congestion and swelling of cervix, profuse leukorrhea with yellow or yellow and green color like pus, or multi-colored leukorrhea with sticky and thick texture and putrid odor, pudendal pruritus, even scorching pain, lower abdominal distending pain, fever and bitter taste in the mouth, yellow and scanty urine, retention of dry feces, red tongue with yellow and greasy fur as well as slippery and rapid pulse.

Therapeutic methods: Clearing away heat and removing toxin, resolving dampness and eliminating turbid substance.

Prescription and drugs: Modified Wuwei Xiaodu Yin composed of 10g of Pugongying (*Herba Taraxaci*), 15g of Jinyinhua (*Flos Lonicerae*), 15g of Zihuadiding (*Herba Violae*), 15g of Baijiangcao (*Herba Patriniae*), 15g of Hongteng (*Caulis Sargentodoxae*), 15g of Chungenpi (*Cortex Toonae Sinensis*), 10g of Baihuasheshecao (*Herba Hedyotis Diffusae*), Tiankuizi (*Semen Senecionis*

加　减　若小腹坠胀加枳壳10 g，柴胡6 g；带下赤白加炒槐花10 g，地榆炭10 g；带下腥臭加红藤15 g，鱼腥草10 g；腰痛甚者，加桑寄生10 g，续断10 g。

二、热毒炽盛证

主要证候　子宫颈充血红肿，带下量多，色黄或黄绿如脓，或五色杂下，质稠粘，有腐臭气，外阴瘙痒，甚至灼热疼痛，小腹胀痛，烦热口苦，尿黄短赤，大便干结，舌质红，苔黄腻，脉滑数。

治　法　清热解毒，化湿泄浊。

方　药　五味消毒饮加减：蒲公英10 g，金银花15 g，紫花地丁15 g，败酱草15 g，红藤15 g，椿根皮15 g，白花蛇舌草10 g，天葵子10 g，薏苡仁20 g，怀牛膝10 g。

Nudicaulis), 20g of Yiyiren (*Semen Coicis*) and 10g of Huainiuxi (*Radix Achyranthis Bidentatae*).

Modification: For reddish and sticky leukorrhea like blood, 10g of Mudanpi (*Cortex of Moutan Radicis*) and 10g of roasted Huaihua (*Flos Sophorae*) are added; for bitter taste in the mouth and dry throat, 6g of Zhizi (*Fructus Gardeniae*) and 10g of Huangqin (*Radix Scutellariae*) are added.

(3) Syndrome of asthenia of spleen qi

Main symptoms: Chronic cervicitis, profuse and incessant leukorrhea with white or light-yellow color, thick and sticky texture, no odor, facial dropsy, cold limbs, dispiritedness and lassitude, anorexia and loose stool, light-colored tongue with tooth prints, white or greasy tongue fur, slow and weak pulse.

Therapeutic methods: Strengthening the spleen and nourishing qi, elevating yang and eliminating dampness.

Prescription and drugs: Modified Wandai Tang composed of 10g of Baizhu (*Rhizoma Atractylodis Macrocephalae*), 15g of Shanyao (*Rhizoma Dioscoreae*), 10g of Dangshen (*Radix Codonopsis Pilosulae*), 12g of Baishaoyao (*Radix Paeoniae Alba*), 10g of Cangzhu (*Rhizoma Atractylodis*), 3g of Gancao (*Radix Glycyrrhizae*), 6g of Chenpi (*Pericarpium Citri Reticulatae*), 6g of Chaihu (*Radix Bupleuri*), 10g of Cheqianzi (*Semen Plantaginis*) and 20g of Yiyiren (*Semen Coicis*).

Modification: For longer duration of cervicitis and incessant leukorrhea, 20g of calcined Longgu (*Os Draconis*), 15g of Qianshi (*Semen Euryales*) and 10g of Jinyingzi (*Fructus Rosae Laevigatae*) are added; for accompanied kidney asthenia and lumbago, 10g of Duzhong (*Cortex Eucommiae*), 10g of Fupenzi (*Fructus Rubi*) and 10g of Tusizi (*Semen Cuscutae*) are added; for ac-

加 减 若带下色红,似血非血,质粘稠,加牡丹皮10 g,炒槐花10 g;口苦咽干者,加栀子6 g,黄芩10 g。

三、脾气虚弱证

主要证候 慢性宫颈炎,带下量多,色白或淡黄,质粘稠,无臭味,绵绵不断,面目浮肿,四肢不温,神疲乏力,纳呆便溏,舌质淡,边有齿印,苔白或腻,脉缓弱。

治 法 健脾益气,升阳除湿。

方 药 完带汤加减:白术10 g,山药15 g,党参10 g,白芍药12 g,苍术10 g,甘草3 g,陈皮6 g,柴胡6 g,车前子10 g,薏苡仁20 g。

加 减 若病程较长,带下日久不止,加煅龙骨20 g,芡实15 g,金樱子10 g;兼肾虚腰痛者,加杜仲10 g,覆盆子10 g,菟丝子10 g;兼小腹冷痛者,加艾叶6 g,炮姜6 g,延胡索10 g。

companied cold pain in the lower abdomen, 6g of Aiye (*Folium Artemisiae*), 6g of Paojiang (*baked Rhizoma Zingiberis*) and 10g of Yanhusuo (*Rhizoma Corydalis*) are added.

(4) Syndrome of asthenia of kidney qi

Main symptoms: Chronic cervicitis, profuse leukorrhea with white color and thin texture, no odor, severe lumbago, bright-white complexion, cold limbs, dispiritedness and lassitude, clear and profuse urine, light-colored tongue with white fur, thin and deep pulse.

Therapeutic methods: Nourishing the kidney and strengthening qi.

Prescription and drugs: Modified Dabu yuan Jian composed of 15g of Dangshen (*Radix Codonopsis Pilosulae*), 15g of Shanyao (*Rhizoma Dioscoreae*), 12g of Duzhong (*Cortex Eucommiae*), 10g of Shanzhuyu (*Fructus Corni*), 6g of Chenpi (*Pericarpium Citri Reticulatae*), 10g of Fupenzi (*Fructus Rubi*), 10g of Buguzi (*Fructus Psoraleae*), 20g of Yiyiren (*Semen Coicis*), 10g of Tusizi (*Semen Cuscutae*) and 3g of Gancao (*Radix Glycyrrhizae*).

Modification: For longer duration of cervicitis and incessant leukorrhea, 20g of calcined Longgu (*Os Draconis*), 15g of Qianshi (*Semen Euryales*) and 10g of Jinyingzi (*Fructus Rosae Laevigatae*) are added; for accompanied diarrhea due to spleen asthenia, 10g of Liuqu (*Massa Medicata Fermentata*) and 10g of Muxiang (*Radix Aucklaneliae*) are added; for accompanied cold pain in the lower abdomen, 6g of Aiye (*Folium Artemisiae Argyi*), 6g of Paojiang (*baked Rhizoma Zingiberis*) and 10g of Yanhusuo (*Rhizoma Corydalis*) are added.

[Other therapeutic methods]

(1) Chinese patent drugs

1) **Simiao Pill:** 10g each time and twice a day,

四、肾气虚弱证

主要证候 慢性宫颈炎，带下量多，色白质清稀，无臭味，腰痛如折，面色㿠白，四肢不温、神疲乏力，小便清长，舌质淡，苔白，脉细沉。

治 法 益肾固气。

方 药 大补元煎加减：党参15 g，山药15 g，杜仲12 g，山茱萸10 g，陈皮6 g，覆盆子10 g，补骨脂10 g，薏苡仁20 g，菟丝子10 g，甘草3 g。

加 减 若病程较长，带下日久不止，加煅龙骨20 g，芡实15 g，金樱子10 g；兼脾虚腹泻者，加六曲10 g，木香10 g；兼小腹冷痛者，加艾叶6 g，炮姜6 g，延胡索10 g。

【其他疗法】

1. 中成药

（1）四妙丸 每次服

applicable to the treatment of syndrome of damp-heat accumulation.

2) Longdan Xiegan Pill: 8 g each time and twice a day, applicable to the treatment of syndrome of damp-heat accumulation.

3) Yudai Pill: 5g each time and three times a day, applicable to the treatment of heat transformation from cold-dampness or syndrome with mixed dampness and heat.

(2) Empirical and folk recipes

1) Zhenzhu Powder: 3g of Zhenzhu (*Margarita*), 3g of Qingdai (*Indigo Naturalis*), 5g of Xionghuang (*Realgar*), 9g of Huangbai (*Cortex Phellodendri*), 6g of Ercha (*Catechu*) and 0.03g of Bingpian (*Borneolum Syntheticum*) are ground into powder for external application, applicable to the treatment of kidney qi asthenia syndrome.

2) Proper amount of fig leaves (Folium Fici Caricae): Applicable to the treatment of chronic cervicitis with profuse, yellow or yellow and white leukorrhea, occasionally appearing like pus or multi-colored.

2.4.3 Pelvic inflammation

Pelvic inflammation refers to the inflammation of the interior reproductive organs and the connective tissues and pelvic peritoneum around. Clinically it is either acute or chronic. Pelvic inflammation is usually caused by weakness, improper caring, infection of pathogenic toxin and retention of damp-heat in the uterus and uterine collaterals during menstruation or after delivery. At the early stage it is marked by struggle between damp-heat and blood and qi, constant accumulation and fumigation of damp-heat as well as manifestations of acute inflammation. Prolonged duration will turn into asthenia of the

10 g,1 日 2 次,适用于湿热蕴结证。

（2）龙胆泻肝丸　每次服 8 g,1 日 2 次,适用于湿热蕴结证。

（3）愈带丸　每次服5 g,1 日 3 次,适用于寒湿化热,或湿热错杂证。

2. 单验方

（1）珍珠散　珍珠3 g,青黛3 g,雄黄5 g,黄柏9 g,儿茶6 g,冰片0.03 g,研细末外用,适用于肾气虚弱证。

（2）无花果叶适量,适用于慢性宫颈炎带下呈量多,色黄,或黄白相兼,时呈脓带或赤白相间者。

第三节　盆腔炎

盆腔炎是指女性内生殖器及其周围的结缔组织、盆腔腹膜发生炎症。临床分为急、慢性期。本病多因月经期或产后体质虚弱,摄生不慎,感染邪毒,湿热瘀滞于子宫、胞脉、胞络所致。初期湿热与血气相搏,蕴蒸不解,呈急性炎症反应,若日久不愈,则正虚邪盛,呈慢性炎症反应,常可急性发作。临证常有下腹痛、

healthy qi and sthenia of pathogenic factors, marked by manifestations of chronic inflammation and acute seizure. The clinical manifestations are frequent lower abdominal pain, fever, leukorrhea and even pyogenic mass. Pelvic inflammation pertains to the conceptions of abdominal pain, invasion of heat into the blood chamber, leukorrhagia and abdominal mass in TCM.

[Key points for diagnosis]

(1) The main symptoms are constant pain in the lower abdomen and increased vaginal discharge.

(2) The accompanied symptoms at the acute stage are fever, aversion to cold and headache, increase of the total number of white blood cells and neutrophilic granulocyte.

(3) The accompanied symptoms at the chronic stage are abdominal pain, irregular menstruation, dysmenorrhea or sterility.

(4) Gynecological examination: Lower abdominal tenderness, tenderness in the uterus, thickening of the appendage or formation of mass, accompanied by obvious tenderness. At the acute stage there appear rebound tenderness in the lower abdomen and tenderness in the cervix.

[Syndrome differentiation and treatment]

The main symptom in pelvic inflammation is lower abdominal pain. So syndrome differentiation should be done in light of the nature and degree of pain as well as the accompanied symptoms. Usually the syndrome with sudden onset and severe pain accompanied by chills and high fever pertains to heat and sthenia; while the syndrome with incomplete treatment, lingering duration or slow onset is marked by a mixture of cold and heat as well as asthenia and sthenia.

发热、带下,甚者出现脓性包块等症状,故中医归属于"腹痛"、"热入血室"、"带下"、"癥瘕"之范畴。

【诊断要点】

(1) 主要症状为下腹部持续性疼痛,以及阴道分泌物增多。

(2) 急性期伴有发热、畏寒、头痛等症状。白细胞总数及中性粒细胞增多。

(3) 慢性期伴有腹痛、月经不调、痛经或不孕等症状。

(4) 妇科检查:下腹部压痛;子宫体压痛,附件增厚或有包块形成,伴有明显压痛。急性期下腹部可有反跳痛,子宫颈有触痛。

【辨证论治】

本病的主症是下腹部疼痛,临证应当根据疼痛的性质、程度及其伴有症状进行辨证论治。一般情况下,凡起病急,疼痛剧烈,伴寒战高热者,多属热属实;若未能彻底治疗,而病状缠绵不愈,或起病较缓者,往往寒热虚实混杂可见,临床当仔细审证。

The frequent manifestations at the acute stage are accumulation and exuberance of damp-heat in the lower energizer which should be treated mainly by clearing away damp-heat and removing toxin to resolving stagnation; the usual manifestations at the chronic stage are qi stagnation and blood stasis or asthenia of both the spleen and kidney, the former should be treated by promoting qi flow and activating blood, while the latter by dealing with both the asthenia and sthenia. For the treatment of frequent relapse and abscess or formation of cyst that cannot be effectively treated with drugs, operation has to be resorted to.

(1) Syndrome of accumulation and exuberance of damp-heat

Main symptoms: Fever, aversion to cold, sweating, unpressable pain in the lower abdomen and sides of the lower abdomen, yellowish and pus-like leukorrhea, red tongue with yellow and greasy fur as well as slippery and rapid pulse.

Therapeutic methods: Clearing away heat and draining dampness, resolving toxin and stasis.

Prescription and drugs: Modified Dahuang Mudanpi Tang combined with Hongteng Jian composed of 30g of Baijiangcao (*Herba Patriniae*), 30g of Hongteng (*Caulis Sargentodoxae*), 30g of Zihuadiding (*Herba Violae*), 15g of Jinyinhua (*Flos Lonicerae*), 15g of Lianqiao (*Fructus Forsythiae*), 10g of Dahuang (*Radix et Rhizoma Rhei*), 15g of Yiyiren (*Semen Coicis*), 10g of Mudanpi (*Cortex Moutan Radicis*), 10g of Chishaoyao (*Radix Paeoniae Rubra*) and 10g of Taoren (*Semen Persicae*).

Modification: For severe damp-heat marked by thirst without desire to drink water, chest oppression, nausea, yellow urine and yellow and greasy tongue fur, 5g of

急性期常见下焦湿热壅盛,当以清利湿热、解毒化滞为治法;慢性期常见气滞血瘀或脾肾两虚证,前者当以行气活血为主,清热利湿为佐,后者则当虚实兼顾;若反复发作,脓肿或包块形成,经药物治疗乏效者,可考虑手术治疗。

一、湿热壅盛证

主要证候　发热、畏寒、有汗,下腹部及少腹两侧疼痛、拒按,带下色黄如脓,苔黄腻质红,脉滑数。

治　法　清热利湿,解毒化瘀。

方　药　大黄牡丹皮汤合红藤煎加减:败酱草30 g,红藤30 g,紫花地丁30 g,金银花15 g,连翘15 g,大黄10 g,薏苡仁15 g,牡丹皮10 g,赤芍药10 g,桃仁10 g。

加　减　湿热甚,见口渴不欲饮、胸闷、恶心、尿黄、苔黄腻等症状者,酌加苍术5 g,

Cangzhu （ *Rhizoma Atractylodis* ）, 10g of Huangbai （ *Cortex Phellodendri* ）, 10g of Cheqianzi （ *Semen Plantaginis* ）, 10g of Zhuling （ *Polygorus* ） and 10g of Zexie （ *Rhizoma Alismatis* ） are added; for formation of mass, 5g of Zhechong （ *Eupolyphaga* ）, 5g of Ruxiang （ *Olibanum* ） and 5g of Moyao （ *Myrrha* ） are added.

（2） Syndrome of qi stagnation and blood stasis

Main symptoms: Stabbing pain in the lower abdomen and sides of lower abdomen, even formation of mass, aching pain in the loins, irregular menstruation, profuse leukorrhea, lassitude, purplish tongue or with ecchymoses, whitish thin tongue fur and taut and unsmooth pulse.

Therapeutic methods: Regulating qi, activating blood and stopping pain.

Prescription and drugs: Modified Juhe Wan composed of 10g of Juhe （ *Semen Citri Reticulatae* ）, 10g of Lizhihe （ *Semen Litchi* ）, 10g of Danshen （ *Radix Salviae Miltiorrhizae* ）, 10g of Chishaoyao （ *Radix Paeoniae Rubra* ）, 10g of Tianxianteng （ *Herba Aristolochiae* ）, 10g of Xiangfu （ *Rhizoma Cyperi* ）, 10g of Chuanlianzi （ *Fructus Toosendan* ） and 10g of stir-baked Yanhusuo （ *Rhizoma Corydalis* ）.

Modification: For formation of mass, 10g of Taoren （ *Semen Persicae* ）, 5g of Honghua （ *Flos Carthami* ）, 10g of Sanleng （ *Rhizoma Sparganii* ）, 10g of Ezhu （ *Rhizoma Curcumae* ）, 10g of Fuling （ *Poria* ）, 10g of Zexie （ *Rhizoma Alismatis* ） and 12g of Mutouhui （ *Radix Patriniae* ） are added.

（3） Syndrome of asthenia of both spleen and kidney

Main symptoms: Dull pain in the lower abdomen and both sides of lower abdomen, even aching pain in the

黄柏10 g, 车前草10 g, 猪苓10 g, 泽泻10 g; 有包块者, 酌加䗪虫5 g, 乳香5 g, 没药5 g。

二、气滞血瘀证

主要证候　下腹部及少腹两侧疼痛如针刺, 甚至有包块, 腰脊酸痛, 月经失调, 带下量多, 精神疲惫, 舌质紫气或瘀斑, 苔薄白, 脉弦涩。

治　法　理气活血止痛。

方　药　橘核丸加减: 橘核10 g, 荔枝核10 g, 丹参10 g, 赤芍药10 g, 天仙藤10 g, 香附10 g, 川楝子10 g, 炒延胡索10 g。

加　减　有包块者, 酌加桃仁10 g, 红花5 g, 三棱10 g, 莪术10 g, 茯苓10 g, 泽泻10 g, 墓头回12 g。

三、脾肾两虚证

主要证候　下腹部及少腹两侧隐隐作痛, 甚至牵及腰

lumbosacral region, profuse and thin leukorrhea, spiritual lassitude, cold limbs, loose stool, thin and greasy tongue fur as well as thin and deep pulse.

Therapeutic methods: Nourishing the kidney and strengthening the spleen, harmonizing the collaterals and stopping pain.

Prescription and drugs: Modified Yougui Wan composed of 20g of Shanyao (*Rhizoma Dioscoreae*), 15g of Duzhong (*Cortex Eucommiae*), 10g of Bajitian (*Radix Morindae Officinalis*), 10g of stir-baked Mudanpi (*Cortex Moutan Radicis*), 10g of Fuling (*Poria*), 10g of Lujiaopian (*sliced Cornu Cervi*), 10g of Xiangfu (*Rhizoma Cyperi*), 12g of Chuanduan (*Radix Dipsaci*) and 12g of Sangjisheng (*Ramulus Taxilli*).

Modification: For profuse leukorrhea, 10g of Qianshi (*Semen Euryales*), 10g of Jinyingzi (*Fructus Rosae Laevigatae*) and 20g of Wuzeigu (*Os Sepiae*) are added; for lower abdominal mass, 10g of Sanleng (*Rhizoma Sparganii*), 10g of Ezhu (*Rhizoma Curcumae*) and 12g of Zaojiaoci (*Spina Gleditsiae*) are added.

[Other therapeutic methods]

(1) Chinese patent drugs

1) Fuke Qianjin Tablet: 6 tablets each time and three times a day, applicable to the treatment of accumulation and exuberance of damp-heat syndrome.

2) Nüjin Bolus: 1 bolus each time and twice a day, applicable to the treatment of asthenia cold syndrome.

(2) External therapy

1) Enema: 30g of Jinyinhua (*Flos Lonicerae*), 20g of Pugongying (*Herba Taraxaci*), 20g of Zihuadiding (*Herba Violae*), 30g of Hongteng (*Caulis Sargentodoxae*), 20g of Baijiangcao (*Herba Patriniae*), 20g of Lianqiao (*Fructus Forsythiae*), 15g of Sanleng (*Rhizoma Sparganii*), 15g of Ezhu (*Rhizoma Curcumae*), 20g of

骶酸痛,带下量多清稀,精神疲倦,四肢不温,大便溏薄,舌苔薄腻,脉细沉。

治　法　益肾健脾,和络止痛。

方　药　右归丸加减:山药20 g,杜仲15 g,巴戟天10 g,炒牡丹皮10 g,茯苓10 g,鹿角片10 g,香附10 g,川断12 g,桑寄生12 g。

加　减　带下量多加芡实10 g,金樱子10 g,乌贼骨20 g;下腹部有包块,加三棱10 g,莪术10 g,皂角刺12 g。

【其他疗法】

1. 中成药

(1) 妇科千金片　每次服6片,1日3次,适用于湿热壅盛证。

(2) 女金丹　每次服1丸,1日2次,适用于虚寒证。

2. 外治法

(1) 灌肠疗法　金银花30 g,蒲公英20 g,紫花地丁20 g,红藤30 g,败酱草20 g,连翘20 g,三棱15 g,莪术15 g,丹参20 g,赤芍药15 g,浓煎至100 ml,冷却至 30～35℃ ,保

Danshen (*Radix Salviae Miltiorrhizae*) and 15g of Chi-shaoyao (*Radix Paeoniae Rubra*) are decocted in water into 100ml of decoction. When cooled down to 30 – 35℃, it is used for enema. This treatment is given once a day and 10 times make up one course of treatment.

2) External application: 20g of Ruxiang (*Olibanum*), 20g of Moyao (*Myrrha*), 20g of Jiangxiang powder (*Lignum Dalbergiae Odoriferae*), 20g of Chuanjiao (*Pericarpium Zanthoxyli*), 20g of Dahuixiang (*Fructus Anisi Stellati*) and 20g of Xiaohuixiang (*Fructus Foeniculi*) are ground into fine powder which is mixed up with flour into paste. In application, the paste is added with a little sorghum wine, spread on a piece of gauze and fixed on the affected part of the abdomen. Then hot-water bag is compressed on it. This treatment is given twice a day and 10 days make up one course of treatment.

留灌肠,每日 1 次,10 次为 1 个疗程。

（2）**外敷疗法** 乳香 20 g,没药20 g,降香末20 g,川椒20 g,大茴香20 g,小茴香 20 g,上药细末,用面粉和匀,用时以高粱酒少许,调湿摊于纱布上,置于腹部痛处,其上用热水袋外敷,每日 2 次,10 天为 1 个疗程。

2.5 Leukorrhea diseases

Leukorrhea, vaginal discharge composed of mucous exudate and secreta of uterine cervical gland and endometrium, contains vaginal exfoliated cells, white blood cells and some non-pathogenic bacteria. Normally the texture and quantity of leukorrhage vary in accordance with the menstrual cycle. When menstruation has cleared, vaginal discharge is scanty, whitish and pasty. During ovulation, leukorrhea increases, appearing transparent and sticky like the egg white. Two or three days after ovulation, vaginal discharge appears turbid, sticky and scanty. Leukorrhea increases before and after menstruation. The abnormal change of leukorrhea in color, texture and volume is called leukorrhea disease in TCM, including profuse and scanty menstruation as well as multi-colored menstruation, reddish-whitish menstruation, gonorrhea and leukorrhagia.

2.5.1 Leukorrhagia

Leukorrhagia refers to profuse vaginal discharge with abnormal changes of color, texture and odor. Clinically white leukorrhea, yellow leukorrhea and multi-colored leukorrhea are frequently encountered. The incidence of this disease is high. It is usually due to various inflammation of the reproductive organs. But sometimes leukorrhagia occurs without inflammation, such as leukorrhagia seen in submucosal myoma of uterus and cervical cancer.

第五章 带下病

白带是指阴道排出液,由阴道黏膜渗出物、宫颈腺体及子宫内膜分泌物混合而成,内含阴道脱落细胞、白细胞和一些非致病性细菌。在正常情况下,白带的质和量可随月经的周期而变化;月经净后,阴道排液量少、色白,呈糊状;排卵期白带增多,呈透明微黏而似蛋清状;排卵2~3天后,阴道排出液较混浊,黏稠而量少;经行前后,白带又增多。如果白带的颜色、质地和排泄量发生异常改变,中医称为"带下病",包括带下过多和过少两大类,以及赤白带下、五色带、白浊、白淫等病症。

第一节 带下过多

带下过多是指女性阴道排出液超过正常量,同时伴有色、质、气味的异常。临床上以白带、黄带、赤白带为多见。本病发病率较高,与女性各种生殖器炎症有关,但也有非炎症性带下过多者,如子宫黏膜下肌瘤、宫颈癌等均可见带下量多。

According to the clinical manifestations, leukorrhagia pertains to the conception of leukorrhea disease in TCM, the cause of which is various. TCM believes that leukorrhagia is mainly due to dampness, but it is also related to the disorder of the belt vessel. Dampness either exogenous or endogenous is due to dysfunction of the viscera. Leukorrhagia is caused either by dysfunction of the spleen in transformation and transportation that accumulate cereal nutrients into dampness, the downward migration of which affects the belt vessel; or by loss of essential fluid due to dysfunction of the kidney in storage and in dredging the thoroughfare and conception vessels; or by disorder of the conception and belt vessels due to stagnation of liver qi affecting the transformation of the spleen; or by invasion of exogenous dampness and virulent and turbid pathogenic factors into the conception and belt vessels due to asthenia of the uterine vessels or water contamination in bathing or prolonged living in damp area. Prolonged leukorrhea will certainly consume body fluid, the manifestation of which is a mixture of asthenia and sthenia.

[Key points for diagnosis]

(1) Profuse leukorrhea appears whitish or light-yellow, or multi-colored, or yellowish and bluish like pus, or turbid like rice swill; the texture of leukorrhea appears thin like water, or sticky and thick like pus, or like bean dregs and coagulated milk, or frothy; the leukorrhea appears odorless, or foul or stinky; the accompanied symptoms are vulva or vaginal pruritus, prolapsing sensation or pain.

(2) Gynecological examination finds vaginitis, pelvic inflammation, cervicitis and tumor.

(3) Laboratory test may find acute or subacute pelvic inflammation and increase of white blood cells. The vaginal

带下过多发生的原因很多,中医认为主要与湿有关,且与任带失约有联系。湿有内湿、外湿之别,内湿因脏腑功能失调所致,有脾虚运化失健,水谷精微反聚而成湿浊,湿浊下注,任脉失约者;或因肾虚既不能行其封藏之职,又不能通任带等行其约制固纳作用,精液滑脱者;或因肝郁气机郁滞,影响脾运,土湿下陷,任带失约者;外湿因经行产后,胞脉空虚,或因洗澡水污,久居湿地,湿毒秽浊之邪乘虚而入,损伤任带,发为带下。带下日久,必耗阴液,表现为虚实夹杂之证。

【诊断要点】

(1) 带下量多,色白或淡黄,或赤白相兼,或黄绿如脓,或浑浊如米泔;质或清稀如水,或稠粘如脓,或如豆渣凝乳,或如泡沫状;气味无臭,或有臭气,或臭秽难闻;可伴有外阴、阴道灼热瘙痒、坠胀或疼痛等。

(2) 妇科检查可见各类阴道炎、宫颈炎、盆腔炎的体征,也可发现肿瘤。

(3) 实验室检查可见急性或亚急性盆腔炎,白细胞计数

cleaning degree is Ⅲ. Vaginoscopy may find trichomonad, fungus and other specific or non-specific pathogen.

(4) Type B-Ultrasonic examinaiton is necessary for pelvic inflammation and pelvic tumor.

[**Syndrome differentiation and treatment**]

Syndrome differentiation of leukorrhagia concentrates on the analysis of the quantity, color, texture and odor of leukorrhea. Profuse leukorrhea without odor is usually due to damp encumbrance caused by hypofunction of the spleen or unconsolidation resulting from kidney deficiency; yellowish or whitish and turbid leukorrhea is often caused by downward migration of damp-heat, and more damp-heat, the stronger odor; bloody leukorrhea is frequently caused by fire transformed from damp-heat or damage of collaterals by asthenia-fire; frequent occurrence of bloody leukorrhea in middle-aged or old women may suggest cancer of uterus or uterine cervix. Leukorrhagia is usually marked by mixture of asthenia and sthenia, simple asthenia syndrome is seldom seen. The treatment focuses on elimination of dampness. Exogenous dampness is treated mainly by clearing and draining therapy, while endogenous dampness is dealt with mainly by regulating the kidney, liver, spleen and stomach by means of elevating yang, drying dampness, astringing therapy and clearing-draining method. If it is accompanied by genital pruritus, it can be treated with the combination of external therapy for clearing away heat, eliminating dampness and removing toxin.

(1) Syndrome of spleen asthenia and dampness encumbrance

Main symptoms: Whitish or light yellow, profuse,

增高。阴道炎阴道清洁度检查Ⅲ度。镜检可查到滴虫、真菌及其他特异性或非特异性病原体。

(4) B超检查对盆腔炎症及盆腔肿瘤有意义。

【辨证论治】

带下过多的辨证,重在对量、色、质、气味的分析:白带津津,量多无臭,多属脾虚湿困或肾虚不固;带下色黄,或白而腐浊,多属湿热下注所致,湿热愈盛,则多夹有臭秽异味;若兼见血性白带,往往由湿热化火,或虚火灼伤脉络所致,中老年女性出现血性白带,应警惕子宫或宫颈癌变的可能。临床上往往是虚实夹杂者多,全虚者少。治疗上着眼于"湿",外湿者以清利为主,内湿者以调理肾肝脾胃为要,分别采用升阳、燥湿、固涩、清利诸法,伴有阴痒者可结合外治法,清热除湿解毒,才能提高疗效。

一、脾虚湿困证

主要证候 带下色白或

odorless and incessant leukorrhea, nausea and anorexia, spiritual lassitude, light-colored and bulgy tongue with white and greasy fur as well as slow and weak pulse.

Therapeutic methods: Strengthening the spleen and nourishing qi, elevating yang and eliminating dampness.

Prescription and drugs: Modified Wandai Tang composed 10g of stir-baked Baizhu (*Rhizoma Atractylodis Macrocephalae*), 10g of stir-baked Shanyao (*Rhizoma Dioscoreae*), 10g of Dangshen (*Radix Codonopsis Pilosulae*), 10g of Baishaoyao (*Radix Paeoniae Alba*), 10g of stir-baked Cangzhu (*Rhizoma Atractylodis*), 4g of roasted Gancao (*Radix Glycyrrhizae*), 6g of Chenpi (*Pericarpium Citri Reticulatae*), 10 g of Heijiesui (*Spica Schizonepetae*), 5g of Chaihu (*Radix Bupleuri*) and 10g of Cheqianzi (*Semen Plantaginis*) (to be wrapped for decocting).

Modification: For spleen asthenia involving the kidney accompanied by severe lumbago, 10g of Xuduan (*Radix Dipsaci*), 10g of Duzhong (*Cortex Eucommiae*) and 10g of Tusizi (*Semen Cuscutae*) are added for warming and invigorating kidney yang as well as strengthening the conception vessel and stopping leukorrhea; for cold coagulation and abdominal pain, 10g of Xiangfu (*Rhizoma Cyperi*) and 10g of Aiye (*Folium Artemisiae Argyi*) are added; for prolonged and incessant leukorrhea, 10g of Qianshi (*Semen Euryales*), 10g of calcined Muli (*Caro Ostreae*), 12g of roasted Wuzeigu (*Os Sepiae*) and 10g of Jinyingzi (*Fructus Rosae Laevigatae*) are added; for transformation of heat from stagnation of damp due to spleen asthenia marked by yellowish, sticky, thick and foul leukorrhea, the treatment should concentrate on strengthening the spleen to eliminate dampness and clearing away heat to stop leukorrhea with Yihuang Tang com-

淡黄,量多如涕,无臭,绵绵不断,恶心纳少,神倦,舌淡胖,苔白腻,脉缓弱。

治　法　健脾益气,升阳除湿。

方　药　完带汤加减:炒白术10 g,炒山药10 g,党参10 g,白芍药10 g,炒苍术10 g,炙甘草 4 g,陈皮6 g,黑芥穗10g,柴胡5 g,车前子(包煎)10 g。

加　减　若脾虚及肾,兼腰痛者,酌加续断10 g,杜仲10 g,菟丝子10 g,温补肾阳,固任止带;若寒凝腹痛者,酌加香附10 g,艾叶10 g,温经理气止痛;若带下日久,滑脱不止者,酌加芡实10 g,煅龙骨10 g,煅牡蛎10 g,炙乌贼骨12 g,金樱子10 g等固涩止带之品。若脾虚湿郁化热,带下色黄粘稠,有臭味者,宜健脾除湿,清热止带,方选易黄汤,药用山药10 g,芡实10 g,车前子(包煎)10 g,白果10 g,黄柏10 g。

posed of 10g of Shanyao (*Rhizoma Dioscoreae*), 10g of
Qianshi (*Semen Euryales*), 10g of Cheqiancao (*Herba
Plantaginis*) (to be wrapped for decocting), 10g of Baiguo (*Semen Ginkgo*) and 10g of Huangbai (*Cortex Phellodendri*).

(2) Syndrome of kidney yin asthenia

Main symptoms: Yellowish or yellowish and reddish
leukorrhea with sticky texture and without odor, burning
sensation in the vagina, feverish sensation over the
palms, soles and chest, aching in the loins and tinnitus,
dizziness and palpitation, red tongue with scanty fur, thin
and rapid pulse.

Therapeutic methods: Nourishing the kidney yin,
clearing away heat and eliminating dampness.

Prescription and drugs: Enriched Zhibai Dihuang
Tang composed of 10g Shudihuang (*Rhizoma Rehmanniae Praeparata*), 10g of Shanzhuyu (*Fructus Corni*),
10g of Shanyao (*Rhizoma Dioscoreae*), 10g of Zexie
(*Rhizoma Alismatis*), 10g of Fuling (*Poria*), 10g of
Mudanpi (*Cortex Moutan Radicis*), 10g of Zhimu (*Rhizoma Anemarrhenae*), 10g of Huangbai (*Cortex Phellodendri*), 10g of Qianshi (*Semen Euryales*) and 10g of
Jinyingzi (*Fructus Rosae Laevigatae*).

Modification: For yin asthenia and fire exuberance,
10g of roasted Guiban (*Plastrum Testudinis*) (to be decocted first) and 10g of roasted Digupi (*Cortex Lycii*) are
added for nourishing yin to reduce fire; for accompanied
damp-heat, 15g of Baijiangcao (*Herba Patriniae*) and
12g of Yiyiren (*Semen Coicis*) are added for clearing
away heat and draining dampness.

(3) Syndrome of kidney yang asthenia

Main symptoms: Profuse, thin, or transparent and

二、肾阴亏虚证

主要证候 带下色黄或
兼赤,质粘无臭,阴户灼热,五
心烦躁,腰酸耳鸣,头晕心悸,
舌红,苔少,脉细数。

治 法 益肾滋阴,清热
祛湿。

方 药 知柏地黄汤加
味:熟地黄10g,山茱萸10g,
山药10g,泽泻10g,茯苓10g,
牡丹皮10g,知母10g,黄柏
10g,芡实10g,金樱子10g。

加 减 若偏于阴虚火
旺者,加炙龟版(先煎)10g,炙
地骨皮10g以滋阴降火。若夹
有湿热者,加败酱草15g,薏苡
仁12g以清热利湿。

三、肾阳亏虚证

主要证候 带下量多,清

incessant leukorrhea, aching sensation in the loins, cold sensation in the abdomen, clear and profuse urine, especially in the night, light-colored tongue with thin and white fur, deep and slow pulse.

Therapeutic methods: Warming the kidney and assisting yang, astringing essence and stopping leukorrhea.

Prescription and drugs: Modified Neibu Wan composed of 10g of Lurong (*Cornu Cervi Pantotrichum*), 10g of Tusizi (*Semen Cuscutae*), 10g of Tongjili (*Semen Astragali Complanati*), 10g of Huangqi (*Radix Astragali*), 10g of Baijili (*Fructus Tribuli*), 5g of Rougui (*Cortex Cinnamomi*) (to be decocted later), 10g of Sangpiaoxiao (*Ootheca Mantidis*), 10g of Roucongrong (*Herba Cistanches*) and 5g of prepared Fuzi (*Radix Aconiti Praeparata*).

Modification: For diarrhea and loose stool, Roucongrong (*Herba Cistanches*) is deleted, while 10g of Buguzhi (*Fructus Psoraleae*) and 10g of Roudoukou (*Semen Myristicae*) are added for warming the spleen and kidney; for fulminant leukorrhea due to kidney deficiency, Gujing Wan is used to nourish the spleen and kidney as well as to consolidate the extraordinary vessels, composed of 10g of Muli (*Caro Ostreae*) (to be decocted first), 10g of Sangpiaoxiao (*Ootheca Mantidis*), 10g of Longgu (*Os Draconis*) (to be decocted first), 10g of Baifuling (*Poria*), 10g of Wuweizi (*Fructus Schisandrae*), 10g of Tusizi (*Semen Cuscutae*) and 10g of Jiucaizi (*Semen Allii Tuberosi*).

(4) Syndrome of downward migration of damp-heat

Main symptoms: Profuse, or yellow, or yellowish and reddish leukorrhea like bean dregs or frothy leukorrhea with foul odor, burning sensation and pruritus in the

稀如水,或透明如鸡子清,绵绵不绝,腰酸腹冷,小便频数清长,夜间尤甚,舌质淡,苔薄白,脉沉迟。

治　法　温肾助阳,涩精止带。

方　药　内补丸加减:鹿茸10g,菟丝子10g,潼蒺藜10g,黄芪10g,白蒺藜10g,肉桂(后下)5g,桑螵蛸10g,肉苁蓉10g,制附子5g。

加　减　若腹泻便溏者,去肉苁蓉,酌加补骨脂10g,肉豆蔻10g以温脾肾。若肾虚不固,带下如崩,方选固精丸以补脾肾、固奇经,药用牡蛎(先煎)10g,桑螵蛸10g,龙骨(先煎)10g,茯苓10g,五味子10g,菟丝子10g,韭菜子10g。

四、湿热下注证

主要证候　带下量多,色黄或兼见赤带,质粘稠,或如豆渣,或似泡沫气秽或臭,阴

vagina, scanty and brown urine, or accompanied by spasmodic pain in the abdomen, red tongue with yellow and greasy fur, soft and rapid pulse.

Therapeutic methods: Clearing away heat, draining dampness and stopping leukorrhea.

Prescription and drugs: Modified Zhidai Fang composed of 10g of Zhuling (*Polygorus*), 10g of Fuling (*Poria*), 10g of Cheqianzi (*Semen Plantaginis*) (to be wrapped for decocting), 10g of Zexie (*Rhizoma Alismatis*), 10g of Yinchen (*Herba Artemisiae*), 10g of Chishaoyao (*Radix Paeoniae Rubra*), 10g of Mudanpi (*Cortex Moutan Radicis*), 10g of Zhizi (*Fructus Gardeniae*), 10g of Huangbai (*Cortex Phellodendri*) and 10g of Niuxi (*Radix Achyranthis Bidentatae*).

Modification: Longdan Xiegan Tang can be used to treat downward migration of damp-heat from the liver meridian marked by profuse leukorrhea, yellow or yellow and green color like pus, sticky or frothy texture with foul odor, accompanied by pudendal pruritus and pain, dizziness, bitter taste in the mouth and dry throat, restlessness and susceptibility to rage, retention of dry feces, brown urine, red tongue with yellow and greasy fur, taut, slippery and rapid pulse. This prescription is composed of 3g of Longdancao (*Radix Gentianae*), 5g of Chaihu (*Radix Bupleuri*), 10g of Zhizi (*Fructus Gardeniae*), 10g of Huangqin (*Radix Scutellariae*), 10g of Cheqiancao (*Herba Plantaginis*) (to be wrapped for decocting), 6g of Mutong (*Caulis Akebiae*), 10g of Zexie (*Rhizoma Alismatis*), 10g of Shengdihuang (*Radix Rehmanniae*), 10g of Danggui (*Radix Angelicae Sinensis*), 4g of Gancao (*Radix Glycyrrhizae*), 10g of Kushen (*Radix Sophorae Flavescentis*) and 3g of Huanglian (*Rhizoma Coptidis*). For relative predominance of dampness marked by profuse leukorrhea with white color

户灼热瘙痒,小便短赤,或伴有腹部抽掣痛,舌质红、苔黄腻、脉濡数。

治 法 清热利湿止带。

方 药 止带方加减:猪苓10 g,茯苓10 g,车前子(包煎)10 g,泽泻10 g,茵陈10 g,赤芍药10 g,牡丹皮10 g,栀子10 g,黄柏10 g,牛膝10 g。

加 减 若肝经湿热下注者,症见带下量多,色黄或黄绿如脓,质粘稠或呈泡沫状,有臭气,伴阴部痒痛,头晕目眩,口苦咽干,烦躁易怒,便结尿赤,舌红,苔黄腻,脉弦滑而数,宜用龙胆泻肝汤清热除湿,药用龙胆草3 g,柴胡5 g,栀子10 g,黄芩10 g,车前子(包煎)10 g,木通6 g,泽泻10 g,生地黄10 g,当归10 g,甘草4 g,苦参10 g,黄连3 g。若湿浊偏甚者,症见带下量多,色白,如豆渣状或凝乳状,阴部瘙痒,胸闷纳差,舌红,苔黄腻,脉滑数。宜用萆薢渗湿汤以清热利湿,疏风化浊,药用萆薢10 g,薏苡仁10 g,黄柏10 g,赤茯苓10 g,牡丹皮10 g,泽泻10 g,滑石10 g,通草6 g, like bean dregs or coagulated milk, pudendal pruritus, chest oppression and anorexia, red tongue with yellow and greasy fur, slippery and rapid pulse, Bixie Shenshi Tang can be used to clear away heat and drain dampness as well as to expel wind and resolve turbid substance. This prescription is composed of 10g of Bixie (*Rhizoma Dioscoreae Hypoglaucae*), 10g of Yiyiren (*Semen Coicis*), 10g of Huangbai (*Cortex Phellodendri*), 10g of Chifuling (*Poria Rubra*), 10g of Mudanpi (*Cortex Moutan Radicis*), 10g of Zexie (*Rhizoma Alismatis*), 10g of Huashi (*Talcum*), 6g of Tongcao (*Medulla Tetrapanacis*), 10g of Cangzhu (*Rhizoma Atractylodis*) and 10g of Huoxiang (*Herba Agastaches seu Pogostemonis*).

[Other therapeutic methods]

(1) Chinese patent drugs

1) Ermiao Pill: 6g each time and twice a day, applicable to the treatment of downward migration of damp-heat.

2) Qianjin Zhidai Pill: 9g each time and twice a day, applicable to the treatment of asthenia of the spleen and kidney complicated by dampness.

3) Baidai Pill: 6g each time and twice a day, applicable to the treatment of cold dampness syndrome.

4) Wuji Baifeng Pill: 9g each time and twice a day, applicable to the treatment of leukorrhagia due to asthenia of both qi and blood.

(2) Empirical and folk recipes

1) 15g of Baijiguanhua (*Flos Celosiae Cristatae*) is decocted for oral taking, applicable to the treatment of leukorrhagia due to spleen asthenia complicated by dampness.

2) 60g of Yiyiren (*Semen Coicis*) and 60g of Qianshi (*Semen Euryales*) are decocted in water with rice, sesame oil and salt for oral taking, applicable to the treat-

苍术10 g,藿香10 g。

【其他疗法】

1. 中成药

（1）二妙丸　每次服6 g, 1 日 2 次,适用于湿热下注证。

（2）千金止带丸　每次服9 g,1 日 2 次,适用于脾肾虚夹湿证。

（3）白带丸　每次服6 g, 1 日 2 次,适用于寒湿证。

（4）乌鸡白凤丸　每次服9 g,1 日 2 次,适用于气血两虚证带下过多。

2. 单验方

（1）白鸡冠花15 g,水煎服,适用于脾虚夹湿带下证。

（2）薏苡仁 60 g,芡实 60 g,米适量共煮,加麻油、食盐调味,适用于脾虚寒湿证。

ment of spleen asthenia syndrome with cold and dampness.

   3) Guanzhong (*Rhizoma Dryopteris Gassirhizo-mae*) and Haipiaoxiao (*Os Sepiellae seu Sepiae*) of the same dosage are ground into powder for oral taking with millet wine, 10g each time and twice a day. This treatment is applicable to the treatment of damp-heat and spleen asthenia syndrome.

   4) 30g of Yimucao (*Herba Leonuri*) and 30g of Dahongzao (*Fructus Jujubae Rubra*) are decocted for oral taking, applicable to the treatment of spleen asthenia syndrome.

   5) 50g of Huaishanyao (*Rhizoma Dioscoreae*) and 30g of Jinyingzi (*Fructus Rosae Laevigatae*) are decocted for oral taking, applicable to the treatment of spleen asthenia and retention of dampness syndrome.

(3) External therapy

   1) Fumigation and washing lotion: 15g of Heshi (*Herba Carotae*), 15g of Kushen (*Radix Sophorae Flavescentis*), 15g of Weilingxian (*Radix Clematidis*), 12g of Guiwei (*carda part of Radix Angelicae Sinensis*), 15g of Shechuangzi (*Fructus Cnidii*) and 10g of Langdu (*Radix Euphorbiae Ebracteolatae*) are decocted in 3,000ml of water. After boiling for several times, the residue is removed. The decoction is used to fumigate and wash the pudendum. To improve the effect, the bile of 1 - 2 pig gallbladder can be put into the decoction before washing. This decoction is applicable to the treatment of attack by exogenous dampness and insects. This treatment should not be used if there is pudendal ulceration.

   2) Sitting bathing: 15g of Shechuangzi (*Fructus Cnidii*), 10g of Huajiao (*Pericarpium Zanthoxyli*), 10g of Mingfan (*Alumen*), 15g of Kushen (*Radix Sophorae Flavescentis*) and 15g of Baibu (*Radix Stemonae*) are

（3）贯众、海螵蛸各等分，研细末，每次服10 g，1 日 2 次，黄酒送服，适用于湿热脾虚证。

（4）益母草30 g，大红枣30 g，水煎服，适用于脾虚证。

（5）怀山药50 g，金樱子30 g，水煎服，适用于脾虚湿滞证。

3. 外治法

（1）薰洗法　鹤虱15 g，苦参15 g，威灵仙15 g，归尾12 g，蛇床子15 g，狼毒10 g，加水3 000 ml，煎数沸去渣，乘热薰洗阴部，临洗时加1～2枚猪胆汁更佳。用于外感湿虫者，外阴溃疡者勿用。

（2）坐浴法　蛇床子15 g，花椒10 g，明矾10 g，苦参15 g，百部15 g，煎汤趁热先熏后坐浴，适用于滴虫性阴道

decocted into decoction for fumigation and then bathing in it. This treatment is applicable to trichomonal vaginitis. If pudendal pruritus is ulcerated, Huajiao (*Pericarpium Zanthoxyli*) in the prescription should be deleted.

炎。若阴痒破溃者,则去花椒。

2.5.2　Scanty leukorrhea

Scanty leukorrhea means that the fluid discharged from the vagina is too little to lubricate the vagina, usually seen in the late stage of menstruation and ovulatory period.

This disease is usually caused by congenital defect, excessive sexual life and multiparity as well as deficiency of essence in the liver and kidney; or by constitutional hypofunction of the spleen and stomach, improper diet, overstrain, lack of proper care in cold and warm weather as well as insufficiency of cereal nutrients and body fluid; or by retention of remaining blood due to cold attack during menstruation, or mental depression, unsmooth circulation of qi and blood and prolonged stagnation transforming into stasis; or by invasion of pathogenic dampness into the thoroughfare and conception vessels as well as the uterus, leading to qi stagnation, retention of menstrual blood in the uterus, unsmooth flow of qi and failure of body fluid to distribute. So scanty leukorrhea is usually believed to be caused by asthenia of the liver and kidney, hypofunction of the spleen and stomach as well as interior retention of blood stasis. The clinical manifestations are frequently scanty leukorrhea, dry sensation in the vagina or accompanied by pudendal pruritus.

[**Key points for diagnosis**]

(1) Scanty or even no leukorrhea in the late stage of menstruation and in ovulatory period, or dry sensation in the vagina, dizziness and aching sensation in the loins,

第二节　带下过少

带下过少是指女子阴道内流出的液体过少,甚至不能润泽阴道,主要见于月经后期至排卵期。

带下稀少,多因禀赋不足,房劳多产,大病、久病致肝肾阴精亏乏;或素体脾胃较弱,饮食不当,劳倦过度,寒暖不调,损伤脾胃,水谷之精,不能充养天癸,津液不足所致。亦有因经产感寒,余血留蓄,或情怀抑郁,气机不畅,血行不利,久而积聚成瘀;或湿邪外侵,流注冲任子宫,湿阻气滞,经血留阻致瘀,血瘀内阻,气机不畅,津液不得敷布所致。一般将带下过少的病因病机归纳为肝肾亏虚、脾胃虚弱、血瘀内阻,临证常伴有阴道干涩或阴痒等症状。

【诊断要点】

(1) 月经后期至排卵期带下过少,甚至全无,或伴有阴道干燥,头昏腰酸,胸闷心烦,

chest oppression and dysphoria, sexual frigidity, delayed menstruation and scanty menorrhea.

(2) Vaginal smear or endocrine examination indicates low level of estrin.

(3) Scanty leukorrhea should be differentiated from Sheehan's syndrome, polycystic ovary syndrome and peri-menopausal dryness syndrome.

[**Syndrome differentiation and treatment**]

Scanty leukorreha is either asthenia or sthenia. Asthenia syndrome in scanty leukorrhea results either from the kidney, or the liver or the spleen. Sthenia syndrome is usually due to interior retention of blood stasis. Clinically asthenia syndrome is frequently seen while sthenia syndrome is seldom seen. Scanty leukorrhea is classified into three types: asthenia of the liver and kidney, hypofunction of the spleen and stomach, and interior retention of blood stasis. The therapeutic principles are nourishing yin and replenishing essence. The therapeutic methods are nourishig the liver and kidney, strengthening the spleen and harmonizing the stomach as well as activating blood and resolving stasis.

(1) Syndrome of asthenia of the liver and kidney

Main symptoms: Scanty or even no leukorrhea in the late stage of menstruation or in the ovulatory period, dry sensation in the vagina or accompanied by pudendal pruritus, dizziness and aching sensation in the loins, chest oppression and dysphoria, poor sleep in the night, red tongue with thin and yellow or scanty fur, thin and taut or rapid pulse.

Therapeutic methods: Nourishing the liver and kidney, promoting production of body fluid.

Prescription and drugs: Modified Erjia Dihuang Tang composed of 15g of roasted Guiban (*Plastrum Testudinis*) (to be decocted first), 15g of roasted Biejia (*Carapax*

性功能减退,月经落后,经量偏少等症状。

(2) 阴道涂片或内分泌检查提示雌激素水平较低。

(3) 本病应注意与席汉综合征、多囊卵巢综合征、围绝经期干燥综合征相鉴别。

【辨证论治】

带下过少的辨证,以分清虚实为要,虚者有属肾、属肝、属脾之别,实者以血瘀内阻为主,临床上虚证多见,主要分为肝肾亏损证、脾胃虚弱证及血瘀内阻证。治疗以滋阴填精为原则,分别采用滋补肝肾、健脾和胃、活血化瘀法。

一、肝肾亏损证

主要证候 月经后期至排卵期带下过少,甚或全无,阴道干涩或伴阴痒,头昏腰酸,胸闷心烦,夜寐甚差,舌质偏红,苔薄黄或少苔,脉细弦或数。

治 法 滋补肝肾,生津养液。

方 药 二甲地黄汤加减:炙龟版(先煎)15g,炙鳖甲(先煎)15g,干地黄10g,山

Trionycis) (to be decocted first), 10g of dry Dihuang (*Radix Rehmanniae*), 10g of Shanyao (*Rhizoma Dioscoreae*), 10g of Shanzhuyu (*Fructus Corni*), 10g of stir-baked Mudanpi (*Cortex Moutan Radicis*), 10g of Fuling (*Poria*), 9g of Tianmendong (*Radix Asparagi*), 9g of Maimendong (*Radix Ophiopogonis*), 15g of Yejiaoteng (*Caulis Polygoni Multiflori*) and 3g of Lianzixin (*Plumula Nelumbinis*).

Modification: For severe stagnation of heart and liver fire, 15g of Gouteng (*Ramulus Uncariae cum Uncis*), 10g of Heishanzhi (*Fructus Gardeniae*), 6g of Jingjie (*Herba Schizonepetae*) and 6g of Guangyujin (*Radix Curcumae*) are added; for relative exuberance of heart fire, 3g of Huanglian (*Rhizoma Coptidis*), 6g of stir-baked Zaoren (*Semen Ziziphi Spinosae*) and 10g of Qinglongchi (*Dens Draconis*) (to be decocted first) are added; for disharmony between the spleen and stomach, Gandihuang (*Radix Rehmanniae*) and Tianmendong (*Radix Asparagi*) and Maimendong (*Radix Ophiopogonis*) are deleted, 10g of Baizhu (*Rhizoma Atractylodis Macrocephalae*), 10g of Stir-baked Baibiandou (*Semen Lablab Album*), 10 g of crispy Shanzha (*Fructus Crataegi*), 6g of stir-baked Zhuru (*Caulis Bambusae in Taeniam*), 6g of Chenpi (*Pericarpium Citri Reticulatae*), 10g of Taizishen (*Radix Pseudostellariae*) and 9g of Liuqu (*Massa Medicata Fermentata*) are added.

(2) Syndrome of hypofunction of the spleen and stomach

Main symptoms: Scanty or even no leukorrhea in the late stage of menstruation and ovulatory period, dry sensation in the vagina or accompanied by pudendal pruritus, poor appetite, spiritual lassitude, epigastric and abdominal distension, frequent flatus, or loose stool, light-red tongue with thin, white and greasy fur, and thin

药10 g,山茱萸10 g,炒牡丹皮10 g,茯苓10 g,天门冬9 g,麦门冬9 g,夜交藤15 g,莲子心3 g。

加　减　如心肝郁火甚者,加钩藤15 g,黑山栀10 g,荆芥6 g,广郁金6 g;心火偏甚者,加黄连3 g,炒枣仁6 g,青龙齿(先煎)10 g;若脾胃失和者,去干地黄、天门冬、麦门冬,加白术10 g,炒白扁豆10 g,焦山楂10 g,炒竹茹6 g,陈皮6 g,太子参10 g,六曲9 g。

二、脾胃虚弱证

主要证候　月经后期至排卵期带下过少,甚或全无,自觉阴道内干燥或兼阴痒,纳欠神疲,脘腹作胀,矢气频频,大便或溏,舌淡红,苔薄白腻,脉细。

pulse.

Therapeutic methods: Strengthening the spleen and stomach, nourishing qi and promoting the production of body fluid.

Prescription and drugs: Modified Shenling Baizhu San composed of 10g of Dangshen (*Radix Codonopsis Pilosulae*), 10g of stir-baked Baizhu (*Rhizoma Atractylodis Macrocephalae*), 10g of Fuling (*Poria*), 10g of Shanyao (*Rhizoma Dioscoreae*), 6g of roasted Gancao (*Radix Glycyrrhizae*), 6g of Chenpi (*Pericarpium Citri Reticulatae*), 6g of Jiegeng (*Radix Platycodi*), 5g of roasted Muxiang (*Radix Aucklaneliae*), 12g of stir-baked Guya (*Fructus Oryzae Germinatus*), 9g of crispy Shanzha (*Fructus Crataegi*) and 9g of Lianzirou (*Semen Nelumbinis*).

Modification: For frequent loose stool, 5g of Sharen (*Fructus Amomi*) (to be decocted later), 10g of Shenqu (*Massa Medicata Fermentata*) and 6g of Paojiang (*Processed Rhizoma Zingiberis*) are added; for poor appetite and thick and greasy tongue fur, 10g of Peilan (*Herba Eupatorii*) and 5g of prepared Chuanpo (*Cortex Magnoliae Officinalis*) are added; for dysphoria and restless sleep, 6g of roasted Yuanzhi (*Radix Polygalae*), 10g of Hehuanpi (*Cortex Albiziae*) and 5g of stir-baked Zaoren (*Semen Ziziphi Spinosae*) are added.

(3) Syndrome of interior retention of blood stasis

Main symptoms: Scanty or even no leukorrhea, abdominal pain during menstruation, with purplish and blackish color and large blood clot, lower abdominal pain, chest oppression, dysphoria, thirst with no desire to drink water, dry and squamous skin, deep-red tongue with ecchymoses on the margin, and thin and unsmooth pulse.

Therapeutic methods: Activating blood and resol-

治 法 健脾和胃,益气生津。

方 药 参苓白术散加减:党参10 g,炒白术10 g,茯苓10 g,山药10 g,炙甘草6 g,陈皮6 g,桔梗6 g,煨木香5 g,炒谷芽12 g,焦山楂9 g,莲子肉9 g。

加 减 便溏较频者,加砂仁(后下)5 g,神曲10 g,炮姜6 g;纳欠,苔厚腻者,加佩兰10 g,制川朴5 g;心烦寐差者,加炙远志6 g,合欢皮10 g,炒枣仁5 g。

三、血瘀内阻证

主要证候 带下过少,甚或全无,经行腹痛,色紫黑有血块,下腹疼痛,胸闷烦躁,口渴不欲饮,肌肤甲错干燥,舌暗红,边有瘀斑或瘀点,脉细涩。

治 法 活血化瘀,滋阴

ving stasis, nourishing yin and promoting production of body fluid.

Prescription and drugs: Modified Huoxue Runzao Shengjin Tang composed of 10g of Danggui (*Radix Angelicae Sinensis*), 10g of Chishaoyao (*Radix Paeoniae Rubra*), 10g of Baishaoyao (*Radix Paeoniae Alba*), 10g of Shengdihuang (*Radix Rehmanniae*), 6g of Tianmendong (*Radix Asparagi*), 6g of Maimendong (*Radix Ophiopogonis*), 9g of Tianhuafen (*Radix Trichosanthis*), 9g of Taoren (*Semen Persicae*), 9g of Honghua (*Flos Carthami*), 15g of roasted Biejia (*Carapax Trionycis*) and 10g of Shanzha (*Fructus Crataegi*).

Modification: For retention of dry feces and constipation, 5g of Dahuang (*Radix et Rhizoma Rhei*) is added; for chest oppression and abdominal distension, 10g of Goujuli (*Fructus Ponciri Trifoliatae*), 6g of Qingpi (*Pericarpium Citri Reticulatae Viride*), 6g of Chenpi (*Pericarpium Citri Reticulatae*) and 5g of stir-baked Chaihu (*Radix Bupleuri*) are added; for obvious lower abdominal pain, 10g of Wulingzhi (*Faeces Trogopterorum*) and 10g of Yanhusuo (*Rhizoma Corydalis*) are added.

[Other therapeutic methods]
(1) Chinese patent drugs

1) Dahuang Zhechong Pill: 3g each time and three times a day, applicable to the treatment of scanty leukorrhea due to blood stasis.

2) Qiju Dihuang Liquid: 10ml each time and twice a day, applicable to the treatment of scanty leukorrhea due to asthenia of liver and kidney yin.

(2) Empirical and folk recipes

1) Heiguipi Tang composed of 15g of Huangqi (*Radix Astragali*), 15g of Dangshen (*Radix Codonopsis Pilosulae*), 10g of Baizhu (*Rhizoma Atractylodis Macro-*

生津。

方　药　活血润燥生津汤加减：当归10 g，赤芍药10 g，白芍药10 g，生地黄10 g，天门冬6 g，麦门冬6 g，天花粉9 g，桃仁9 g，红花9 g，炙鳖甲15 g，山楂10 g。

加　减　大便干结难解者，加大黄5 g；胸闷腹胀者，加枸橘李10 g，青皮6 g，陈皮6 g，炒柴胡5 g；小腹疼痛明显者，加五灵脂10 g，延胡索10 g。

【其他疗法】
1. 中成药

（1）大黄䗪虫丸　每次服3 g，1 日 3 次，适用于血瘀之带下过少。

（2）杞菊地黄口服液　每次10 ml，1 日 2 次，适用于肝肾阴虚之带下过少。

2. 单验方

（1）黑归脾汤　黄芪15 g，党参15 g，白术10 g，茯苓10 g，当归10 g，木香6 g，炙远

cephalae）, 10g of Fuling（*Poria*）, 10g of Danggui（*Radix Angelicae Sinensis*）, 6g of Muxiang（*Radix Aucklaneliae*）, 6g of roasted Yuanzhi（*Radix Polygalae*）, 10g of stir-baked Zaoren（*Semen Ziziphi Spinosae*）, 6g of Chenpi（*Pericarpium Citri Reticulatae*）and 10g of Shudihuang （ *Rhizoma Rehmanniae Praeparata* ）. These herbs are decocted for oral taking, applicable to the treatment of scanty leukorrhea due to spleen asthenia and deficiency of blood.

2) Modified Maiwei Dihuang Tang composed of 60g of Maimendong（*Radix Ophiopogonis*）, 60g of Wuweizi （*Fructus Schisandrae*）, 10g of Shudihuang（*Rhizoma Rehmanniae Praeparata*）, 10g of Huaishanyao（*Rhizoma Dioscoreae*）, 10g of Shanzhuyu（*Fructus Corni*）, 10g of stir-baked Mudanpi（*Cortex Moutan Radicis*）, 10g of Fuling（*Poria*）, 10g of Zexie（*Rhizoma Alismatis*）, 12g of Xuanshen（*Radix Scrophulariae*）and 10g of Huainiuxi （ *Radix Achyranthis Bidentatae* ）. These herbs are decocted for oral taking, applicable to the treatment of scanty leukorrhea due to yin asthenia.

志6 g,炒枣仁10 g,陈皮6 g,熟地黄10 g。水煎服,适用于脾虚血少之带下过少。

（2）麦味地黄汤加减
麦门冬60 g,五味子60 g,熟地黄10 g,山药10 g,山茱萸10 g,炒牡丹皮10 g,茯苓10 g,泽泻10 g,玄参12 g,怀牛膝10 g,水煎服,适用于阴虚证之带下过少。

2.6 Pregnancy diseases

2.6.1 Abortion

Abortion refers to stoppage of pregnancy within 28 weeks and with the weight of the fetus less than 1,000g. Abortion occurring within 12 weeks after pregnancy is called early abortion, while abortion occurring from 12 weeks to less than 28 weeks is known as late abortion. Abortion may be either natural or artificial. The incidence of abortion is 10%-18%, most of which is early abortion.

The clinical manifestations of threatened abortion are slight and occasional bleeding from vagina after pregnancy, or dripping vaginal bleeding, or aching sensation in the loins and abdominal pain as well as prolapsing sensation and distension in the lower abdomen. Abortion is due to either the maternal body or the fetus itself. Abortion is caused either by deficiency of essence in both the wife and husband failing to keep the fetus though able to conceive it; or by weakness of the body and insufficiency of kidney qi; or by intemperance of sexual life and consumption of kidney essence; or by asthenia of both qi and blood; or by pathogenic heat disturbing the fetus; or by other diseases after pregnancy. Besides, falling, sprain, contusion, operation and certain drugs may also lead to abortion.

第六章 妊娠病

第一节　流产

流产是指妊娠不足 28 周、胎儿体重不足 1 000 g 而终止者。流产发生在妊娠 12 周前者称为早期流产,发生在妊娠 12～28 周者称晚期流产;流产又可分自然流产和人工流产。本病发病率较高,约占所有妊娠的 10%～18%,且多数为早期流产。

先兆流产属中医"胎漏"、"胎动不安"等病症范畴。临床表现为妊娠后出现少量阴道流血,时下时止,或淋漓不断,或腰酸腹痛,下腹坠胀等症状。本病的发生有母体与胎儿两方面原因。胎元方面:夫妇之精气不足,两精虽能结合,但胎元不固,以致流产。若因胎元有缺陷,胎多不能成实而易殒堕。母体方面:因素体虚弱,肾气不足,或因房事不节,耗损肾精,或由气血虚弱,或因邪热动胎,或受孕之后兼患其他疾病,干扰胎气,以致流产。此外,跌仆闪挫、

[Key points for diagnosis]

(1) Slight occasional vaginal bleeding occurs during pregnancy. Restless movement of the fetus is marked by aching sensation in the loins, abdominal distension and prolapsing sensation and pain in the abdomen, or accompanied by slight vaginal bleeding. If abortion occurs frequently and the examination of the husband is normal, it is known as habitual abortion.

(2) Pregnancy test is positive. Type B ultrasonic examination indicates normal fetal movement, fetal heart beat and normal size of fetus. Vaginal bleeding with those results above is helpful for determining diagnosis.

(3) Chromosome examination excludes hereditary factors.

[Syndrome differentiation and treatment]

Clinically abortion is classified into four types: syndrome of insufficiency of kidney qi, syndrome of asthenia of qi and blood, syndrome of interior disturbance of blood heat and syndrome of external injury impairing collaterals. The basic therapeutic principles are preventing miscarriage, nourishing kidney qi and protecting fetus. The therapeutic methods include nourishing qi and blood, tranquilizing the heart and quieting the mind, strengthening the spleen and harmonizing the stomach as well as clearing away heat and calming the fetus. After proper treatment with Chinese herbs, vaginal bleeding will be controlled and abdominal pain will disappear. In most cases, pregnancy is successfully protected. If vaginal bleeding continues with worsened aching in the loins and abdominal pain, measures should be taken to remove the fetus to protect the mother.

手术和药物的影响也可引起流产。

【诊断要点】

（1）妊娠期间，阴道少量下血，时下时止为"胎漏"；腰酸腹部胀坠作痛，或伴有少量出血称为"胎动不安"。屡孕屡堕，男方检查正常者为"滑胎"。

（2）妊娠试验呈阳性反应，B超检查胎动、胎心搏动正常，并与停经月份相符而见阴道出血者，有助于确立诊断。

（3）染色体检查排除遗传因素所致。

【辨证论治】

流产临床上主要分为肾气不足证、气血亏虚证、血热内扰证及外伤损络证。本病的治疗，以安胎为主，补益肾气、固摄胎元为基本治则，并根据不同情况分别采用补气养血、宁心安神、健脾和胃、清热安胎等法。经过中医药治疗，阴道出血迅速控制，腹痛消失，多能继续妊娠。若继续出血量多、腰酸、腹痛加剧则胎元难安，又当急以去胎益母。

(1) Syndrome of insufficiency of kidney qi

Main symptoms: Slight vaginal bleeding with light color during pregnancy, aching sensation in the loins and prolapsing sensation in the abdomen, or accompanied by dizziness and tinnitus, frequent urination, or experience of abortion, light-colored tongue with white fur, deep and slippery or weak pulse over chi region.

Therapeutic methods: Nourishing the kidney and strengthening the thoroughfare vessel, stopping bleeding and calming the fetus.

Prescription and drugs: Modified Shoutai Wan composed of 10g of Tusizi (*Semen Cuscutae*), 15g of Sangjisheng (*Ramulus Taxilli*), 10g of stir-baked Xuduan (*Radix Dipsaci*), 10g of Duzhong (*Cortex Eucommiae*), 9g of Shanyao (*Rhizoma Dioscoreae*), 9g of Baizhu (*Rhizoma Atractylodis Macrocephalae*), 15g of Zhumagen (*Radix Boehmeriae Niveae*), 10g of Ejiao (*Colla Corii Asini*) (to be melted for decocting) and 5g of Sharen (*Fructus Amomi*) (to be decocted later).

Modification: For accompanied serious qi asthenia with prolapsing sensation, 10g of Dangshen (*Radix Codonopsis Pilosulae*) and 10g of Huangqi (*Radix Astragali*) are added; for insufficiency of the spleen and stomach accompanied by abdominal distension, flatus and loose stool, 10g of Dangshen (*Radix Codonopsis Pilosulae*), 5g of Zisugeng (*Caulis Perillae*) and 3g of roasted Muxiang (*Radix Aucklaneliae*) are added; for dysphoria and insomnia, 15g of Gouteng (*Ramulus Uncariae cum Uncis*), 6g of stir-baked Zaoren (*Semen Ziziphi Spinosae*) and 10g of Fushen (*Sclerotium Poriae Circum Radicem Pini*) are added.

(2) Syndrome of qi and blood asthenia

Main symptoms: Slight vaginal bleeding with light

一、肾气不足证

主要证候　妊娠期阴道漏红,量少色淡,腰酸腹坠,或伴头晕耳鸣,小便频数,或有流产史,舌淡,苔白,脉沉滑尺弱。

治　法　补肾固冲,止血安胎。

方　药　寿胎丸加减:菟丝子10g,桑寄生15g,炒续断10g,杜仲10g,山药9g,白术9g,苎麻根15g,阿胶(烊冲)10g,砂仁(后下)5g。

加　减　兼气虚下坠甚者,酌加党参10g,黄芪10g;脾胃不足,兼见腹胀矢气,大便偏溏者,加党参10g,紫苏梗5g,煨木香3g;心烦不得眠者,加钩藤15g,炒枣仁6g,茯神10g。

二、气血亏虚证

主要证候　妊娠期阴道

color and thin texture, aching sensation in the loins and prolapsing sensation in the abdomen, spiritual lassitude, flaccidity of limbs, palpitation, shortness of breath, lusterless complexion, light-colored tongue, white and thin tongue fur, thin and slippery pulse.

Therapeutic methods: Nourishing qi and invigorating blood, strengthening the kidney and calming the fetus.

Prescription and drugs: Modified Taiyuan Yin composed of 10g of Dangshen (*Radix Codonopsis Pilosulae*), 10g of Baizhu (*Rhizoma Atractylodis Macrocephalae*), 10g of Baishaoyao (*Radix Paeoniae Alba*), 10g of Shudihuang (*Rhizoma Rehmanniae Praeparata*), 10g of Ejiao (*Colla Corii Asini*) (to be melted for decocting), 10g of Duzhong (*Cortex Eucommiae*), 15g of Huangqi (*Radix Astragali*), 6g of Chenpi (*Pericarpium Citri Reticulatae*) and 5g of roasted Gancao (*Radix Glycyrrhizae*).

Modification: For profuse vaginal bleeding, 10g of Wuzeigu (*Os Sepiae*) and 10g of charred Aiye (*Folium Artemisiae Argyi*) are added; for loose stool and diarrhea, 5g of Sharen (*Fructus Amomi*) (to be decocted later), 5g of roasted Muxiang (*Radix Aucklaneliae*) and 15g of roasted Guya (*Fructus Oryzae Germinatus*) are added; for palpitation and insomnia, 6g of roasted Yuanzhi (*Radix Polygalae*), 6g of stir-baked Zaoren (*Semen Ziziphi Spinosae*) and 9g of Hehuanpi (*Cortex Albiziae*) are added.

(3) Syndrome of interior disturbance of blood-heat

Main symptoms: Fresh vaginal bleeding during pregnancy, or prolapsing sensation and pain in the abdomen, dysphoria and restlessness, scorching sensation over

漏红,量少,色淡质薄,腰酸腹坠,神疲肢软,心悸气短,面色少华,舌淡,苔薄白,脉细滑。

治　法　补气养血,固肾安胎。

方　药　胎元饮加减:党参10 g,白术10 g,白芍药10 g,熟地黄10 g,阿胶(烊冲)10 g,杜仲10 g,黄芪15 g,陈皮6 g,炙甘草5 g。

加　减　若阴道下血量多者,酌加乌贼骨10 g,艾叶炭10 g;大便溏泄者,加砂仁(后下)5 g,煨木香5 g,炒谷芽15 g;心悸失眠者,加炙远志6 g,炒枣仁6 g,合欢皮9 g。

三、血热内扰证

主要证候　妊娠期阴道漏红色鲜,或腹痛下坠,心烦不安,手心灼热,口干咽燥,大

palms, dry mouth and throat, constipation, red tongue, yellow and dry tongue fur, taut and slippery or slippery and rapid pulse.

Therapeutic methods: Clearing away heat and cooling blood, strengthening the thoroughfare vessel and calming the fetus.

Prescription and drugs: Modified Baoyin Jian composed of 10g of Shengdihuang (*Radix Rehmanniae*), 10g of Shudihuang (*Rhizoma Rehmanniae Praeparata*), 10g of Shanyao (*Rhizoma Dioscoreae*), 10g of Baishaoyao (*Radix Paeoniae Alba*), 10g of Huangqi (*Radix Astragali*), 10g of Xuduan (*Radix Dipsaci*), 6g of stir-baked Huangbai (*Cortex Phellodendri*), 9g of Diyutan (*Charred Radix Sanguisorbae*) and 15g of Zhumagen (*Radix Boehmeriae Niveae*).

Modification: For profuse vaginal bleeding, 10g of Ejiao (*Colla Corii Asini*) (to be melted for decocting), 10g of Hanliancao (*Herba Ecliptae*), 6g of charred Diyu (*Radix Sanguisorbae*) and 15g of roasted Guiban (*Plastrum Testudinis*) (to be decocted first) are added; for dysphoria and insomnia, 3g of Huanglian (*Rhizoma Coptidis*), 1g of Lianzixin (*Plumula Nelumbinis*), 15g of Gouteng (*Ramulus Uncariae cum Uncis*) and 5g of Wuweizi (*Fructus Schisandrae*).

(4) Syndrome of external injury impairing collaterals

Main symptoms: Prolapsing sensation and pain in the loins and abdomen, vaginal bleeding with purplish red color or with small blood clot after pregnancy, light-red tongue, thin, slippery and weak pulse.

Therapeutic methods: Nourishing qi and invigorating blood, strengthening the kidney and calming the fetus.

便秘结,舌红,苔黄而干,脉弦滑或滑数。

治　法　清热凉血,固冲安胎。

方　药　保阴煎加减:生地黄10 g,熟地黄10 g,山药10 g,白芍药10 g,黄芪10 g,续断10 g,炒黄柏6 g,地榆炭9 g,苎麻根15 g。

加　减　若下血较多者,酌加阿胶(烊冲)10 g,旱莲草10 g,地榆炭6 g,炙龟版(先煎)15 g;心烦失眠者,加黄连3 g,莲子心1 g,钩藤15 g,五味子5 g。

四、外伤损络证

主要证候　妊娠外伤后,腰腹坠作痛,阴道漏红,色紫红,或有小血块,舌淡红,脉细滑无力。

治　法　益气养血,固肾安胎。

Prescription and drugs: Enriched Shengyu Tang composed of 10g of Danggui (*Radix Angelicae Sinensis*), 10g of Baishaoyao (*Radix Paeoniae Alba*), 10g of Shudihuang (*Rhizoma Rehmanniae Praeparata*), 15g of Dangshen (*Radix Codonopsis Pilosulae*), 15g of Huangqi (*Radix Astragali*), 10g of Duzhong (*Cortex Eucommiae*), 10g of Xuduan (*Radix Dipsaci*), 5g of Sharen (*Fructus Amomi*) (to be decocted later), 10g of Ejiao (*Colla Corii Asini*) (to be melted for decocting) and 10g of charred Aiye (*Folium Artemisiae Argyi*).

Modification: For abdominal distension and flatus as well as chest oppression and restlessness, 5g of Zisugeng (*Caulis Perillae*), 10g of crispy Shanzha (*Fructus Crataegi*) and 6g Chenpi (*Pericarpium Citri Reticulatae*) are added; for restless fever and thirst as well as yellow and dry tongue fur, 3g of Huanglian (*Rhizoma Coptidis*) and 15g of Gouteng (*Ramulus Uncariae cum Uncis*) are added; for aching sensation in the loins and spiritual lassitude, 10g of Sangjisheng (*Ramulus Taxilli*) is added.

[**Other therapeutic methods**]

(1) Chinese patent drugs

1) Zishen Yutai Pill: 6g each time and twice a day, applicable to the treatment of threatened abortion due to kidney asthenia.

2) Taichan Jindan: 1 bolus each time and twice a day, applicable to the treatment of threatened abortion due to asthenia of qi and blood.

3) Antai Yimu Pill: 9g each time and twice a day, applicable to the treatment of abortion due to asthenia of both the spleen and kidney as well as insufficiency of both qi and blood.

4) Qianjin Baoyun Pill: 10g each time and three times a day, applicable to the treatment of abortion due to asthenia of both qi and blood as well as insufficiency of the

方　药　加味圣愈汤:
炒当归10 g,白芍药10 g,熟地黄10 g,党参15 g,黄芪15 g,杜仲10 g,续断10 g,砂仁(后下)5 g,阿胶(烊冲)10 g,艾叶炭10 g。

加　减　腹胀矢气,胸闷烦躁者,加紫苏梗5 g,焦山楂10 g,陈皮6 g;烦热口渴,苔黄燥者,加黄连3 g,钩藤15 g;腰酸神疲乏力者,加桑寄生10 g。

【其他疗法】

1. 中成药

(1) 滋肾育胎丸　每次服6 g,1 日 2 次,适用于肾虚证先兆流产。

(2) 胎产金丹　每次服1丸,1 日 2 次,适用于气血亏虚之先兆流产。

(3) 安胎益母丸　每次服9 g,1 日 2 次,适用于脾肾两虚,气血不足证流产。

(4) 千金保孕丸　每次服10 g,1 日 3 次,适用于气血两亏,肝肾不足证流产。

liver and kidney.

5) Yunfu Qinghuo Pill: 6g each time and twice a day, applicable to the treatment of abortion due to superabundance of heat and fire in the fetus.

(2) Empirical and folk recipes

1) Taire Tang: 30g of Zhumagen (*Radix Boehmeriae Niveae*), 12g of Heyedi (*Basis Folii Nelumbinis*) and 9g of Cebaiye (*Cacumen Platydadi*) are decocted for oral taking, applicable to the treatment of threatened abortion due to blood heat.

2) Baotai San: 6g of Duzhong (*Cortex Eucommiae*), 6g of Xuduan (*Radix Dipsaci*), 6g of Tusizi (*Semen Cuscutae*), 6g of Sangjisheng (*Ramulus Taxilli*) and 6g of Aiye (*Folium Artemisiae Argyi*) are ground into fine powder for oral taking, 3g each time and twice a day in the morning and evening, applicable to the treatment of threatened abortion due to asthenia of the liver and kidney.

3) Baotai Fang: 15g of Dangshen (*Radix Codonopsis Pilosulae*), 15g of Huangqi (*Radix Astragali*), 15g of Baizhu (*Rhizoma Atractylodis Macrocephalae*), 15g of Xuduan (*Radix Dipsaci*), 15g of Fupenzi (*Fructus Rubi*), 15g of Tusizi (*Semen Cuscutae*), 15g of Duzhong (*Cortex Eucommiae*), 10g of Shengma (*Rhizoma Cimicifugae*) and 10g of Lujiaojiao (*Colla Cornus Cervi*) are decocted for oral taking, applicable to the treatment of threatened abortion due to asthenia of the spleen and kidney.

4) 15g of Heye (*Folium Nelumbinis*) and 6g of Baifan (*Alumen*) are decocted with 3 eggs with reddish shell for oral taking, applicable to the treatment of abortion due to fetal heat.

（5）孕妇清火丸　每次服6g，1日2次，适用于胎热火盛证流产。

2. 单验方

（1）胎热汤　苎麻根30g，荷叶蒂12g，侧叶柏9g，水煎服，适用于血热证先兆流产。

（2）保胎散　杜仲6g，续断6g，菟丝子6g，桑寄生6g，艾叶6g，共为细末，每服3g，每日早、晚各1次，适用于肝肾亏损证先兆流产。

（3）保胎方　党参15g，黄芪15g，白术15g，续断15g，覆盆子15g，菟丝子15g，杜仲15g，升麻10g，鹿角胶10g，水煎服，适用于脾肾亏虚证先兆流产。

（4）荷叶15g，白矾6g，红皮鸡蛋3个，水煎煮，去药渣分服，适用于胎热证流产。

2.6.2　Heterotopic pregnancy

Heterotopic pregnancy refers to nidation of the fertilized ovum outside the uterus. Clinically heterotopic pregnancy is classified into oviducal pregnancy, ovary pregnancy, abdominal pregnancy and cervical pregnancy, among which oviducal pregnancy is the most commonly encountered one and occupies about 90% of heterotopic pregnancy and about 50% is on the right side.

According to acute sharp pain and abdominal massive hemorrhage, heterotopic pregnancy is similar to abdominal pain during pregnancy, blood stasis in the lower abdomen and abdominal mass in TCM. Heterotopic pregnancy is usually caused by retention of stasis in the lower abdomen, unsmooth circulation of qi and blood in the thoroughfare and conception vessels that lead to fertilized ovum to stay in the lower abdomen; or by weakness of the viscera and consumption of qi and blood failing to transport the fertilized ovum to the uterus. Both conditions will lead to development of the fertilized ovum in the oviduct that dilates and ruptures the vessels, resulting in hemorrhage in the lower abdomen and blockage of the vessels.

[Key points for diagnosis]

(1) History of amenorrhea and early pregnancy manifestations; positive pregnancy test, acute reduction of hematochrome and emptiness of the uterus indicated by ultrasonic B examination.

(2) Abdominal pain, irregular vaginal bleeding, syncope and coma due to acute abdominal hemorrhage and sharp abdominal pain, tenderness and rebound pain in the lower abdomen as well as mobile dull sound in percussion.

(3) Gynecological examination: Fullness and tender-

第二节　异位妊娠

异位妊娠是指受精卵在子宫体腔以外着床发育。临床上分为输卵管妊娠、卵巢妊娠、腹腔妊娠、宫颈妊娠等,以输卵管妊娠为最常见。约占异位妊娠发生率的90%左右,其中50%发生在右侧。

根据本病急性剧烈腹痛及腹腔大出血的特点,与中医学"妊娠腹痛"、"少腹蓄血"、"癥瘕"等病症相似。其发病多因少腹有宿瘀,冲任不畅,以致孕卵凝聚在少腹,不得达于子宫;或脏腑虚弱,气血劳伤,不能运孕卵于胞宫,使受精卵在输卵管内着床发育,以致涨破脉络,阴血内溢于少腹,阻滞血脉,不通则痛。

【诊断要点】

(1) 有停经史及早妊反应,妊娠试验阳性,急性期血色素下降,B超显示宫腔空虚。

(2) 腹痛,阴道不规则出血,由腹腔内急性出血和剧烈腹痛引起昏厥与休克。下腹部有压痛及反跳痛,叩诊有移动性浊音。

(3) 妇科检查:阴道后穹

ness in the posterior fornix, evident pain in raising and shaking the uterus, slight enlargement and softness of the uterus, floating sensation in the uterus, tumescent mass palpable in one side or in the posterior side of the uterus and withdrawal of uncoagulated blood from the posterior fornix by puncture.

(4) Heterotopic pregnancy should be differentiated from uterine pregnancy abortion, rupture of yellow body, acute appendicitis and torsion of ovarian cyst.

[Syndrome differentiation and treatment]

Heterotopic pregnancy mainly manifests as the sthenia syndrome of blood stasis in the lower abdomen. So the therapeutic principle is activating blood and resolving stasis. Clinically it is divided into syndrome of blood loss due to qi asthenia, stagnation and stasis syndrome and blood stasis syndrome. It can be treated with blood transfusion and fluid infusion according to the development of the pathological conditions. Treatment should be monitored carefully in light of the complications when operation is not resorted to. The most commonly encountered complication is sthenia syndrome of fu organs, the manifestations of which are constipation, abdominal distension, epigastric discomfort, unpressable abdominal pain and reduction or disappearance of borborygmus. Sthenia syndrome of fu organs is either heat-sthenia or cold-sthenia or mixture of cold and heat.

(1) Syndrome of blood loss due to qi asthenia

Main symptoms: Rupture of oviducal pregnancy or abortion of oviducal pregnancy, pale complexion, cold limbs, lowering of blood pressure, unpressable lower abdominal pain, light-colored tongue with thin and white fur, deep, thin and indistinct pulse.

Therapeutic methods: Restoring yang and arresting

穹窿饱满,触痛;宫颈有明显举痛和摇摆痛;子宫稍大而软,有漂浮感;子宫一侧或后方可触及肿块;后穹窿穿刺可抽出不凝血。

四、须与宫内妊娠流产、黄体破裂、急性阑尾炎及卵巢囊肿蒂扭转鉴别。

【辨证论治】

本病主要病机属"少腹蓄血"实证,治疗上以活血化瘀为原则。临床辨证一般分为气虚血脱证、瘀滞证及血瘀证。确诊患者应全过程密切观察病情发展,必要时采取输血、输液及手术治疗。非手术治疗过程中,必须重视对兼证的处理。最常见的兼证是腑实证,表现为腹胀便秘,胃脘不适,腹痛拒按,肠鸣减弱或消失。腑实证有属热实、寒实及寒热夹杂之分,临证须明辨之。

一、气虚血脱证

主要证候　输卵管妊娠破裂或输卵管妊娠流产,面色苍白,四肢发冷,血压降低,少腹剧痛拒按,舌淡苔薄,脉沉细而微。

治　法　回阳固脱,活血

prostration or loss, activating blood and resolving stasis.

Prescription and drugs: Modified Shenfu Tang combined with Huoluo Xiaoling Dan composed of 9g of prepared slice of Fuzi (*Radix Aconiti Praeparata*), 6g of Hongshen (*Radix Ginseng Destillata*) (to be decocted separately), 5g of roasted Gancao (*Radix Glycyrrhizae*), 3g of roasted Guizhi (*Ramulus Cinnamomi*), 10g of Fuling (*Poria*), 10g of Mudanpi (*Cortex Moutan Radicis*), 10g of Danshen (*Radix Salviae Miltiorrhizae*), 10g of Chishaoyao (*Radix Paeoniae Rubra*), 6g of roasted Ruxiang (*Olibanum*) and 6g of roasted Moyao (*Myrrha*).

Modification: For constipation and abdominal distension as well as yellow and greasy tongue fur, 6g of crude Daihuang (*Radix et Rhizoma Rhei*) (to be decocted later), 9g of Xuanmingfen (*Natrii Sulfas Exsiccatus*) (to be mixed in boiled water for oral taking) and 9g of Zhishi (*Fructus Aurantii Immaturus*) are added; for complication with cold and heat with yellow, white, greasy and thick tongue fur, 6g of crude Dahuang (*Radix et Rhizoma Rhei*) (to be decocted later), 9g of Xuanmingfen (*Natrii Sulfas Exsiccatus*) (to be mixed in boiled water for oral taking) and 3g of Rougui (*Cortex Cinnamomi*) (to be decocted later) are added.

(2) Syndrome of stagnation and stasis

Main symptoms: Abortion and rupture of oviducal pregnancy, mild interior hemorrhage, stable blood pressure, unpressable distending pain in the lower abdomen, tenderness and rebound pain, slight vaginal bleeding and thin and slow pulse.

Therapeutic methods: Activating blood and resolving stasis, regulating qi and stopping pain.

Prescription and drugs: Modified Gongwaiyun No.1

化瘀。

方　药　参附汤合活络效灵丹加减：制附片9 g,红参(另煎)6 g,炙甘草5 g,炙桂枝3 g,茯苓10 g,牡丹皮10 g,丹参10 g,赤芍药10 g,炙乳香6 g,炙没药6 g。

加　减　大便秘结、鼓肠腹胀,苔黄腻,加生大黄(后下)6 g,玄明粉(冲服)9 g,枳实9 g;寒热夹杂,苔黄白腻厚者,加生大黄(后下)6 g,玄明粉(冲服)9 g,肉桂(后下)3 g。

二、瘀滞证

主要证候　输卵管妊娠流产或破裂,内出血量不多,血压平稳,腹痛腹胀拒按,有压痛及反跳痛,有少量阴道流血,脉细缓。

治　法　活血化瘀,理气止痛。

方　药　宫外孕Ⅰ号方

(No. 1 prescription for heterotopic pregnancy) composed of 15g of Danshen (*Radix Salviae Miltiorrhizae*), 10g of Chishaoyao (*Radix Paeoniae Rubra*), 9g of Taoren (*Semen Persicae*), 10g of Chuanniuxi (*Radix Cyathulae*), 3g of Wugong (*Scolopendra*), 10g of Wulingzhi (*Faeces Trogopterorum*) and 9g of prepared Xiangfu (*Rhizoma Cyperi*).

Modification: For massive hemorrhage, 0.5g of Yunnan White Powder (for oral taking) or 3g of Shensanqi (*Radix Notoginseng*) powder (to be taken orally) are added, twice or three times a day.

(3) Syndorme of blood stasis

Main symptoms: Hematoma and mass in the abdomen, gradual alleviation of abdominal pain, prolapsing sensation and distension in the lower abdomen or desire for defecation, stoppage of vaginal bleeding and thin and unsmooth pulse.

Therapeutic methods: Breaking stasis and eliminating abdominal mass.

Prescription and drugs: Modified Gongwaiyun No. 2 (No. 2 prescription for heterotopic pregnancy) composed of 12g of Danshen (*Radix Salviae Miltiorrhizae*), 10g of Chishaoyao (*Radix Paeoniae Rubra*), 6g of Ruxiang (*Olibanum*), 6g of Moyao (*Myrrha*), 9g of Taoren (*Semen Persicae*), 10g of Sanleng (*Rhizoma Sparganii*), 10g of Ezhu (*Rhizoma Curcumae*) and 6g of Zhechong (*Eupolyphaga seu Steleophaga*).

Modification: For infection, 15 g of Jinyinhua (*Flos Lonicerae*), 10g of Lianqiao (*Fructus Forsythiae*), 30g of Hongteng (*Caulis Sargentodoxae*) and 30g of Baijiangcao (*Herba Patriniae*) are added; for constipation, 6 - 9g of crude Dahuang (*Radix et Rhizoma Rhei*) or 9g of Fanxieye (*Folium Sennae*) are added.

加减：丹参15 g，赤芍药10 g，桃仁9 g，川牛膝10 g，蜈蚣3 g，五灵脂10 g，制香附9 g。

　加　减　出血多者，加云南白药(吞服)0.5 g，或参三七粉(吞服)3 g，每日 2～3 次。

三、血瘀证

　主要证候　腹腔血肿包块形成，腹痛逐渐减轻，有下腹坠胀或便意感，阴道出血停止，脉细涩。

　治　法　破瘀消癥。

　方　药　宫外孕Ⅱ号方加减：丹参12 g，赤芍药10 g，乳香6 g，没药6 g，桃仁9 g，三棱10 g，莪术10 g，䗪虫6 g。

　加　减　有感染者，加金银花15 g，连翘10 g，红藤30 g，败酱草30 g；便秘加生大黄(后下)6 g或番泻叶9 g。

[Other therapeutic methods]

(1) Chinese patent drugs

1) Dahuang Zhechong Pill: 1 pill each time and twice a day, applicable to the treatment of heterotopic pregnancy.

2) Shixiao Powder: 6 - 9g each time and once or twice a day (mixed with vinegar or millet wine for oral taking), applicable to the treatment of heterotopic pregnancy without rupture or old heterotopic pregnancy.

3) Huazheng Huisheng Bolus: 6g each time and twice a day, applicable to the treatment of heterotopic pregnancy without rupture or old heterotopic pregnancy.

(2) Empirical and folk recipes

1) Huoluo Xiaoling Bolus composed of 9 - 15g of Danshen (*Radix Salviae Miltiorrhizae*), 6 - 9g of Chishaoyao (*Radix Paeoniae Rubra*), 3 - 6g of Ruxiang (*Olibanum*), 3 - 6g of Moyao (*Myrrha*) and 6 - 9g of Taoren (*Semen Persicae*). These herbs are decocted for oral taking, applicable to the treatment of heterotopic pregnancy without rupture due to blood stasis.

2) Enriched Huoluo Xiaoling Bolus composed of 15g of Danshen (*Radix Salviae Miltiorrhizae*), 12g of Chishaoyao (*Radix Paeoniae Rubra*), 6g of Ruxiang (*Olibanum*), 6g of Moyao (*Myrrha*), 6g of Sanleng (*Rhizoma Sparganii*), 6g of Ezhu (*Rhizoma Curcumae*), 30g of Niuxi (*Radix Achyranthis Bidentatae*), 9g of Taoren (*Semen Persicae*), 18g of Dongkuizi (*Semen Malvae*), 2 Wugong (*Scolopendra*) and 10g of Zhechong (*Eupolyphaga seu Steleophaga*). These ingredients are decocted for oral taking, applicable to the treatment of heterotopic pregnancy without rupture due to blood stasis.

3) 3 - 6g of Hongshen (*Radix Ginseng Destillata*) slices or powder for oral taking, applicable to the treatment of ruptured heterotopic pregnancy due to qi as-

【其他疗法】

1. 中成药

（1）大黄䗪虫丸　每服1丸,每日2次,适用于血瘀证之异位妊娠。

（2）失笑散　每服6～9g,每日1～2次,醋或黄酒冲服,适用于未破损期或陈旧性异位妊娠。

（3）化癥回生丹　每服6g,每日1～2次,适用于未破损期或陈旧性异位妊娠。

2. 单验方

（1）活络效灵丹　丹参9～15g,赤芍药6～9g,乳香3～6g,没药3～6g,桃仁6～9g,水煎服,适用于未破损期血瘀证异位妊娠。

（2）加味活络效灵丹　丹参15g,赤芍药12g,乳香6g,没药6g,三棱6g,莪术6g,牛膝30g,桃仁9g,冬葵子18g,蜈蚣2条,䗪虫10g,水煎服,适用于未破损期血瘀证异位妊娠。

（3）红参片或红参粉3～6g,吞服,适用于已破损期气虚血脱证异位妊娠。

thenia and blood loss.

4) 3g of Sanqi (*Radix Notoginseng*) powder for oral taking, applicable to the treatment of ruptured heterotopic pregnancy with massive bleeding.

(3) External therapy

1) 6g of Zhangnao (*Camphora*), 9g of Xuejie (*Resina Draconis*), 9g of Songxiang (*Colophonium*) and 9g of Yinzhu (*Hydrargyrum Sulfuratum*) are ground into powder and heated into paste. The paste is spread over a piece of cloth and applied to the part of abdomen where pain is located.

2) 60g of Qiannianjian (*Rhizoma Homalomenae*), 120g of Xuduan (*Radix Dipsaci*), 60g of Zuandifeng (*Cortex Schizophragmatis Integrifolii Radicis*), 60g of Huajiao (*Pericarpium Zanthoxyli*), 120g of Wujiapi (*Cortex Acanthopanacis Radicis*), 120g of Baizhi (*Radix Angelicae*), 120g of Sangjisheng (*Ramulus Taxilli*), 500g of Aiye (*Folium Artemisiae Argyi*), 250g of Tougucao (*Herba Speranskiae Tuberculatae*), 60g of Qianghuo (*Rhizoma seu Radix Notopterygii*), 60g of Duhuo (*Radix Angelicae Pubescentis*), 120g of Chishaoyao (*Radix Paeoniae Rubra*), 120g of Guiwei (*the carda part of Radix Angelicae Sinensis*), 60g of Xuejie (*Resina Draconis*), 60g of Ruxiang (*Olibanum*) and 60g of Moyao (*Myrrha*). These herbs are ground into powder which is wrapped in a piece of gauze and heated for 15 minutes and then applied to the affected part. This treatment is given once or twice a day, applicable to the treatment of heterotopic pregnancy of mass type. Ten days make up one course of treatment.

(4) Enema with Chinese medicinal herbs

1) 15g of Shanyangxue (*Sanguis Naemorhedi*), 15g of Taoren (*Semen Persicae*), 15g of Danshen (*Radix*

（4）三七粉 3 g，吞服，适用于已破损期出血多之异位妊娠。

3. 外敷法

（1）樟脑6 g，血蝎9 g，松香9 g，银珠9 g，研细加热成糊状，涂于布上，趁热贴于腹部疼痛处。

（2）千年健60 g，续断120 g，钻地风60 g，花椒60 g，五加皮120 g，白芷120 g，桑寄生120 g，艾叶500 g，透骨草250 g，羌活60 g，独活60 g，赤芍药120 g，归尾120 g，血竭60 g，乳香60 g，没药60 g，上药共研为末，纱布包，蒸15分钟，趁热外敷，每日 1～2 次，10 天为 1 个疗程。适用于包块型异位妊娠。

四、中药保留灌肠法

（1）山羊血15 g，桃仁15 g，丹参15 g，赤芍药15 g，延

Salviae Miltiorrhizae), 15g of Chishaoyao (*Radix Paeoniae Rubra*), 15g of Yanhusuo (*Rhizoma Corydalis*), 9g of Sanleng (*Rhizoma Sparganii*), 9g of Ezhu (*Rhizoma Curcumae*) and 9g of Zhechong (*Eupolyphaga seu Steleophaga*) are decocted in water into 150 – 200ml decoction for retention enema under low pressure, applicable to the treatment of heterotopic pregnancy without rupture or old heterotopic pregnancy.

2) 15g of Taoren (*Semen Persicae*), 15g of Danshen (*Radix Salviae Miltiorrhizae*), 15g of Pugongying (*Herba Taraxaci*), 30g of Yuxingcao (*Herba Houttuyniae*) and 30g of Yazhicao (*Herba Commelinae*) are decocted in water into 150 – 200ml decoction added with 10ml procaine of 1% for retention enema, applicable to the treatment of heterotopic pregnancy without rupture or old heterotopic pregnancy.

2.6.3 Morning sickness

Morning sickness refers to nausea, vomiting, dizziness and anorexia or even postcibal vomiting in the early period of pregnancy.

Morning sickness is usually caused by upward adverse flow of qi from the thoroughfare vessel and failure of gastric qi to descend in the early period of pregnancy; or by frequent asthenia of gastric qi, or frequent restlessness and susceptibility to rage and transformation of fire from liver depression; or by asthenia of spleen yang leading to interior retention of phlegm and fluid as well as invasion of qi from the thoroughfare vessel with liver fire into the stomach; or by upward adverse flow of qi from the thoroughfare vessel with phlegm and fluid.

[**Key points for diagnosis**]

(1) Vomiting, anorexia and postcibal vomiting,

胡索15 g,三棱9 g,莪术9 g,䗪虫9 g,浓煎成 150～200 ml,低压保留灌肠,适用于未破损期或陈旧性异位妊娠。

（2）桃仁15 g,丹参15 g,蒲公英15 g,鱼腥草30 g,鸭跖草30 g,浓煎成 150～200 ml,加入 1% 普鲁卡因10 ml,低压保留灌肠,适用于未破损期或陈旧性异位妊娠。

第三节 妊娠恶阻

妊娠恶阻是指妊娠早期出现严重的恶心呕吐、头晕厌食等反应,严重者食入即吐。

本病多因妊娠早期冲脉之气上逆,胃失和降所致。若胃气素虚,或平素性躁多怒,肝郁化热,或脾阳素虚,痰饮内停,冲气挟肝火上逆犯胃,或冲气挟痰饮上逆所致。

【诊断要点】

（1）呕吐厌食或食入即

usually occurring in the first three months of pregnancy.

(2) Nausea, vomiting of saliva or preference for sour taste are signs of early pregnancy.

(3) Morning sickness should be differentiated from hepatitis, gastritis and appendicitis in pregnancy.

[Syndrome differentiation and treatment]

Clinically morning sickness is classified into syndrome of stomach asthenia, syndrome of liver heat and syndrome of phlegm stagnation. The therapeutic principles are regulating qi to harmonize the middle energizer and descending adverse flow of qi to stop vomiting. Usually the therapeutic methods of strengthening the stomach, clearing away heat from the liver, resolving phlegm and descending adverse flow of qi can be used according to the clinical manifestations. Integrated traditional Chinese and western medical therapy can be used if necessary.

(1) Syndrome of stomach asthenia

Main symptoms: Nausea, vomiting, postcibal vomiting, epigastric and abdominal fullness and distension, anorexia, dizziness, lassitude, somnolence, light-colored tongue with white fur, slow and weak pulse.

Therapeutic methods: Strengthening the stomach and harmonizing the middle energizer, descending adverse flow of qi to stop vomiting.

Prescription and drugs: Modified Xiangsha Liujunzi Tang composed of 10g of Dangshen (*Radix Codonopsis Pilosulae*), 10g of Baizhu (*Rhizoma Atractylodis Macrocephalae*), 3g of Gancao (*Radix Glycyrrhizae*), 6g of prepared Banxia (*Rhizoma Pinelliae*), 6g of Chenpi (*Pericarpium Citri Reticulatae*), 10g of Fuling (*Poria*), 5g of Guanghuoxiang (*Herba Agastaches seu Pog-*

吐,一般发生于妊娠早期的 3 个月内。

（2）若仅见恶心吐涎,择食嗜酸者,称早孕反应。

（3）须与妊娠肝炎、胃炎、阑尾炎相鉴别。

【辨证论治】

本病临床主要分为胃虚证,肝热证及痰滞证。治疗以调气和中、降逆止呕为原则,根据辨证分别采用健胃、清肝、化痰降逆法,必要时,采用中西医结合方法治疗。

一、胃虚证

主要证候　妊娠早期,恶心呕吐,吐出食物,甚则食入即吐,脘腹胀闷,不思饮食,头晕体倦,怠懒思睡,舌淡,苔白,脉缓慢无力。

治　法　健胃和中,降逆止呕。

方　药　香砂六君子汤加减:党参10 g,白术10 g,甘草 3 g,制半夏6 g,陈皮6 g,茯苓10 g,广藿香 5 g,砂仁 5 g,紫苏叶 5 g,炒竹茹9 g,生姜 3 片,大枣 3 枚。

ostemonis), 5g of Sharen (*Fructus Amomi*), 5g of
Zisuye (*Folium Perillae*), 9g of roasted Zhuru (*Caulis
Bambusae in Taeniam*), 3 slices of Shengjiang (*Rhizo-
ma Zingiberis Recens*) and 3 Dazao (*Fructus Jujubae*).

Modification: For asthenia-cold of the spleen and
stomach, 5g of Dingxiang (*Flos Caryophylli*) and 10g of
Baidoukou (*Fructus Amomi Rotundus*) are added to
warm the middle and descend adverse flow of qi; for severe vomiting that impairs yin with the symptoms of dry
mouth and constipation, Muxiang (*Radix Aucklandiae*),
Sharen (*Fructus Amomi*) and Fuling (*Poria*) are deleted, 10g of Yuzhu (*Rhizoma Polygonati Odorati*), 10g
of Maimendong (*Radix Ophiopogonis*), 10g of Shihu
(*Herba Dendrobii*) and 10g of Humaren (*Semen Sesami*) are added; for abnormal increase of saliva and frequent drooling, 10g of Yizhiren (*Fructus Alpiniae
Oxyphyllae*) and 10g of Baidoukou (*Fructus Amomi Rotundus*) are added.

(2) Liver-heat syndrome

Main symptoms: Vomiting of acid fluid or bitter fluid, fullness and oppression in the chest and hypochondri-
um, belching and sighing, dizziness, bitter taste in the
mouth and dry throat, thirst with preference for cold
drinks, constipation and reddish urine, reddish tongue
with yellowish dry coating, taut, slippery and rapid pulse.

Therapeutic methods: Clearing the liver and harmonizing the stomach, descending adverse flow of qi and
stopping vomiting.

Prescription and drugs: Jiawei Wendan Decoction
composed of 6g of Chenpi (*Pericarpium Citri Reticulatae*), 6g of prepared Banxia (*Rhizoma Pinelliae*), 6g of
fried Zhuru (*Caulis Bambusae Taeniam*), 10g of Fuling
(*Poria*), 3g of Gancao (*Radix Glycyrrhizae*), 9g of

加 减 若脾胃虚寒者,
酌加丁香5 g,白豆蔻10 g,以
增强温中降逆之力;若吐甚伤
阴,症见口干便秘者,宜去木
香、砂仁、茯苓等温燥或淡渗
之品,酌加玉竹10 g,麦门冬
10 g,石斛10 g,胡麻仁10 g;若
孕妇唾液分泌量异常增多,时
时流涎者,加益智仁10 g,白豆
蔻10 g。

二、肝热证

主要证候 妊娠早期,
呕吐酸水或苦水,胸胁满闷,
嗳气叹息,头晕目眩,口苦咽
干,渴喜冷饮,便秘溲赤,舌
红,苔黄燥,脉弦滑数。

治 法 清肝和胃,降逆
止呕。

方 药 加味温胆汤:
陈皮6 g,制半夏6 g,炒竹茹
6 g,茯苓10 g,甘草3 g,炒枳实
9 g,黄芩9 g,黄连5 g,麦门冬
10 g,芦根15 g,生姜 3 片。

fried Zhishi (*Fructus Aurantii Immaturus*), 9g of Huangqin (*Radix Scutellariae*), 5g of Huanglian (*Rhizoma Coptidis*), 10g of Maimendong (*Radix Ophiopogonis*), 15g of Lugen (*Rhizoma Phragmitis*) and 3 slices of Shengjiang (*Rhizoma Zingiberis Recens*).

Modification: For consumption of body fluid due to excessive vomiting, feverish sensation over the palms, soles and chest, red tongue and dry mouth, 10g of Shihu (*Herba Dendrobii*) and 10g of Yuzhu (*Rhizoma Polygonati Odorati*) are added for nourishing yin and clearing away heat; for constipation, 10g of Humaren (*Semen Sesami*) is added for lubricating intestines to promote defecation.

加 减 若呕甚伤津,五心烦热,舌红口干者,酌加石斛10 g,玉竹10 g,以养阴清热;便秘者,酌加胡麻仁10 g,以润肠通便。

(3) Syndrome of phlegm stagnation

Main symptoms: Vomiting of phlegm and drool, chest and diaphragm fullness and oppression, anorexia, bland and greasy taste in the mouth, dizziness, palpitation and shortness of breath, light-colored and bulgy tongue, white and greasy tongue fur, and slippery pulse.

Therapeutic methods: Resolving phlegm and eliminating dampness, descending adverse flow of qi and stopping vomiting.

Prescription and drugs: Modified Xiaobanxia Plus Fuling Tang composed of 6g of prepared Banxia (*Rhizoma Pinelliae*), 6g of Chenpi (*Pericarpium Citri Reticulatae*), 10g of Fuling (*Poria*), 3 slices of Shengjiang (*Rhizoma Zingiberis Recens*), 6g of Guanghuoxiang (*Herba Agastaches seu Pogostemonis*), 9g of roasted Zhuru (*Caulis Bambusae in Taeniam*), 6g of Chuanpohua (*Flos Magnoliae Officinalis*), 10g of roasted Guya (*Fructus Oryzae Germinatus*) and 10g of roasted Maiya (*Fructus Hordei Germinatus*).

Modification: For hypofunction of the spleen and

三、痰滞证

主要证候 妊娠早期,呕吐痰涎,胸膈满闷,不思饮食,口中淡腻,头晕目眩,心悸气短,舌淡胖,苔白腻,脉滑。

治 法 化痰除湿,降逆止呕。

方 药 小半夏加茯苓汤加减:制半夏6 g,陈皮6 g,茯苓10 g,生姜 3 片,广藿香6 g,炒竹茹9 g,川朴花6 g,炒谷牙10 g,炒麦芽10 g。

加 减 若脾胃虚弱痰

stomach and interior exuberance of phlegm and dampness, 10g of Cangzhu (*Rhizoma Atractylodis*) and 10g of Baizhu (*Rhizoma Atractylodis Macrocephalae*) are added; for vomiting of clear fluid, cold sensation in the body and limbs as well as pale complexion, 5g of Dingxiang (*Flos Caryophylli*) and 10g of Baidoukou (*Fructus Amomi Rotundus*) are added; for vomiting yellowish fluid, dizziness, dysphoria and preference for sour and cold foods due to heat, 10g of Huangqin (*Radix Scutellariae*), 10g of Zhimu (*Rhizoma Anemarrhenae*) and 10g of Qianhu (*Radix Peucedani*) are added.

[Other therapeutic methods]

(1) Chinese patent drugs

1) Zuojin Pill: 1.5g each time and 3 – 4 times a day, applicable to the treatment of morning sickness due to liver heat syndrome.

2) Xiangsha Liujunzi Pill: 6 - 9g each time and twice a day, applicable to the treatment of morning sickness due to hypofunction of the spleen and stomach.

3) Shengmai Liquid: 10ml each time and twice a day, applicable to the treatment of morning sickness due to asthenia of both qi and yin.

(2) Empirical and folk recipes

1) Pibaye Tea: 15g of Pipaye (*Folium Eriobotryae*) (removal of the fur) and 30g of Fulonggan (*Terra Flava Usta*) (to be wrapped) are decocted in water. The decoction is taken orally as tea, applicable to the treatment of morning sickness due to stomach asthenia.

2) 9g of Zhuru (*Caulis Bambusae in Taeniam*) and 3g of Chenpi (*Pericarpium Citri Reticulatae*) are decocted in water for oral taking, applicable to the treatment of morning sickness due to phlegm and dampness.

3) 30 - 90g of Fulonggan (*Terra Flava Usta*) (to be wrapped) is decocted in water. The clear decoction is for

湿内盛者,酌加苍术10 g,白术10 g;兼寒者,症见呕吐清水,形寒肢冷,面色苍白,宜加丁香5 g,白豆蔻10 g;若挟热者,症见呕吐黄水,头晕心烦,喜食酸冷,酌加黄芩10 g,知母10 g,前胡10 g。

【其他疗法】

1. 中成药

（1）左金丸 每服1.5 g,每日 3～4 次,适用于肝热证之妊娠恶阻。

（2）香砂六君子丸 每次服6～9 g,每日 2 次,适用于脾胃虚弱证恶阻。

（3）生脉饮 每次服10 ml,每日 2 次,适用于气阴两亏证恶阻。

2. 单验方

（1）枇杷叶茶 生枇杷叶(去毛)15 g,伏龙肝(布包)30 g,水煎后代茶频呷,适用于胃虚证之妊娠恶阻。

（2）竹茹9 g,陈皮3 g,水煎服,适用于痰湿证恶阻。

（3）伏龙肝 30～90 g,布包水煎,澄清液分 3～5 次服,

oral taking for 3 - 5 times, applicable to the treatment of morning sickness due to asthenia-cold in the spleen and stomach.

4) 1 cup of Ganzhe (*Truncus Sacchari*) juice and 4 - 5 drops of Shengjiang (*Rhizoma Zingiberis Recens*) juice are mixed together and taken a little each hour, applicable to the treatment of morning sickness due to hypofunction of the spleen and stomach.

5) 10g of Huangqin (*Radix Scutellariae*) and 50g of Gouqizi (*Fructus Lycii*) are soaked in boiling water for oral taking, applicable to the treatment of morning sickness due to various factors.

(3) External therapy

1) Cupping therapy: This therapy is applied to Zhongwan (CV 12) for the treatment of morning sickness due to asthenia of the stomach.

2) Scraping therapy: This therapy is applied to the regions of Pishu (BL 20), Weishu (BL 21), Ganshu (BL 18), and Danshu (BL 19). This therapy is applicable to the treatment of morning sickness due to stomach asthenia.

3) Steaming therapy: 50g of fresh Yuansui (*Herba Coriandri*), 3g of Zisuye (*Folium Perillae*), 3g of Huoxiang (*Herba Agastaches seu Pogostemonis*) and 6g of Chenpi (*Pericarpium Citri Reticulatae*) are boiled in a pot. When vapour comes out of the mouth of the pot, the patient is asked to breathe in the vapour. This treatment is applicable to the treatment of morning sickness due to hypofunction of the spleen and stomach.

2.6.4　Pregnancy-induced hypertension syndrome

Pregnancy-induced hypertension syndrome refers to the syndrome of hypertension, edema and proteinuria oc-

适用于脾胃虚寒证恶阻。

（4）甘蔗汁 1 杯,生姜汁 4～5 滴,每隔 1 小时服少许,适用于脾胃虚弱证恶阻。

（5）黄芩 10 g,枸杞子 50 g,沸水泡后频饮,适用于各证恶阻。

3. 外治法

（1）火罐治疗法　取中脘穴拔火罐,适用于胃虚证妊娠恶阻。

（2）刮痧疗法　取背部脾俞、胃俞、肝俞、胆俞刮痧,使被刮皮肤呈红色,适用于胃虚证之妊娠恶阻。

（3）蒸气法　鲜芫荽 50 g,紫苏叶 3 g,藿香 3 g,陈皮 6 g,放入壶内水煮,气从壶口出,令患者吸其气,适用于脾胃虚弱证恶阻。

第四节　妊娠高血压综合征

妊娠高血压综合征是指妊娠 20 周以后发生高血压、

curring 20 weeks after pregnancy. This syndrome is commonly seen among the gravida of younger or elder age. The incidence in cities and among the educated people is higher than that in the rural areas. This syndrome is easy to occur among those with the history of primary hypertension, chronic nephritis, diabetes, twin fetuses and polyhydramnios. In serious cases, this syndrome may lead to spasm, unconsciousness and failure of the heart and kidney, or even death of both the gravida and fetus. So this syndrome is one of the acute, urgent and severe gynecological diseases. This disease pertains to "edema in pregnancy", "dizziness in pregnancy" and "eclampsia gravidarum" in TCM.

This syndrome is usually caused by worsened weakness of the body after pregnancy; or by constitutional asthenia of the spleen and kidney yang, dysfunction of the spleen and liver, lack of enough warmth to transform and transport dampness, leading to retention of fluid and dampness and edema in the skin and the four limbs; or by growth of the fetus hindering the flow of qi, blocking the circulation of fluid and causing edema; or by frequent asthenia of liver and kidney yin as well as worsened deficiency of essence and blood after pregnancy, leading to hyperactivity of liver yang due to failure of yin to control yang; or by malnutrition of the liver and endogenous liver wind; or by phlegm-fire invading the upper part of the body or asthenia-wind attacking the upper orifices, resulting in eclampsia gravidarum.

[Key points for diagnosis]

(1) Symptoms gradually occurring after 20 weeks of pregnancy, such as hypertension, edema or proteinuria; gradual dizziness, distension of head and headache, blurred vision, edema above the ankle and scanty urine; sudden syncope or coma, staring eyes, lockjaw, spasm of

水肿、蛋白尿的综合征。本病易发生于年轻或高龄初产妇,其城市发病率高于农村,文化程度高者发病率高;有原发性高血压、慢性肾炎、糖尿病、双胎及羊水过多者好发。本病严重时可出现抽搐、昏迷、心肾功能衰竭,甚至可导致母婴死亡。属妇产科危、急、重症之一。中医将本病归属于"子肿"、"子晕"、"子痫"范畴。

因脏气本虚,受孕后愈虚;或因素体脾肾阳虚,肝脾失调,不能温煦、运化水湿,以致水湿停滞,泛于肌肤、四肢,脾虚肝旺;胎体渐长,则可阻碍气机升降,水道不利,水湿泛于肌肤,发为"子肿"。如若素体肝肾阴虚,精血不足,妊娠后血聚以养胎,精血愈虚,阴不敛阳,肝阳上亢而谓之"子晕";甚则肝失所养,肝风内动,或挟痰火上扰,或虚风上犯清窍而成"子痫"。

【诊断要点】

(1) 妊娠 20 周后逐渐出现头晕目眩,头胀而痛,视物昏花,踝部以上水肿,小便短少;妊娠晚期及新产后,可突然眩晕仆倒,昏不知人,两目

limbs, opisthotonos or even unconsciousness during labor or after labor.

(2) Pregnancy 20 weeks later accompanied by varied hypertension, edema or proteinuria of mild, medium and severe degrees.

(3) Other examination: Blood and urine tests, test of liver functions, fundus examination, electrocardiography and examination of placenta functions and the growth of the fetus are helpful for diagnosis.

(4) This syndrome should be differentiated from complication of primary hypertension, chronic nephritis and pheochromocytoma in pregnancy; eclampsia gravidarum should be differentiated from epilepsy, cerebral hemorrhage, hysteria and convulsion of hands and feet.

[Syndrome differentiation and treatment]

Clinically this syndrome is classified into syndrome of yin asthenia and liver hyperactivity, syndrome of spleen asthenia and liver hyperactivity, wind-fire syndrome and phlegm-fire syndrome. The therapeutic principle is soothing the liver and suppressing yang. The therapeutic methods used are nourishing yin and descending adverse flow of qi, regulating qi and resolving phlegm, and nourishing qi and invigorating blood.

(1) Syndrome of yin asthenia and liver hyperactivity

Main symptoms: Dizziness, poor sleep, aching sensation in the loins, palpitation, shortness of breath, hypertension, proteinuria, edema of lower limbs, red or deep-red tongue, taut and rapid pulse in the late stage of pregnancy.

Therapeutic methods: Fostering yin and suppressing yang, soothing the liver and clearing away heat.

Prescription and drugs: Modified Qiju Dihuang

上视,牙关紧闭,四肢抽搐,角弓反张,甚至昏迷不醒等。

(2) 妊娠 20 周后伴不同程度的高血压、水肿或蛋白尿,分为轻、中、重三度。

(3) 其他检查:如血液、尿液检查,肝肾功能测定,眼底检查,心电图,胎盘功能,胎儿成熟度检查等有助于诊断。

(4) 本病须与妊娠合并原发性高血压、慢性肾炎、嗜酪细胞瘤等相鉴别;子痫还应与癫痫、脑溢血、癔病、手足搐搦症相鉴别。

【辨证论治】

本病临床主要分为阴虚肝旺证、脾虚肝旺证、风火证及痰火证。治疗以平肝潜阳为基本治则,根据病情分别采用滋阴潜降、理气化痰、益气养血法等。

一、阴虚肝旺证

主要证候 妊娠晚期头晕目眩,寐差,腰酸,心悸气短,面色潮红,伴见高血压,蛋白尿,下肢浮肿,舌红或绛,脉弦数。

治 法 育阴潜阳,平肝清心。

方 药 杞菊地黄汤:

Tang composed of 10g of Gouqizi (*Fructus Lycii*), 6g of Ganjuhua (*sweet Flos Chrysanthemi*), 10g of crude Dihuang (*Radix Rehmanniae*), 10g of Shanyao (*Rhizoma Dioscoreae*), 10g of Shanzhuyu (*Fructus Corni*), 10g of stir-baked Mudanpi (*Cortex Moutan Radicis*), 10g of roasted Fuling (*Poria*), 10g of Zexie (*Rhizoma Alismatis*), 10g of Baishaoyao (*Radix Paeoniae Alba*), 20g of roasted Guiban (*Plastrum Testudinis*), 20g of crude Muli (*Caro Ostreae*) and 15g of Gouteng (*Ramulus Uncariae cum Uncis*) (to be decocted later).

Modification: For constipation, 6g of crude Dahuang (*Radix et Rhizoma Rhei*) (to be decocted later) and 9g of Baiziren (*Semen Platycladi*) are added; for evident heat, 10g of Zhimu (*Rhizoma Anemarrhenae*) and 10g of Huangbai (*Cortex Phellodendri*) are added; for bitter taste in the mouth and dysphoria, 10g of Huangqin (*Radix Scutellariae*) and 10g of Zhuru (*Caulis Bambusae in Taeniam*) are added; for dizziness and syncope, 9g of Tianma (*Rhizoma Gastrodiae*) is added.

(2) Syndrome of spleen asthenia and liver hyperactivity

Main symptoms: Facial dropsy, edema of limbs, headache and dizziness, anorexia, chest oppression and nausea, spiritual lassitude and flaccidity of limbs, loose stool, hypertension, proteinuria, light-red color of the tongue with greasy fur, weak, taut and slippery pulse in the late stage of pregnancy.

Therapeutic methods: Strengthening the spleen and draining dampness, soothing the liver and suppressing yang.

Prescription and drugs: Modified Banxia Baizhu Tianma San composed of 9g of roasted Tianma (*Rhizoma Gastrodiae*), 6g of prepared Banxia (*Rhizoma Pinelliae*), 15g of Fuling (*Poria*), 6g of Chenpi (*Pericarpium*

枸杞子10 g,甘菊花6 g,生地黄10 g,山药10 g,山茱萸10 g,炒牡丹皮10 g,茯苓10 g,泽泻10 g,白芍药10 g,炙龟版20 g,生牡蛎(先煎)20 g,钩藤(后下)15 g。

加　减　大便秘结者加生大黄(后下)6 g,柏子仁9 g;若热象明显者,酌加知母10 g,黄柏10 g;口苦心烦者,酌加黄芩10 g,竹茹10 g;眩晕昏仆者,酌加天麻9 g。

二、脾虚肝旺证

主要证候　妊娠晚期,面浮肢肿,头痛头晕,纳食不馨,胸闷泛恶,神疲肢软,大便偏溏,血压高,蛋白尿,舌淡红,苔腻,脉虚弦而滑。

治　法　健脾利湿,平肝潜阳。

方　药　半夏白术天麻散:煨天麻9 g,白术10 g,制半夏6 g,茯苓15 g,陈皮6 g,大腹皮9 g,钩藤(后下)15 g,防已

Citri Reticulatae), 9g of Dafupi (*Pericarpium Are-cae*), 15g of Gouteng (*Ramulus Uncariae cum Uncis*) (to be decocted later), 10g of Fangji (*Radix Stephaniae Tetrandrae*), 10g of Kudingcha (*Folium Ilicis*), 10g of Baijili (*Fructus Tribuli*) and 10g of Chixiaodou (*Semen Phaseoli*).

Modification: For evident proteinuria, 10g of Zhul-ing (*Polygorus*), 10g of Tufuling (*Rhizoma Smilacis Glabrae*) and 10g of Baimaogen (*Rhizoma Imperatae*) are added; for severe hypertension, 15g of Zhenzhumu (*Concha Margaritifera*) and 15g of crude Muli (*Caro Ostreae*) (to be decocted later) are added.

(3) Disturbance of liver-wind syndrome

Main symptoms: Sudden dizziness, convulsion of limbs, lockjaw, staring eyes, opisthotonos, feverish palms and soles, flushed cheeks and rough breathing, red or deep-red tongue with thin yellow fur, taut, thin and rapid or taut and powerful pulse.

Therapeutic methods: Stopping wind and suppress-ing yang, soothing the liver and clearing away heat from the heart.

Prescription and drugs: Modified Lingjiao Gouteng Tang composed of 0.3 - 0.6g of Lingyangjiao (*Cornu Saigae Tatarricae*) powder (for oral taking) [use 15 - 30g, of Shuiniujiao (*Cornu Bubali*) instead] 20g of Gouteng (*Ramulus Uncariae cum Uncis*), 6g of Sangye (*Folium Mori*), 6g of Chuanbeimu (*Bulbus Frityllari-ae Cirrhosae*), 10g of fresh and crude Dihuang (*Radix Rehmanniae*), 10g of Baishaoyao (*Radix Paeoniae Al-ba*), 10g of Zhuru (*Caulis Bambusae in Taeniam*), 10g of Fushen (*Sclerotium Poriae Circum Radicem Pini*), 10g of Baijili (*Fructus Tribuli*), 5g of Ganjuhua (*sweet*

10 g,苦丁茶10 g,白蒺藜10 g,赤小豆10 g。

　　加　减　蛋白尿明显者,加猪苓10 g,土茯苓10 g,白茅根10 g;血压甚高者,加珍珠母15 g,生牡蛎(先煎)15 g。

三、肝风内动证

　　主要证候　妊娠晚期或临产及新产后,突然眩晕,四肢抽搐,牙关紧闭,目睛直视,腰背反张,手足心热,颧赤息粗,舌红或绛,苔薄黄,脉弦细而数或弦劲有力。

　　治　法　熄风潜阳,平肝清心。

　　方　药　羚角钩藤汤:羚羊角粉(吞服)0.3~0.6 g(水牛角 15~30 g代),钩藤(后下)20 g,桑叶6 g,川贝母6 g,鲜生地黄 10 g,白芍药10 g,竹茹10 g,茯神10 g,白蒺藜10 g,甘菊花 5 g,珍珠母20 g,生牡蛎(先煎)15 g。

Flos Chrysanthemi), 20g of Zhenzhumu (Concha Margaritifera) and 15g of crude Muli (Caro Ostreae) (to be decocted first).

Modification: For exuberant fire in the liver and heart, 6g of Longdancao (Radix Gentianae), 3g of Huanglian (Rhizoma Coptidis), 10g of Kudingcha (Folium Ilicis) and 10g of Xiakucao (Spica Prunellae) are added; for syncope and profuse phlegm, 10g of Tianzhuhuang (Concretio Silicea Bambusae), 10g of Chendanxing (Arisaema cum Bile) and 6g of roasted Yuanzhi (Radix Polygalae) are added.

加 减　如心肝火旺盛者,加龙胆草6 g,黄连3 g,苦丁茶10 g,夏枯草10 g;挟有昏迷痰多者,加天竺黄10 g,陈胆星10 g,炙远志6 g。

(4) Phlegm-fire syndrome

四、痰火证

Main symptoms: Headache, chest oppression, sudden syncope, lockjaw, frothy drooling, rough breathing, sputum rale, restlessness, palpitation, nervousness, poor sleep at night, red tongue with yellow, greasy and thick fur, slippery and rapid pulse.

主要证候　妊娠晚期,或临产及新产后,头痛胸闷,突然昏仆不知人,牙关紧闭,口流痰涎,息粗痰鸣,烦躁不已,惊悸不安,入夜寐差,舌偏红,舌苔黄腻而厚,脉滑数。

Therapeutic methods: Clearing away heat and expelling phlegm, resuscitating brain and tranquilizing spirit.

治 法　清热豁痰,开窍安神。

Prescription and drugs: Modified Qinggong Tang combined with Niuhuang Qingxin Wan composed of 6g of Lianqiao (Fructus Forsythiae), 3g of Xuanshen, 3g of Lianzixin, 0.3 - 0.6g of Lingyangjiao (Cornu Saigae Tataricae) powder (for oral taking) [use 15 - 30g of Shuiniujiao (Cornu Bubali) instead], 10g of Mudanpi (Cortex Moutan Radicis), 9g of Fanyujin (Radix Curcumae), 6g of roasted Juhong (Exocarpium Citri Tangerinae), 5g of Shichangpu (Rhizoma Acori Graminei), 10g of Tianzhuhuang (Concretio Silicea Bambusae), 1 spoonful of Zhulishui (Succus Phyllostachydis Henonis) and 0.3g of Niuhuang powder (Calculus Bovis) (for oral taking).

方 药　清宫汤合牛黄清心丸:连翘6 g,玄参6 g,莲子心3 g,羚羊角粉(吞)0.3～0.6 g(水牛角 15～30 g代),牡丹皮10 g,矾郁金9 g,炙橘红6 g,石菖蒲5 g,陈胆星10 g,天竺黄10 g,竹沥水1 匙,牛黄粉(吞)0.3 g。

Modification: For occasional convulsion, 15g of Gouteng (*Ramulus Uncariae cum Uncis*) and 3g of Quanxie powder (*Resina Draconis*) are added; for syncope, 1 pill of Zhibao Pellet or 1 pill of Suhexiang Pill are added for oral taking, twice a day.

[Other therapeutic methods]

(1) Chinese patent drugs

1) Qiju Dihuang Pill: 10g each time and twice a day, applicable to the treatment of vertigo during pregnancy due to yin asthenia and liver hyperactivity.

2) Zhibai Dihuang Pill: 10g each time and twice a day, applicable to the treatment of vertigo during pregnancy due to yin asthenia and liver hyperactivity.

3) Jiawei Xiaoyao Pill: 6 - 9g each time and twice a day, applicable to the treatment of vertigo during pregnancy due to yin asthenia and liver hyperactivity.

4) Angong Niuhuang Pill: 1 pill each time and twice a day, applicable to the treatment of eclampsia gravidarum of coma type.

5) Niuhuang Qingxin Pill: 9g each time and twice a day, applicable to the treatment of eclampsia gravidarum due to phlegm-fire attacking the brain.

6) Zixue Pellet: 1.5 - 3g each time and once or twice a day, applicable to the treatment of vertigo eclampsia gravidarum due to endogenous liver wind.

(2) Empirical and folk recipes

1) 9g of Tianma (*Rhizoma Gastrodiae*) is decocted together with two eggs. The decoction is applicable to the treatment of premonitrory signs of eclampsia gravidarum due to yin asthenia and yang hyperactivity.

2) 250g of Baijuhua (*White Flos Chrysanthemi*) is decocted. The decoction is taken orally as tea, applicable to the treatment of premonitory signs of eclampsia gravidarum due to yin asthenia and liver hyperactivity.

加　减　有时抽搐者,加钩藤15 g,全蝎粉(吞)3 g;昏迷者,加服至宝丹 1 粒,或苏合香丸,每次 1 丸,日服 2 次。

【其他疗法】

1. 中成药

(1) 杞菊地黄丸　每次服10 g,1 日 2 次,适用于阴虚肝旺证子晕。

(2) 知柏地黄丸　每次服10 g,1 日 2 次,适用于阴虚肝旺证子晕。

(3) 加味逍遥丸　每次服 6~9 g,1 日 2 次,适用于脾虚肝旺证子晕。

(4) 安宫牛黄丸　每次服 1 粒,1 日 2 次,适用于昏迷型子痫。

(5) 牛黄清心丸　每次服9 g,1 日 2 次,适用于痰火上扰证子痫。

(6) 紫雪丹　每次服1.5~3 g,1 日 1~2 次,适用于肝风内动证子痫。

2. 单验方

(1) 天麻9 g水煎炖鸡蛋 2个。适用于阴虚阳亢证先兆子痫。

(2) 白菊花250 g,泡茶饮。适用于阴虚肝旺证先兆子痫。

3) 15ml of Zhulishui (*Succus Phyllostachydis Henonis*) is mixed with water for oral taking, applicable to the treatment of eclampsia gravidarum due to phlegm heat.

4) 500g of carp, 6g of scallion and ginger, 15g of Fuling (*Poria*) and 15g of Cheqianzi (*Semen Plantaginis*) (to be wrapped for decocting) are decocted in water for oral taking, applicable to the treatment of various types of edema during pregancy.

5) 400g of Zaodaogen (*rice root*) is decocted for oral taking, applicable to the treatment of edema during pregancy due to asthenia of spleen and kidney yang.

2.6.5 Intrahepatic cholestasis in pregnancy

Intrahepatic cholestasis refers to general pruritus, abnormal changes of liver function, mild increase of jaundice and cholic acid during the middle and late stages of pregnancy. These symptoms tend to recur in future pregnancy. It is also called specific jaundice during pregnancy or recurrent jaundice during pregnancy. The incidence in China is 0.3% – 4.4% with obvious regional and racial differences. Intrahepatic cholestasis during pregnancy may lead to retardation of fetus development, polyhydraminios, premature delivery and fetal distress. It is one of the factors responsible for perinatal death.

Intrahepatic cholestasis during pregnancy pertains to pruritus during pregnancy and jaundice during pregnancy in TCM. The exogenous cause is multiparity that consumes blood. The endogenous causes are asthenia of yin, consumption of body fluid and deficiency of blood and accumulation of blood in the uterus to nourish the fetus after

（3）竹沥水15 ml冲服。适用于痰热子痫。

（4）鲤鱼500 g，葱姜6 g，茯苓15 g，白术20 g，车前子（包煎）15 g，水煎服。适用于各证妊娠水肿。

（5）早稻根 400 g，水煎服。适用于脾肾阳虚证妊娠水肿。

第五节　妊娠期肝内胆汁淤积症

妊娠期肝内胆汁淤积症是孕妇特有的疾病。临床表现为在妊娠中、晚期出现全身瘙痒、肝功能异常、轻度黄疸、胆酸等升高，并在继续妊娠过程中有复发倾向，故又称妊娠特发性黄疸或妊娠期复发性黄疸。本病国内发病率为0.3%～4.4%，有明显的地区和种族差异。可导致宫内发育迟缓、羊水过少、早产，胎儿窘迫，是导致围生儿死亡的原因之一。

根据本病的临床表现，可归属于中医学"妊娠瘙痒证"、"妊娠黄疸"范畴。其外因为多产房劳，阴血暗耗，内因与素体阴虚，津亏血少，加之怀孕后阴血下聚以养胎元，营阴

pregnancy, leading to deficiency of blood and giving rise to dryness transformed from endogenous wind and pruritus due to malnutrition of the skin. Asthenia of yin will result in malnutrition of the liver, dysfunction of the liver and failure of bile to convey which, in turn, lead to jaundice. Intrahepatic cholestasis during pregnancy may also be caused by obesity and retention of dampness and fluid; or by retention of dampness due to dysfunction of the spleen and hyperactivity of yang due to deficiency of blood after pregnancy. The combination of heat transformed from exuberance of yang with dampness, together with gradual enlargement of the fetus, hinders the flow of qi and the conveyance of bile, and eventually leading to the onset of intrahepatic cholestasis.

[Key points for diagnosis]

(1) The disease may involve family history, personal pregnancy history and history of contraception with oral contraceptives.

(2) Pruritus, jaundice, nausea, reduced appetite, lassitude, diarrhea and abdominal distension in the middle and late stages of pregnancy.

(3) Increase of serum bilirubin over 17.1 μmol/L, increase of SGPT, evident increase of serum cholic acid with 9.64 mol/L which has earlier appearance than the symptoms.

[Syndrome differentiation and treatment]

Clinically intrahepatic cholestasis is classified into syndrome of yin asthenia and blood dryness and syndrome of stagnation and accumulation of damp-heat. The therapeutic principles are nourishing yin to invigorate blood, expelling wind to relieve pruritus, clearing away heat and draining dampness as well as eliminating jaundice and protecting the fetus. In nourishing yin to invigorate blood, cares should be taken to avoid excessive use of nutritive

亏乏,生风化燥,肌肤失养,故呈瘙痒症;阴虚肝木失养,疏泄失常,胆汁不得宣泄而发为黄疸。或因素体肥胖、水湿内停,或脾虚运化失司水湿内聚,孕后阴血不足,阳气偏旺,阳盛则热,湿与热结,加之胎体渐大,阻碍气机,以致宣泄失常,滞于肌肤或体内,碍及胆汁宣泄,而发为本病。

【诊断要点】

(1) 本病可追及家族史、个人妊娠史及口服避孕药后发生史等。

(2) 妊娠中、晚期,出现瘙痒、黄疸、恶心、食欲减退、乏力、腹泻、腹胀等症状。

(3) 血清胆红素升高,≥17.1 μmol/L;SGPT升高;血清胆酸明显升高,≥9.64 mol/L,且较症状出现早。

【辨证论治】

本病临床主要分为阴虚血燥证、湿热郁结证。治疗以滋阴养血、疏风止痒、清热利湿、退黄安胎为原则,根据不同证型有所偏重。谱方用药应注意滋阴养血不可过于滋腻,适当加入理气行滞之品,以免阻碍气机,加重黄疸;利

herbs and proper amount of herbs for regulating qi and eliminating stagnation can be added lest the flow of qi be blocked and jaundice be worsened. In draining dampness, measures should be taken to add some ingredients for nourishing blood, invigorating kidney and protecting the fetus lest the fetus be damaged.

(1) Syndrome of yin asthenia and blood dryness

Main symptoms: Dryness and pruritus of the skin during pregnancy, or accompanied by mild yellow coloration of the sclera, dysphoria, restless sleep at night, aching and weak sensation in the loins and knees, feverish palms and soles, dry mouth and throat, yellow and scanty urine, red tongue with scanty or thin and yellow fur, thin, slippery and rapid pulse.

Therapeutic methods: Nourishing yin and invigorating blood, expelling wind and stopping pruritus.

Prescription and drugs: Enriched Danggui Yinzi composed of 10g of Danggui (*Radix Angelicae Sinensis*), 3g of Chuanxiong (*Rhizoma Chuanxiong*), 10g of Baishaoyao (*Radix Paeoniae Alba*), 10g of Shengdi huang (*Radix Rehmanniae*), 10g of Heshouwu (*Radix Polygoni Multiflori*), 10g of Baijili (*Fructus Tribuli*), 6g of Jingjie (*Herba Schizonepetae*), 6g of Fangfeng (*Radix Ledebouriellae*), 10g of Huangqin (*Radix Scutellariae*), 15g of Yinchen (*Herba Artemisiae*), 10g of Huangqi (*Radix Astragali*) and 3g of Gancao (*Radix Glycyrrhizae*).

Modification: For severe pruritus, 6g of Chantui (*Periostracum Cicadae*) and 10g of Baijiangcan (*Bombyx Batryticatus*) are added for dispersing wind and heat as well as stopping endogenous wind and relieving pruritus.

湿不可过于滑利,以免伤及胎元,还当加入养血、补肾安胎之品。

一、阴虚血燥证

主要证候 妊娠期间,皮肤干燥瘙痒,或伴轻度巩膜黄染,心烦,夜寐不安,腰膝酸软,手足心热,口干咽燥,小便黄少,舌质红,少苔或薄黄苔,脉细滑数。

治 法 滋阴养血,疏风止痒。

方 药 当归饮子加味:当归10 g,川芎3 g,白芍药10 g,生地黄10 g,何首乌10 g,白蒺藜10 g,荆芥6 g,防风6 g,黄芩10 g,茵陈15 g,黄芪10 g,甘草3 g。

加 减 瘙痒甚者,加蝉蜕6 g,白僵蚕10 g,以加强疏散风热、熄风止痒之功。

(2) Syndrome of damp-heat stagnation

Main symptoms: Yellow coloration of the sclera and skin during pregnancy, pruritus, poor appetite, epigastric and abdominal distension and fullness, frequent nausea, yellowish and brownish urine like strong tea, yellow and greasy tongue fur, taut, slippery and rapid pulse.

Therapeutic methods: Clearing away heat and draining dampness, eliminating jaundice and relieving pruritus.

Prescription and drugs: Modified Yangxue Tuihuang Zhiyang Tang composed of 15g of Yinchen (*Herba Artemisiae*), 10g of Huangqin (*Radix Scutellariae*), 10g of Zhizi (*Fructus Gardeniae*), 10g of Fuling (*Poria*), 10g of Zexie (*Rhizoma Alismatis*), 15g of Zhuling (*Polygorus*), 10g of Dangshen (*Radix Codonopsis Pilosulae*), 10g of Baizhu (*Rhizoma Atractylodis Macrocephalae*), 6g of Mudanpi (*Cortex Moutan Radicis*), 10g of Chaihu (*Radix Bupleuri*), 10g of Baixianpi (*Cortex Dictamni*) and 10g of Jingjie (*Herba Schizonepetae*).

Modification: For manifestations of severe heat like thirst, dysphoria and constipation, Fuling (*Poria*) and Zexie (*Rhizoma Alismatis*) are deleted, while 10g of prepared Dahuang (*Radix et Rhizoma Rhei*) and 15g of Pugongying (*Herba Taraxaci*) are added; for manifestations of severe dampness like sticky sensation in the mouth, abdominal distension, loose stool and thick and white tongue fur with yellowish color on the surface, Zhizi (*Fructus Gardeniae*) and Huangqin (*Radix Scutellariae*) are deleted, while 5g of Cangzhu (*Rhizoma Atractylodis*), 5 g of Houpo (*Cortex Magnoliae Officinalis*) and 3g of Baikouren (*Fructus Amomi Rotundus*) are added.

二、湿热郁结证

主要证候 妊娠期间,巩膜及皮肤黄染,瘙痒,食纳不佳,脘腹胀满,时时欲呕,小便黄赤如浓茶,舌苔黄腻,脉弦滑数。

治 法 清热利湿,退黄止痒。

方 药 养血退黄止痒汤:茵陈15 g,黄芩10 g,栀子10 g,茯苓10 g,泽泻10 g,猪苓15 g,党参10 g,白术10 g,牡丹皮6 g,柴胡10 g,白鲜皮10 g,荆芥10 g。

加 减 热偏重,见口渴、心烦、便秘者,去茯苓、泽泻,加制大黄6 g,蒲公英15 g;湿偏重,口粘、腹胀、大便稀溏、苔底厚白罩黄者,去栀子、黄芩,加苍术5 g,厚朴5 g,白蔻仁3 g。

[Other therapeutic methods]

(1) Chinese patent drugs

1) Yinchen Wuling Pill: 6g each time and twice a day, applicable to the treatment of the syndrome due to accumulation of damp heat.

2) Longdan Xiegan Pill: 6g each time and three times a day, applicable to the treatment of the syndrome due to stagnant heat in the liver and gallbladder.

3) Ganlu Xiaodu Bolus: 9g each time and three times a day, applicable to the treatment of the syndrome due to accumulation of damp heat.

4) Yinzhihuang Injection: Each ampule contains 2ml or 10ml. 2 - 4ml each time for intramuscular injection. Or 250 - 500ml of 10% glucose infusion added with 10ml of Yinzhihuang injection is used for intravenous drip.

(2) Empirical and folk recipes

1) Yinchen (*Herba Artemisiae*), Xiakucao (*Spica Prunellae*), Pugongying (*Herba Taraxaci*), Chuipencao (*Herba Sedi*), Fengweicao (*Herba Pteridis Multifidae*), Cheqiancao (*Herba Plantaginis*), Jigucao (*Herba Abri*) and Baimaogen (*Rhizoma Imperatae*). Any two of the herbs of 30 - 60g each can be used to decoct together with 10 Chinese dates for oral taking, one dose a day.

2) Yinchen Tang composed of 10g of Yinchen (*Herba Artemisiae*), 10g of Chaihu (*Radix Bupleuri*), 10g of Danshen (*Radix Salviae Miltiorrhizae*), 9g of Zhizi (*Fructus Gardeniae*), 9g of Baijiangcan (*Bombyx Batryticatus*), 9g of Chantui (*Periostracum Cicadae*), 15g of Pugongying (*Herba Taraxaci*), 15g of Yiyiren (*Semen Coicis*) and 6g of Zhuru (*Caulis Bambusae in Taeniam*) are decocted for oral taking, applicable to the treatment of jaundice during pregnancy due to damp heat.

3) 30g of Yinchenhao (*Cacumen Artemisiae Scop-*

【其他疗法】

1. 中成药

（1）茵陈五苓丸　每次服6 g,1 日 2 次,适用于湿热蕴结证。

（2）龙胆泻肝丸　每次服6 g,1 日 3 次,适用于肝胆郁热证。

（3）甘露消毒丹　每次服9 g,1 日 3 次,适用于湿热蕴结证。

（4）茵栀黄注射液　每支2 ml或10 ml,肌肉注射,每日 2～4 ml。或用 10% 葡萄糖注射液 250～500 ml加入10 ml茵栀黄注射液静脉滴注。

2. 单验方

（1）茵陈、夏枯草、蒲公英、垂盆草、凤尾草、车前草、鸡骨草、白茅根等,任选两种,用30～60 g,加大枣 10 枚,煎服,每日 1 剂。

（2）茵陈汤 茵陈10 g,柴胡10 g,丹参10 g,栀子9 g,白僵蚕9 g,蝉蜕9 g,蒲公英15 g,薏苡仁15 g,竹茹6 g,水煎服。适用于湿热蕴结证妊娠黄疸。

（3）茵陈蒿30 g,水煎服。

ariae) is decocted for oral taking, applicable to the treatment of jaundice during pregnancy due to damp heat.

4) 50g of Cheqiancao is ground and the juice is taken orally, applicable to the treatment of jaundice during pregnancy due to damp heat.

2.6.6　Diabetes in pregnancy

Diabetes during pregnancy is due to relative insufficiency of insulin secreted by pancreas to maintain a balanced metabolism of sugar. This disease is mainly caused by intemperance of food, and excessive intake of greasy and rich food that accumulates in the middle energizer and impairs the spleen and stomach, leading to endogenous heat and consumption of fluid; or by psychological factors, transformation of fire from qi stagnation, consumption of gastric fluid, generation of dryness from fire accumulation that consumes body fluid and deprives the lung and kidney of proper nutrition; or by constitutional weakness of the body, early marriage and multiparity, loss of kidney essence and endogenous asthenia-fire that steams the lung and stomach.

[**Key points for diagnosis**]

（1）Family history of diabetes and faulty delivery (dead fetus, still birth, macrosomia and teratism without evident cause).

（2）Polydipsia, polyphagia and polyuria or accompanied by recurrent monilial infection in the vagina.

（3）Glucose in urine is positive. Blood sugar tests indicate blood sugar on empty stomach is ≥7.8 mmol/L. Or glucose tolerance test for one hour and two hours ≥ 11.1 mmol/L is the evidence of accurate diagnosis of dia-

适用于湿热证妊娠黄疸。

（4）车前草50 g,捣汁冲服。适用于湿热证妊娠黄疸。

第六节　妊娠期糖尿病

妊娠期糖尿病主要由于妊娠导致胰腺分泌胰岛素相对不足,不能维持糖代谢平衡,以致糖耐量试验异常甚或合并糖尿病。本病多因饮食不节,长期过食肥甘厚味,壅滞中焦,损伤脾胃,中焦失于运化,酿生内热,消谷耗液;或因精神因素,气郁化火,消灼胃之津液,蕴结化燥,燥热耗伤阴液,不能滋养肺肾;或素体虚弱,早婚多产,肾精耗损,虚火内生,上蒸肺胃而致。中医归属"消渴"范畴。

【诊断要点】

（1）有糖尿病家族史、不良生育史(不明原因的死胎、死产、巨大儿、畸形儿等)。

（2）孕期有多饮、多食、多尿症状,或伴见反复发作的外阴阴道念珠菌感染体征。

（3）尿糖阳性;多次空腹血糖测定≥7.8 mmol/L,或糖耐量试验1小时及2小时血糖≥11.1 mmoI/L, 即 可 明 确

betes.

[Syndrome differentiation and treatment]

Clinically this disease is classified into syndrome of lung heat and fluid consumption, syndrome of stomach dryness and yin consumption and syndrome of kidney asthenia and essence loss. Yin asthenia is the primary cause and dryness heat is the secondary cause. At the beginning of the disease, the main symptom is dryness-heat. After longer duration, yin asthenia and dryness heat appear simultaneously. With the development of the pathological conditions, asthenia of yin involves yang and leads to asthenia of both yin and yang. The basic therapeutic principle is clearing away heat and nourishing yin. The therapeutic methods usually used are clearing the lung, clearing the stomach and nourishing the kidney,

(1) Syndrome of lung heat and fluid consumption

Main symptoms: Polydipsia, dry throat, dry tongue, frequent and profuse urination, red tip and margins of the tongue, thin tongue fur and rapid pulse.

Therapeutic methods: Clearing the lung, moistening dryness and promoting production of body fluid.

Prescription and drugs: Modified Xiaoke Fang composed of 3g of Huanglian (*Rhizoma Coptidis*), 15g of Shengdihuang (*Radix Rehmanniae*), 15g of Beishashen (*Fructus Amomi*), 10g of Maimendong (*Radix Ophiopogonis*), 10g of Shihu (*Herba Dendrobii*), 120g of fresh lotus root (to be ground for extracting juice) and 15g of Baihe (*Bulbus Lilii*).

Modification: For severe heat with the manifestations of restless thirst, polydipsia, yellow and dry tongue fur, full and large pulse, 30g of Shengshigao (*Gypsum Fibrosum*) (to be decocted first), 10g of Zhimu (*Rhizoma Anemarrhenae*) and 5g of Gancao (*Radix Glycyr-*

诊断。

【辨证论治】

本病临床上辨证分为肺热津伤证、胃燥阴伤证及肾虚精亏证。以阴虚为本,燥热为标,病之初多以燥热为主,病程久则阴虚与燥热互见,进而阴损及阳,以致阴阳两虚。治疗以清热养阴为基本治则,根据病情分别采用清肺、清胃、滋肾等法。

一、肺热津伤证

主要证候 妊娠期口渴多饮,咽干,舌燥,小便频多,舌边尖红,苔薄,脉数。

治 法 清肺润燥生津。

方 药 消渴方加减:黄连 3 g,生地黄15 g,天花粉15 g,北沙参10 g,麦门冬10 g,石斛10 g,鲜藕(捣汁和服)120 g,百合15 g。

加 减 若热甚,见烦渴多饮,舌苔黄燥,脉洪大,加生石膏(先煎)30 g,知母10 g,甘草 5 g;若见气短,易汗,疲倦,脉细,加党参10 g,黄芪10 g, *rhizae*) are added; for shortness of breath, susceptibility to sweating, lassitude and thin pulse, 10g of Dangshen (*Radix Codonopsis Pilosulae*), 10g of Huangqi (*Radix Astragali*) and 5g of Wuweizi (*Fructus Schisandrae*) are added.

(2) Syndrome of stomach dryness and yin consumption

Main symptoms: Polyphagia, emaciation during pregnancy, or retention of dry feces, yellow dry tongue fur, slippery and rapid pulse.

Therapeutic methods: Clearing the stomach and nourishing yin.

Prescription and drugs: Modified Yunü Jian composed of 15g of Shengdihuang (*Radix Rehmanniae*), 12g of Xuanshen (*Radix Scrophulariae*), 30g of Shengshigao (*Gypsum Fibrosum*), 3g of Huanglian (*Rhizoma Coptidis*), 15g of Tianhuafen (*Radix Trichosanthis*), 10g of Maimendong (*Radix Ophiopogonis*) and 10g of Zhimu (*Rhizoma Anemarrhenae*).

Modification: For constipation, Maziren (*Fructus Cannabis*) pill is added.

(3) Syndrome of kidney asthenia and essence loss

Main symptoms: Frequent and profuse urination and greasy urine during pregnancy, dizziness, blurred vision, aching loins and flaccidity of knees, dry mouth, red tongue, deep, thin and rapid pulse.

Therapeutic methods: Nourishing the kidney and consolidating essence.

Prescription and drugs: Modified Liuwei Dihuang Tang composed of 12g of Shudihuang (*Rhizoma Rehmanniae Praeparata*), 12g of Shanzhuyu (*Fructus*

五味子 5 g。

二、胃燥阴伤证

　　主要证候　妊娠期多食易饥,消瘦,或大便干结,舌苔黄燥,脉滑数。

　　治　法　清胃养阴。

　　方　药　玉女煎加减:生地黄15 g,玄参12 g,生石膏(先煎)30 g,黄连 3 g,天花粉15 g,麦门冬10 g,知母10 g。

　　加　减　若大便秘结,多日不解,加服麻子仁丸。

三、肾虚精亏证

　　主要证候　妊娠期小便频数、量多,尿如脂膏,头晕目糊,腰酸腿软,口干,舌红,脉沉细而数。

　　治　法　滋肾固精。

　　方　药　六味地黄汤加减:熟地黄12 g,山茱萸12 g,山药15 g,牡丹皮10 g,茯苓

Corni), 15g of Shanyao (*Rhizoma Dioscoreae*), 10g of Mudanpi (*Cortex Moutan Radicis*), 10g of Fuling (*Poria*), 10g of Wuweizi (*Fructus Schisandrae*) and 12g of Gouqizi (*Fructus Lycii*).

Modification: For yin asthenia and fire exuberance with the manifestations of low fever, night sweating and deep-red tongue, Huangbai (*Cortex Phellodendri*) and Zhimu (*Rhizoma Anemarrhenae*) are added; for complication of yang asthenia with aversion to cold, cold limbs, impotence, profuse urine, light-colored tongue, white tongue fur, deep, thin and weak pulse, Mudanpi (Cortex Moutan Radicis) is removed while 3g of Rougui (*Cortex Cinnamomi*), 5g of prepared Fuzi (*Radix Aconiti Praeparata*), 10g of Lujiaopian (*sliced Cornu Cervi*) and 10g of Tusizi (*Semen Cuscutae*) are added; for complication of asthenia of spleen qi with the manifestations of poor appetite, lassitude, light-red tongue, weak and thin pulse, Mudanpi (*Cortex Moutan Radicis*) and Shudihuang (*Rhizoma Rehmanniae Praeparata*) are removed, while 12g of Dangshen (*Radix Codonopsis Pilosulae*), 10g of Huangqi (*Radix Astragali*), 10g of Baizhu (*Rhizoma Atractylodis Macrocephalae*) and 10g of Jineijin (*Endothelium Corneum Gigeriae Galli*) are added.

[**Other therapeutic methods**]

(1) Chinese patent drugs

1) Zengye Granulae: 20g each time and three times a day, applicable to the treatment of lung heat consuming fluid.

2) Xiaokeping Tablet: 6 - 8 tablets each time and three times a day, applicable to the treatment of asthenia of liver and kidney yin.

(2) Empirical and folk recipes

1) 500ml of Maru (*Lac Equiae*) is boiled for oral

10 g,泽泻10 g,五味子 5 g,枸杞子12 g。

加　减　若阴虚火旺,见低热,盗汗,舌绛,加黄柏、知母;兼肾阳虚,见畏寒、肢冷、阳痿、尿量特多,舌淡,苔白,脉沉细无力,去牡丹皮,加肉桂3 g,制附子5 g,鹿角片10 g,菟丝子10 g;兼脾气虚弱,见食少、倦怠、舌淡红,脉虚细,去牡丹皮、熟地黄,加党参12 g,黄芪10 g,白术10 g,鸡内金10 g。

【其他疗法】

1. 中成药

(1) 增液冲剂　每次服20 g,1 日 3 次,适用于肺热津伤证。

(2) 消渴平片　每次服6～8 片,1 日 3 次,适用于肝肾阴虚证。

2. 单验方

(1) 马乳500 ml,煮沸,每

taking, 50ml each time and three times a day.

2) 50g of fresh waxgourd rind, 50g of watermelon rind and 25g of Tianhuafen (*Radix Trichosanthis*) are decocted for oral taking, 20g each time and twice a day.

3) 30g of Shengdihuang (*Radix Rehmanniae*), 30g of Huangqi (*Radix Astragali*) and 90g of Shanyao (*Rhizoma Dioscoreae*) are decocted for oral taking, applicable to the treatment of asthenia of spleen and stomach qi.

次服50 ml,1 日 3 次。

（2）鲜冬瓜皮50 g,西瓜皮50 g,天花粉25 g,浓煎后每次服20 g,1 日 2 次。

（3）生地黄30 g,黄芪30 g,山药90 g,水煎服,适用于脾胃气虚证。

2.7 Puerperalism

第七章
产褥病

2.7.1 Postpartum hemorrhage

第一节　产后出血

Postpartum hemorrhage refers to over 500ml of vaginal bleeding within 24 hours after labor. It is one of the important causes for parturient death and also one of the causes of puerperal infection. It is a severe and acute disease in obstetrics requiring immediate and correct treatment. The prognosis of postpartum hemorrhage is usually unfavourable.

The main symptom of postpartum hemorrhage is sudden massive bleeding from the vagina right after labor, pertaining to the conceptions of sudden profuse uterine bleeding and postpartum blood syncope in TCM. It is usually caused by the weakness of the parturient; or overstrain and consumption of primordial qi due to prolonged labor; or by invasion of exogenous pathogenic cold that coagulates blood and turbid fluid in the thoroughfare and conception vessels; or by injury of the birth canal.

[Key points for diagnosis]

(1) Sudden massive bleeding from the vagina right after labor, especially over 500mlof bleeding from the vagina within 24 hours after labor.

(2) Examination: To see if placenta and fetal membrane is damaged; if the birth canal is injured; whether the uterus is of subinvolution or soft and large or hard and pain. Examination: Routine blood test, blood platelet test, coagulation factors test and type B ultrasonic exami-

产后出血是指胎儿娩出后 24 小时内阴道流血量超过 500 ml以上者。本病是导致产妇死亡的重要原因之一,也是产褥感染的诱因之一,是产科的危重急症,必须及时抢救,正确处置。

中医属"产后血崩"、"产后血晕"范畴。本病多因产妇素体虚弱,或因产程过长,疲劳过度,损伤元气,或感受寒邪,凝滞余血浊液,瘀阻冲任,或产道损伤所致。

【诊断要点】

(1) 新产后突然阴道大量出血。特别是产后 24 小时内出血量达500 ml以上。

(2) 检查:胎盘、胎膜有无缺损;软产道有无损伤;子宫复旧不良,或软而大,或硬而痛。检验血常规、血小板、凝血因子,查 B 超以帮助诊断。

nation are helpful for diagnosis of the illness.

[Syndrome differentiation and treatment]

Clinically postpartum hemorrhage is classified into qi asthenia syndrome, blood stasis syndrome and birth injury syndrome. The therapeutic principle is nourishing qi and resolving stasis. Syndrome differentiation should be made of the asthenia and sthenia. But emergency treatment has to be resorted to in dealing with serious cases. Treatment with integrated traditional Chinese and Western medicine can be taken if necessary.

(1) Syndrome of qi asthenia

Main symptoms: Sudden massive bleeding from the vagina with fresh red color right after labor, dizziness, palpitation, shortness of breath, no desire to speak, cold limbs, sweating, pale complexion, light-colored tongue, weak and rapid pulse.

Therapeutic methods: Replenishing qi and strengthening the thoroughfare vessel, controlling blood and stopping bleeding.

Prescription and drugs: Modified Shengju Dabu Tang composed of 20g of Huangqi (*Radix Astragali*), 10g of Baizhu (*Rhizoma Atractylodis Macrocephalae*), 6g of Renshen (*Radix Ginseng*) (to be decocted separately and then mixed up with the other ingredients), 6g of prepared Gancao (*Radix Glycyrrhizae*), 6g of Shengma (*Rhizoma Cimicifugae*), 10g of Danggui (*Radix Angelicae Sinensis*), 10g of Shudihuang (*Rhizoma Rehmanniae Praeparata*), 10g of Maimendong (*Radix Ophiopogonis*), 10g of Chuanxiong (*Rhizoma Chuanxiong*), 10g of Baizhi (*Radix Angelicae*), 10g of Heijiesui (*Herba Schizonepetae*), 10g of charred Diyu (*Radix Sanguisorbae*) and 15g of Wuzeigu (*Os Sepiae*).

Modification: For coma, cold limbs, sweating and

【辨证论治】

本病临床主要分为气虚证、血瘀证及产伤证。治疗以益气化瘀为原则,除按虚实辨证论治外,危重者均须立即抢救,必要时应予中西医结合治疗,以免延误病情。

一、气虚证

主要证候　新产后,突然阴道大量出血,色鲜红,头晕目眩,心悸怔忡,气短懒言,肢冷汗出,面色苍白,舌淡,脉虚数。

治　法　补气固冲,摄血止崩。

方　药　升举大补汤加减:黄芪20 g,白术10 g,陈皮6 g,人参(另炖兑入)10 g,炙甘草6 g,升麻6 g,当归10 g,熟地黄10 g,麦门冬10 g,川芎10 g,白芷10 g。黑芥穗10 g,地榆炭10 g,乌贼骨15 g。

加　减　若昏不知人,肢

indistinct pulse, Dushen Tang or Shengmai Injection is used to nourish qi and stop bleeding; for incessant cold sweating and cold limbs, Shenfu Tang or Shenfuqing Injection is used to restore yang and stop adverse development.

(2) Blood stasis syndrome

Main symptoms: Sudden massive bleeding with blood clot from the vagina right after labor, unpressable pain in the lower abdomen, alleviation of abdominal pain after removal of blood clot, dull color of the tongue or with ecchymoses, deep and unsmooth pulse.

Therapeutic methods: Activating blood and eliminating stasis, regulating blood and directing blood to flow in the vessels.

Prescription and drugs: Modified Huayu Zhibeng Tang composed 10g of stir-baked Puhuang (*Pollen Typhae*), 10g of Wulingzhi (*Faeces Trogopterorum*), 30g of Yimucao (*Herba Leonuri*), 10g of Nanshashen (*Radix Adenophorae*), 10g of Danggui (*Radix Angelicae Sinensis*), 6g of Chuanxiong (*Rhizoma Chuanxiong*) and 1.5g of Sanqi powder (*Radix Notoginseng*) (to be taken separately).

Modification: For accompanied chest oppression and vomiting, 10g of Jiangbanxia (*Rhizoma Pinelliae*) is added for descending adverse flow of qi and resolving phlegm.

(3) Birth injury syndrome

Main symptoms: Sudden massive and incessant bleeding from the vagina with fresh red blood, laceration of the soft birth canal, pale complexion, light-colored tongue, thin tongue fur, thin and rapid pulse.

Therapeutic methods: Invigorating qi and nouri-

冷汗出,脉微细欲绝者,用独参汤或生脉注射液补气固脱;若冷汗淋漓,四肢厥逆者,用参附汤或参附青注射液回阳救逆。

二、血瘀证

主要证候 新产后,突然阴道大量下血,夹有血块,小腹疼痛拒按,血块下后腹痛减轻,舌淡黯,或有瘀点瘀斑,脉沉涩。

治 法 活血祛瘀,理血归经。

方 药 化瘀止崩汤加减:炒蒲黄10g,五灵脂10g,益母草30g,南沙参10g,当归10g,川芎6g,三七粉(另吞)1.5g。

加 减 若兼胸闷呕哕者,加姜半夏10g以降逆化痰。

三、产伤证

主要证候 新产后,突然阴道大量下血,血色鲜红,持续不止,软产道有裂伤,面色苍白,舌淡,苔薄,脉细数。

治 法 益气养血,生肌

shing blood, promoting granulation and strengthening meridians and vessels.

Prescription and drugs: Muli San composed of 15g of Muli (*Caro Ostreae*), 10g of Shudihuang (*Rhizoma Rehmanniae Praeparata*), 10g of Fuling (*Poria*), 10g of Longgu (*Os Draconis*), 10g of Xuduan (*Radix Dipsaci*), 10g of Danggui (*Radix Angelicae Sinensis*), 10g of stir-baked Aiye (*Folium Artemisiae Argyi*), 10g of Renshen (*Radix Ginseng*), 10g of Wuweizi (*Fructus Schisandrae*), 10g of Diyu (*Radix Sanguisorbae*) and 5g of Gancao (*Radix Glycyrrhizae*).

If the soft birth canal is evidently injured, it must be sutured immediately and then treated with Chinese medicinal herbs.

[**Other therapeutic methods**]

(1) Chinese patent drugs

1) Danggui Buxue Pill: 9g each time and twice or three times a day, applicable to the recuperative treatment of postpartum hemorrhage due to blood asthenia.

2) Buzhong Yiqi Pill: 9g each time and twice a day, applicable to the recuperative treatment of postpartum hemorrhage due to blood asthenia and qi exhaustion.

3) Shiquan Dabu Pill: 9g each time and twice a day, applicable to the recuperative treatment of postpartum hemorrhage due to qi asthenia.

4) Yimucao Paste: One spoon each time and twice or three times a day, applicable to the recuperative treatment of postpartum hemorrhage due to blood stasis.

(2) Empirical and folk recipes

1) Shensanqi (*Radix Notoginseng*) Powder: 1.5g each time and twice or three times a day, applicable to the treatment of postpartum hemorrhage due to blood stasis.

2) Renshen (*Radix Ginseng*) Powder: 1.5 - 2g is taken when hemorrhage occurs, applicable to the treat-

固经。

方　药　牡蛎散：煅牡蛎15 g,熟地黄10 g,茯苓10 g,龙骨(先煎)10 g,续断10 g,当归10 g,炒艾叶10 g,人参10 g,五味子10 g,地榆10 g,甘草5 g。

若软产道裂伤明显,应及时缝合止血,继以中药调治。

【其他疗法】

1. 中成药

（1）当归补血丸　每次服9 g,1 日 2～3 次,适用于血虚证产后出血调理。

（2）补中益气丸　每次服9 g,1 日 2 次,适用于血虚气脱证产后出血调理。

（3）十全大补丸　每次服9 g,1 日 2 次,适用于气虚证产后出血调理。

（4）益母草膏　每次服1匙,1 日 2～3 次,适用于血瘀证产后出血调理。

2. 单验方

（1）参三七粉　每服1.5 g,每日 2～3 次,适用于血瘀证产后出血。

（2）人参粉　每服1.5～2 g,失血时吞服,适用于血虚

ment of postpartum hemorrhage due to blood asthenia and qi exhaustion.

3) 0. 5g of Xuejie (*Resina Draconis*) powder is taken each time and three times a day, applicable to the treatment of postpartum hemorrhage due to blood stasis.

4) 15g of Puhuang (*Pollen Typhae*) is decocted for oral taking, applicable to the treatment of postpartum hemorrhage due to blood stasis.

5) 6g of stir-baked Puhuang (*Pollen Typhae*), 15g of Xianhecao (*Herba Agrimoniae*) and 6g of Danggui (*Radix Angelicae Sinensis*) are decocted for oral taking, applicable to the treatment of postpartum sudden incessant and massive hemorrhage.

2.7.2 Puerperal infection

Puerperal infection refers to infection of the birth canal during labor or puerperium. The incidence of puerperal infection is 1%-7.2%, and it is one of the four essential causes of parturient death.

The main symptoms are fever, abdominal pain and foul lochia, pertaining to the conception of postpartum fever in TCM. The causes of puerperal infection are various. It is usually caused by sexual activity in the late stage of pregnancy, or early rupture of amniotic fluid, prolonged labor, or improper caring during labor, faulty sterilization or injury of birth canal. The main syndrome is interior retention of blood stasis, tending to develop into syndrome of fever due to retention of blood stasis. Though the location is in the pelvic cavity, the pathogenic factors enter nutrient and blood phases from the defensive and qi phases or even invade the pericardium and disturb the mind, leading to a series of symptoms of intoxication.

气脱证产后出血。

（3）血竭末 0.5 g，每日 3 次冲服，适用于血瘀证产后出血。

（4）蒲黄15 g，水煎服，适用于血瘀证产后出血。

（5）炒蒲黄6 g，仙鹤草 15 g，当归6 g，水煎服。适用于产后血崩，出血不止之证。

第二节　产褥感染

产褥感染是指分娩及产褥期生殖道的感染，引起局部和全身的炎性变化。发病率为1%～7.2%，是产妇死亡的四大原因之一。

本病以发热、腹痛、恶露有臭气为主要症状。故中医归属于"产后发热"范畴。多因妊娠后期不禁房事，或有早期破水、产程延长，或产时处理不当、消毒不严或产道损伤等，外邪经产道感染所致。其主要证型为瘀血内阻，且易出现瘀阻发热之证。病位虽在盆腔子宫，但邪毒由卫、气而入营入血，甚则逆传心包，神明失守，出现一系列中毒症状。

[Key points for diagnosis]

(1) Fever lingers for 10 days after labor and maintains over 38℃, accompanied by abdominal pain and abnormal changes of the color, texture, quantity and odor of vaginal secreta or red swelling, distension and pain of perineal wound.

(2) Gynecological examination, blood and urine test as well as culture of cervical secreta are made to differentiate the location of infection and the bacteria responsible for infection.

(3) Puerperal infection should be differentiated from fever due to blood asthenia, exogenous pathogenic factors, mammary inflammation and pyelonephritis.

[Syndrome differentiation and treatment]

Clinically it is classified into syndrome of infection due to virulent factors and syndrome of blood stasis. The therapeutic principle is clearing away heat and eliminating toxin. This disease is quick in transmission. Therapeutically, treatment of integrated traditional Chinese and Western medicine is necessary.

(1) Syndrome of infection due to virulent factors

Main symptoms: High fever, chills, unpressable pain in the lower abdomen, profuse or scanty lochia with purplish and blackish color and foul odor, dysphoria, thirst, scanty and yellow urine, retention of dry feces, red tongue with yellow fur, rapid and powerful pulse.

Therapeutic methods: Clearing away heat and eliminating toxin, cooling blood and resolving stasis.

Prescription and drugs: Modified Jiedu Huoxue Tang composed of 15g of Lianqiao (*Fructus Forsythiae*), 15g of Jinyinhua (*Flos Lonicerae*), 10g of Huangqin (*Radix Scutellariae*), 10g of Gegen (*Radix Puerariae*), 10g of Chaihu (*Radix Bupleuri*), 5g of Gancao

【诊断要点】

(1) 产后 10 天内发热不解,连续 3 天体温在 38℃ 以上,并伴有腹痛及阴道分泌物的色、质、量、气味异常;或有会阴部伤口红肿胀痛。

(2) 作妇科检查,血、尿常规检查,宫颈分泌物培养等,以明确感染部位及致病菌。

(3) 应与血虚、外感及乳腺炎、肾盂肾炎所致发热相鉴别。

【辨证论治】

本病临床主要分为感染邪毒证及血瘀证,治疗以清热解毒为原则。本病传变迅速,治疗上需要中西医结合。

一、感染邪毒证

主要证候　高热寒战,小腹疼痛拒按,恶露量多或少,色紫黯如败酱,有臭气,烦躁口渴,尿少色黄,大便燥结,舌红苔黄,脉数有力。

治　法　清热解毒,凉血化瘀。

方　药　解毒活血汤加减:连翘15 g,金银花15 g,黄芩10 g,葛根10 g,柴胡10 g,甘草 5 g,生地黄10 g,红花10 g,桃仁10 g,当归10 g,赤芍药

(*Radix Glycyrrhizae*), 10g of Shengdihuang (*Radix Rehmanniae*), 10g of Honghua (*Flos Carthami*), 10g of Taoren (*Semen Persicae*), 10g of Danggui (*Radix Angelicae Sinensis*), 10g of Chishaoyao (*Radix Paeoniae Rubra*) and 10g of Zhike (*Fructus Aurantii*).

Modification: For lingering high fever, profuse sweating, restless thirst, polydipsia, weak, large and rapid pulse, Baihu Tang is used with Renshen (*Radix Ginseng*) for clearing away heat to eliminate restlessness and nourishing qi to produce body fluid; for lingering high fever, restless thirst, polydipsia, retention of dry feces, inhibited discharge of lochia with foul odor like pus, unpressable pain in the lower abdomen, or even fullness and pain in the whole abdomen, delirium, purplish and blackish tongue, yellow and dry tongue fur or dry and prickly tongue fur, slippery and rapid pulse, Dahuang Mudanpi Tang is used for sustaining yin in drastic purgation; for high fever, dysphoria and restlessness, latent maculae, deep-red tongue with scanty or patched fur, taut, thin and rapid pulse, Qingying Tang is used for clearing away heat in blood and eliminating toxin as well as dissipating stasis and reducing heat; for lingering high fever and delirium, Angong Niuhuang Pill or Zixue Bolus can be used.

(2) Blood stasis syndrome

Main symptoms: Fever or alternate fever and chills, profuse or unsmooth lochia with purplish color and stagnant clot, unpressable pain in the lower abdomen, aching and distending sensation in the loins, poor appetite, lassitude, purplish and blackish tongue, thin and yellow fur, rapid and weak pulse.

Therapeutic methods: Activating blood and resolving stasis.

Prescription and drugs: Modified Jiawei Shenghua

10 g, 枳壳10 g。

　　加　减　若高热不退,大汗出,烦渴引饮,脉虚大而数者,用白虎加人参汤以清热除烦,益气生津;若高热不退,烦渴引饮,大便燥结,恶露不畅,秽臭如脓,小腹疼痛拒按,甚则全腹满痛,神昏谵语,舌紫黯,苔黄而燥,或焦老芒剥,脉滑数者,用大黄牡丹皮汤以急下存阴;若高热汗出,心烦不安,斑疹隐隐,舌红绛,苔少或花剥,脉弦细数者,方用清营汤以清营解毒,散瘀泻热;若壮热不退,神昏谵语者,可配服安宫牛黄丸或紫雪丹。

二、血瘀证

　　主要证候　产后数日,发热或寒热时作,恶露较多或不畅,色紫黯而有瘀块,少腹阵痛拒按,腰酸而胀,胃纳差,身倦无力,舌质紫黯,苔薄黄,脉数虚大无力。

　　治　法　活血化瘀。

　　方　药　加味生化汤加

Tang composed of 10g of Danggui (*Radix Angelicae Sinensis*), 15g of Yimucao (*Herba Leonuri*), 6g of Chuanxiong (*Rhizoma Chuanxiong*), 6g of Paojiang (*processed Rhizoma Zingiberis*), 9g of Taoren (*Semen Persicae*), 9g of Shanzha (*Fructus Crataegi*), 5g of Gancao (*Radix Glycyrrhizae*), 10g of Jinyinhua (*Flos Lonicerae*), 10g of Lianqiao (*Fructus Forsythiae*), 15g of Baijiangcao (*Herba Patriniae*) and 9g of Guanzhong (*Rhizoma Dryopteris Gassirhizomae*).

Modification: For alternate fever and chills, 10g of Chaihu (*Radix Bupleuri*), 12g of Huangqin (*Radix Scutellariae*), 3 slices of Shengjiang (*Rhizoma Zingiberis Recens*), 9g of Dazao (*Fructus Jujubae*), 9g of Chishaoyao (*Radix Paeoniae Rubra*) and 9g of Mudanpi (*Cortex Moutan Radicis*) are added; for infection due to retention of placenta, 10g of Chuanniuxi (*Radix Cyathulae*), 9g of Qumai (*Herba Dianthi*) and 9g of Dongkuizi (*Semen Malvae*) are added; for poor appetite and greasy and thick tongue fur, 15g of Hongteng (*Caulis Sargentodoxae*), 30g of Yiyiren (*Semen Coicis*) and 10g of Cangzhu (*Rhizoma Atractylodis*) are added.

[Other therapeutic methods]

(1) Chinese patent drugs

1) Niuhuang Qingxin Pill: 1 pill each time and twice a day, applicable to the medium stage of pathogenic heat and virulent fire.

2) Niuhuang Qingre Powder: 1.5g each time and 3-4 times a day, applicable to puerperal infection due to invasion of pathogenic heat in blood.

3) Shuiniujiao Jiedu Pill: 3g each time and three times a day, applicable to puerperal infection due to invasion of pathogenic heat in blood.

4) Niuhuang Jiedu Pill: 3g each time and twice or three times a day, applicable to infection due to virulence

减：当归10 g，益母草15 g，川芎6 g，炮姜6 g，桃仁9 g，山楂9 g，甘草5 g，金银花10 g，连翘10 g，败酱草15 g，贯众9 g。

加　减　寒热往来者，加柴胡10 g，黄芩12 g，生姜3 片，大枣9 g，赤芍药9 g，牡丹皮9 g；胎盘胎膜残留引起感染者，加川牛膝10 g，瞿麦9 g，冬葵子9 g；纳欠、苔腻厚者，加红藤15 g，薏苡仁30 g，制苍术10 g。

【其他疗法】

1. 中成药

（1）牛黄清心丸　每次服1 丸，1 日2 次，适用于邪热火毒证中期。

（2）牛黄清热散　每次服1.5 g，1 日3～4次，适用于热入营血证产褥感染。

（3）水牛角解毒丸　每次服3 g，1 日3 次，适用于热入营血证产褥感染。

（4）牛黄解毒丸　每次服3 g，1 日2～3 次，适用于感

attack.

5）Qingkailing Injection：Each ampule contains 2ml, 2 - 4ml each time for intramuscular injection and twice or three times a day. Or 5% GS 500ml + 2 - 4ml Qingkailing Injection for intravenous drip, applicable to the treatment of puerperal infection due to invasion of heat into the pericardium.

(2) Empirical and folk recipes

1）Tuire Yin composed of 12g of crude Shanzha (*Fructus Crataegi*), 12g of Shengdihuang (*Radix Reh-manniae*), 8g of Chuanxiong (*Rhizoma Chuanxiong*), 15g of Yimucao (*Herba Leonuri*), 9g of Honghua (*Flos Carthami*) and 8g of Huangqin (*Radix Scutellariae*). These ingredients are decocted for oral taking, applicable to the treatment of postpartum stagnation and depression marked by abdominal pain and lingering fever.

2）100g of Machixian (*Herba Portulacae*) and 50g of Pugongying (*Herba Taraxaci*) are decocted for oral taking, applicable to the treatment of puerperal infection due to virulent toxic factors.

2.7.3 Lochiorrhea

Lochiorrhea is marked by incessant discharge of lochia for over three weeks after labor, usually seen in subinvolution of uterus, infectious disease and diseases due to disturbance of blood coagulation.

Lochiorrhea is usually caused by weakness, exhaustion of qi with loss of blood during labor, impairment of the spleen due to puerperal overstrain, sinking of the gastrosplenic qi, weakness of the thoroughfare and conception vessels to control blood; or by excessive intake of

染邪毒证感染。

（5）清开灵注射液 每支2 ml,1 次 2～4 ml,肌肉注射,1 日 2～3 次,或用5％葡萄糖500 ml加 2～4 ml清开灵注射液静脉滴注。适用于产褥感染热陷心包证。

2. 单验方

（1）退热饮 生山楂12 g,生地黄12 g,川芎 8 g,益母草15 g,红花9 g,黄芩 8 g,水煎服,适用于产后瘀郁,腹痛身热不退。

（2）马齿苋 100 g,蒲公英50 g,水煎服,适用于感染邪毒证产褥感染。

第三节 恶露不绝

产后恶露不绝是指产后恶露持续 3 周以上,仍淋漓不尽者,西医妇科疾病如子宫复旧不全、感染性疾病、凝血机能障碍性疾病等均可见恶露淋漓不止。

本病多因素体虚弱,产时气随血耗,或产后操劳过早伤脾,中气虚陷,冲任失固,血失统摄;或产后过食辛辣温燥之品,或肝气郁而化热,热伤冲

pungent and dry foods after labor; or by transformation of heat from depression of liver qi that impairs the thoroughfare and conception vessels as well as drives blood to flow abnormally; or by invasion of pathogenic cold after labor, leading to cold coagulation and blood stasis; or by emotional factors, qi stagnation and blood stasis in the thoroughfare and conception vessels as well as abnormal circulation of qi and blood. The main symptoms are incessant lochiorrhea for over three weeks and distension or pain in the lower abdomen.

[Key points for diagnosis]

(1) Vaginal bleeding with small amount over three weeks after labor.

(2) Gynecological examination is necessary to detect subinvolution, or mild infection of the uterus, or retention of placenta and fetal membrane.

(3) Choriocarcinoma and malignant mole should be excluded.

[Syndrome differentiation and treatment]

Syndrome differentiation is done according to the quantity, color, texture and odor of lochia in order to decide whether it is of cold, heat, asthenia or sthenia nature. The therapeutic principles are to improve asthenia, purge stagnation and clear away heat. Syndrome differentiation should be done in light of disease differentiation. The therapeutic methods usually used are checking blood, clearing away heat and resolving stasis. Lochiorrhea must be controlled as quick as possible lest massive uterine bleeding be caused.

(1) Qi asthenia syndrome

Main symptoms: Postpartum incessant and profuse lochiorrhea with light color, thin texture and no odor, spiritual lassitude, weakness of the limbs, shortness of

任,破血妄行;或产后寒邪乘虚而入,寒凝血瘀,或七情内伤,气滞血瘀,瘀阻冲任所致,主要是冲任为病,气血运行失常。临证以产后恶露逾 3 周仍淋漓不止,小腹或坠或胀或痛为主要症状。

【诊断要点】

(1) 产后 3 周以上,阴道仍有少量出血。

(2) 妇科检查可确诊子宫复旧不良,或子宫轻度感染,或胎盘、胎膜残留。

(3) 应排除绒癌及恶性葡萄胎。

【辨证论治】

本病的辨证,应从恶露的量、色、质、气味等辨别寒、热、虚、实,治疗应宗虚者补之,瘀者攻之,热者清之的原则,且必须辨证与辨病相结合,分别采用摄血、清热、化瘀法 。尽早控制恶露,严防血崩。

一、气虚证

主要证候　产后恶露过期不止,量多,色淡红,质稀,无臭味,精神倦怠,四肢无力,

breath, no desire to speak, empty prolapsing sensation in the abdomen, bright white complexion, thin and white tongue fur, slow and weak pulse.

Therapeutic methods: Nourishing qi and checking blood.

Prescription and drugs: Modified Buzhong Yiqi Tang composed of 20g of Dangshen (*Radix Codonopsis Pilosulae*), 20g of Huangqi (*Radix Astragali*), 10g of Baizhu (*Rhizoma Atractylodis Macrocephalae*), 6g of roasted Gancao (*Radix Glycyrrhizae*), 5g of Chenpi (*Pericarpium Citri Reticulatae*), 6g of Shengma (*Rhizoma Cimicifugae*), 6g of Chaihu (*Radix Bupleuri*) and 10g of Ejiao (*Colla Corii Asini*) (to be melted for decocting).

Modification: For relative predominance of cold, 10g of Lujiaojiao (*Colla Cornus Cervi*) (to be melted for decocting) and 10g of charred Aiye (*Folium Artemisiae Argyi*) are added; for loose stool, 5g of Paojiang (*processed Rhizoma Zingiberis*) and 6g of Sharen (*Fructus Amomi*) (to be decocted later) are added; for sticky lochia with foul odor, 15g of Baijiangcao (*Herba Patriniae*) and 15g of Yiyiren (*Semen Coicis*) are added.

(2) Blood heat syndrome

Main symptoms: Postpartum incessant and profuse lochiorrhea with deep-red color, sticky texture and foul odor, dry mouth and throat, flushed cheeks, red tongue, scanty tongue fur, thin, rapid and weak pulse.

Therapeutic methods: Nourishing yin and clearing away heat, cooling blood and stopping bleeding.

Prescription and drugs: Modified Baoyin Jian composed of 10g of Shengdihuang (*Radix Rehmanniae*), 10g of Baishaoyao (*Radix Paeoniae Alba*), 10g of Shanyao (*Rhizoma Dioscoreae*), 10g of Xuduan (*Radix Dip-*

气短懒言,小腹空坠,面色㿠白,舌淡,苔薄白,脉缓弱。

治　法　益气摄血。

方　药　补中益气汤加减:党参20 g,黄芪20 g,白术10 g,炙甘草6 g,陈皮5 g,升麻6 g,柴胡6 g,阿胶(烊冲)10 g。

加　减　偏寒者加入鹿角胶(烊冲)10 g,艾叶炭10 g;大便偏溏者加入炮姜5 g,砂仁(后下)6 g;若恶露质粘腻,有臭气者,加败酱草15 g,薏苡仁15 g。

二、血热证

主要证候　产后恶露过期不止,量较多,色深红,质稠粘,气臭秽,口燥咽干,面色潮红,舌红,苔少,脉细数无力。

治　法　益阴清热,凉血止血。

方　药　保阴煎加减:生地10 g,白芍药10 g,山药10 g,续断10 g,黄芩6 g,黄柏10 g,熟地黄10 g,甘草6 g。

saci), 6g of Huangqin (*Radix Scutellariae*), 10g of Huangbai (*Cortex Phellodendri*), 10g of Shudihuang (*Rhizoma Rehmanniae Praeparata*) and 6g of Gancao (*Radix Glycyrrhizae*).

Modification: For asthenia of qi, 10g of roasted Huangqi (*Radix Astragali*) and 10g of Taizishen (*Radix Pseudostellariae*) are added; for transformation of fire from liver depression marked by distending pain in hypochondria, dysphoria, bitter taste in the mouth, taut and rapid pulse, Danzhi Xiaoyao Powder can be used; for attack by pathogenic heat with the complication of damp-heat, 30g of Hongteng (*Caulis Sargentodoxae*), 30g of Baijiangcao (*Herba Patriniae*) and 10g of Diyu (*Radix Sanguisorbae*) are added.

(3) Blood stasis syndrome

Main symptoms: Postpartum incessant scanty lochiorrhea with blackish color and blood clot, unpressable pain in the lower abdomen, alleviation of pain after removal of the clot, purplish and blackish tongue or with ecchymoses, taut and unsmooth pulse.

Therapeutic methods: Activating blood and resolving stasis, regulating blood and directing it to flow in the vessels.

Prescription and drugs: Modified Shenghua Tang composed 10g of Danggui (*Radix Angelicae Sinensis*), 6g of Chuanxiong (*Rhizoma Chuanxiong*), 6g of Taoren (*Semen Persicae*), 5g of Paojiang (*Rhizoma Zingiberis*), 10g of Gancao (*Radix Glycyrrhizae*) and 10g of Shixiao Powder (to be wrapped) and 10g of Yimucao (*Herba Leonuri*).

Modification: For qi asthenia with empty prolapsing sensation in the lower abdomen, 20g of Dangshen (*Radix Codonopsis Pilosulae*) and 20g of Huangqi (*Radix*

加　减　兼气虚者,加炙黄芪10g,太子参10g;肝郁化火,两胁胀痛,心烦口苦,脉弦数者,用丹栀逍遥散;感受邪热,兼夹湿热者,加红藤30g,败酱草30g,地榆10g。

三、血瘀证

主要证候　产后恶露过期不止,淋漓量少,色黯有块,小腹疼痛拒按,块下痛减,舌紫黯,或有瘀点,脉弦涩。

治　法　活血化瘀,理血归经。

方　药　生化汤加减:当归10g,川芎6g,桃仁6g,炮姜5g,甘草10g,失笑散(包)10g,益母草10g。

加　减　气虚,小腹空坠者,加党参20g,黄芪20g;肝气郁结,胸胁胀痛,脉弦者,加

Astragali) are added; for depression of liver qi with distending pain in the chest and hypochondria, and taut pulse, 10g of Yujin (*Radix Curcumae*), 10g of Xiangfu (*Rhizoma Cyperi*) and 10g of Chuanlianzi (*Fructus Toosendan*) are added; for relative predominance of cold to be alleviated with warmth, 5g of Rougui (*Cortex Cinnamomi*) and 6g of Xiaohuixiang (*Fructus Foeniculi*) are added, or Shaofu Zhuyu Tang is used; for downward migration of damp heat with sticky and foul lochiorrhea, 15g of Hongteng (*Caulis Sargentodoxae*), 15g of Baijiangcao (*Herba Patriniae*), 10g of Pugongying (*Herba Taraxaci*), 15g of Machixian (*Herba Portulacae*) and 15g of Yiyiren (*Semen Coicis*) are added.

[Other therapeutic methods]

(1) Chinese patent drugs

1) Yimucao (Herba Leonuri): 20ml each time and three times a day, applicable to the treatment of blood stasis syndrome.

2) Shenghua Decoction: 9g each time and three times a day, applicable to the treatment of blood asthenia and cold coagulation syndrome.

3) Yunnan Baiyao (White Powder): 0.2 - 0.3g each time and once four hours, applicable to the treatment of blood stasis syndrome.

4) Fuke Huisheng Bolus: 9g each time and twice a day, applicable to the treatment of qi asthenia and blood stasis syndrome.

5) Baizhen Yimu Pill: 9g each time and three times a day, applicable to the treatment of asthenia of qi and blood syndrome.

(2) Empirical and folk recipes

1) Fufang Shenghua Decoction: 10g of Danggui (*Radix Angelicae Sinensis*), 6g of roasted Chuanxiong (*Rhizoma Chuanxiong*), 9g of Shudihuang (*Rhizoma*

郁金10 g,香附10 g,川楝子10 g;偏寒得热则舒者,加肉桂5 g,小茴香6 g,或用少腹逐瘀汤;兼有湿热下注,恶露粘稠,有秽臭味者,加红藤15 g,败酱草15 g,蒲公英10 g,马齿苋15 g,薏苡仁15 g。

【其他疗法】

1. 中成药

（1）益母草　每次服20 ml,1 日 3 次,适用于血瘀证。

（2）生化汤丸　每次服9 g,1 日 3 次,适用于血虚寒凝证。

（3）云南白药　每次服0.2～0.3 g,每 4 小时 1 次,适用于血瘀证。

（4）妇科回生丹　每次服9 g,1 日 2 次,适用于气虚血瘀证。

（5）八珍益母丸　每次服9 g,1 日 3 次,适用于气血虚弱证。

2. 单验方

（1）复方生化汤　当归10 g,炒川芎6 g,熟地黄9 g,桃仁6 g,炮姜5 g,益母草10 g,牡

Rehmanniae Praeparata), 6g of Taoren (*Semen Persicae*), 5g of Paojiang (*Rhizoma Zingiberis*), 10g of Yimucao (*Herba Leonuri*), 9g of Mudanpi (*Cortex Moutan Radicis*) and 5g of roasted Gancao (*Radix Glycyrrhizae*) are decocted for oral taking, applicable to the treatment of lochiorrhea due to faulty uterine contraction.

2) Shuanghua Decoction: 15g of Jiguanhua (*Inflorescentia Celosiae Cristatae*), 15g of Jinyinhua (*Flos Lonicerae*), 10g of Danggui (*Radix Angelicae Sinensis*) and 10g of Zelan (*Herba Lycopi*) are decocted for oral taking, applicable to the treatment of lochiorrhea after artificial abortion or induced labor.

3) 15g of crispy Shanzha (*Fructus Crataegi*), 5g of Zelan (*Herba Lycopi*) and 10g of Yimucao (*Herba Leonuri*) are decocted together with proper amount of brown sugar for oral taking, applicable to the treatment of postpartum lochiorrhea due to blood asthenia and blood stasis.

2.7.4　Sunstroke in puerperium

Sunstroke in puerperium refers to dysfunction of central system in regulating body temperature when the parturient is staying in high temperature. Sunstroke in puerperium is usually caused by invasion of summer-heat or summer-heat and dampness and turbid pathogenic factors into the body and consumption of body fluid due to asthenia of meridians and vessels in the parturient; or by transmission of pathogenic heat into the heart blood due to wrong treatment or delayed treatment. The main symptoms of this disease are fever, dizziness, unconsciousness, convulsion, profuse sweating, shallow breath and indistinct pulse, pertaining to the conception of summer febrile disease in TCM.

丹皮9 g,炙甘草 5 g,水煎服,适用于产后子宫收缩不良之恶露不绝。

（2）双花汤　鸡冠花15 g,金银花15 g,当归10 g,泽兰10 g,水煎服,适用于人流或引产后恶露不绝。

（3）焦山楂15 g,泽兰5 g,益母草10 g,红糖适量,水煎服,适用于血虚血瘀证产后恶露不绝。

第四节　产褥中暑

产褥中暑是指产妇在高温环境中引起的中枢性体温调节功能障碍。本病多因产妇产后百脉空虚,暑热或暑湿秽浊之邪乘虚侵袭,耗气伤津;若误治失治,则可内传心营。临证以发热、头昏、胸闷、神志昏迷、抽搐、多汗、呼吸浅促、脉微为主要症状。故中医归属"暑温病"范畴。

[Key points for diagnosis]

(1) Premonitory signs of sun-stroke: Early symptoms are headache, vertigo, palpitation, thirst and chest oppression, occasionally accompanied by fever, lassitude of limbs and profuse sweating.

(2) Mild sunstroke: Gradual increase of body temperature, aggravation of headache and chest oppression, nausea and vomiting, flushed cheeks, rapid heart beating, dyspnea, restlessness and decrease of blood pressure.

(3) Severe sunstroke: High fever (41 - 42℃), no sweating, delirium, convulsion, coma, miosis, hyporeflexia, dyspnea, thin and rapid pulse and death due to heart and lung failure.

(4) Sunstroke in puerperium should be differentiated from eclampsia gravidarum and hematosepsis due to puerperal infection.

[Syndrome differentiation and treatment]

This disease is classified into syndrome of summer-heat consuming qi and fluid as well as syndrome of summer-heat invading heart blood. The therapeutic methods are clearing away summer-heat and invigorating qi, nourishing yin and promoting production of body fluid, cooling nutrient blood and reducing heat as well as clearing the heart and resuscitating brain.

(1) Syndrome of summer-heat consuming qi and fluid

Main symptoms: Puerperium in summer tends to develop such symptoms like fever, profuse sweating, thirst, dysphoria, lassitude, red tongue with scanty fluid and weak and rapid pulse.

Therapeutic methods: Clearing away summer-heat and nourishing qi, nourishing yin and promoting produc-

【诊断要点】

(1) 中暑先兆：早期出现头痛、头晕、心悸、口渴、胸闷，有时伴发热、四肢无力、大量出汗。

(2) 轻度中暑：体温渐升高，头痛胸闷渐加重，恶心呕吐，面色潮红，心率快，呼吸急促，烦躁，血压下降。

(3) 重度中暑：高热，体温达 41～42℃，无汗，谵妄，抽搐，昏迷，瞳孔缩小，反射减弱，呼吸急促，脉搏细数，心肺衰竭死亡。

(4) 须与产后子痫、产褥感染导致的败血症相鉴别。

【辨证论治】

本病临床主要分为暑伤气津证及暑入心营证。治疗以清暑益气、养阴生津、凉营泻热、清心开窍为主。

一、暑伤气津证

主要证候　产褥期正值盛夏之时，身热多汗，口渴心烦，倦怠乏力，舌红少津，脉虚数。

治　法　清暑益气，养阴生津。

tion of body fluid.

Prescription and drugs: Modified Qingshu Yiqi
Tang composed of 10g of Xiyangshen (*Radix Panacis
Quinquefolii*), 10g of Shihu (*Herba Dendrobii*), 10g of
Maimendong (*Radix Ophiopogonis*), 5g of Huanglian
(*Rhizoma Coptidis*), 10g of Zhuye (*Herba Lophan-
theri*), 10g of Hegeng (*Petiolus Nelumbinis*), 10g of
Zhimu (*Rhizoma Anemarrhenae*), 5g of Gancao (*Radix
Glycyrrhizae*), 30g of Jingmi (*Fructus Oryzae Sati-
vae*) and 30g of Xiguapi (*Exocarpium Citrulli*).

Modification: For no sweating, 10g of Xiangru
(*Herba Elsholtziae*) is added; for nausea and vomiting,
10g of Zhuru (*Caulis Bambusae in Taeniam*) and 6g of
Chenpi (*Pericarpium Citri Reticulatae*) are added; for
heavy sensation in the body, epigastric stiffness, nausea,
vomiting, yellow and greasy tongue fur, 10g of Huashi
(*Talcum*), 10g of Tongcao (*Medulla Tetrapanacis*)
and 10g of Zhuling (*Polygorus*) are added for reducing
summer-heat and eliminating dampness.

(2) Syndrome of summer-heat invading heart blood

Main symptoms: High fever, restlessness,
disturbed sleep in the night, occasional delirium, or even
coma, deep-red tongue, thin and rapid pulse; or sudden
syncope, unconsciousness, feverish sensation in the body,
cold limbs, dyspnea, inability to speak, mild lockjaw,
deep-red tongue and rapid pulse.

Therapeutic methods: Cooling blood and reducing
heat, clearing the heart and resuscitating brain.

Prescription and drugs: Qingying decoction composed of 10g of Xijiao (*Cornu Rhinocerotis*) (substituted
by buffalo horn), 15g of Shengdihuang (*Radix Rehmanniae*), 10g of Xuanshen (*Radix Scrophulariae*), 3g

方 药 清暑益气汤：
西洋参10 g，石斛10 g，麦门冬
10 g，黄连 5 g，竹叶10 g，荷梗
10 g，知母10 g，甘草 5 g，粳米
30 g，西瓜皮30 g。

加 减 无汗加香薷
10 g；恶心呕吐，加竹茹10 g，
陈皮6 g；若身重，脘痞呕恶，苔
黄腻者，加滑石 10 g，通 草
10 g，猪苓10 g以消暑渗湿。

二、暑入心营证

主要证候 灼热烦躁，夜
寐不宁，时有谵语，甚或昏迷
不语，舌红绛，脉细数；或猝然
昏倒，不省人事，身热肢厥，气
喘不语，舌关微紧，舌绛脉数。

治 法 凉营泄热，清心
开窍。

方 药 清营汤：犀角
（现以水牛角代）10 g，生地黄
15 g，玄参10 g，竹叶心3 g，麦
门冬10 g，牡丹皮6 g，黄连3 g，

of Zhuyexin (*Plumula Lophantheri*), 10g of Maimen-dong (*Radix Ophiopogonis*), 6g of Mudanpi (*Cortex Moutan Radicis*), 10g of Jinyinhua (*Flos Lonicerae*) and 10g of Lianqiao (*Fructus Forsythiae*). One or two pills of Angong Niuhuang Wan can be taken.

Modification: For convulsion of limbs, 3g of Quan-xie (*Scorpio*), 5g of Wugong (*Scolopendra*), 10g of Shuizhi (*Hirudo*) and 10g of Gouteng (*Ramulus Uncariae cum Uncis*) are added.

[Other therapeutic methods]

(1) Chinese patent drugs

1) Qingshu Yiqi Pill: 9g each time and twice a day, applicable to the treatment of syndrome due to invasion of pathogenic summer-heat.

2) Shidishui: 0.5 - 1mleach time and twice or three times a day, applicable to the treatment of interior retention of summer-heat.

3) Rendan: 10 - 15 pills each time without time restriction, applicable to the treatment of interior stagnation of pathogenic summer-heat.

4) Huoxiang Zhengqi Liquid (Pill): For the pills, 1g each time and twice a day; for the liquid, (each bottle contains 10ml) 10ml each time and twice a day.

(2) Empirical and folk recipes

1) One piece of lotus leaf, 30 - 60g of Qinghao (*Herba Artemisiae Annuae*), Lüdou (*Semen Phaseoli Radiati*), watermelon rind, Peilan (*Herba Eupatorii*) and Jinyinhua (*Flos Lonicerae*) respectively: Select one or two of these ingredients to soak in boiling water or decoct and take as tea.

2) The patient is moved to a shadow and cool place and is treated with cold compress. Then juice of ginger, Chinese chives and 3 - 5 garlic cloves is taken orally, ap-

金银花10 g,连翘10 g。送服安宫牛黄丸1~2 丸。

加　减　若伴四肢抽搐者,加全蝎3 g,蜈蚣 5 g,水蛭10 g,钩藤10 g。

【其他疗法】

1. 中成药

（1）清暑益气丸　每次服9 g,1 日 2 次,适用于暑邪侵袭证。

（2）十滴水　每服0.5~1 ml,1 日 2~3 次,适用于暑热内困证。

（3）人丹　每服 10~15粒,不拘时间,适用于暑邪内闭证。

（4）藿香正气水（丸）丸剂,每次服 1 g,1 日 2 次;滴水 剂, 每 支 10 ml, 每 次 服10 ml,1 日 2 次。

2. 单验方

（1）荷叶 1 张,青蒿、绿豆、西瓜皮、藿香、佩兰、金银花各 30~60 g,任选 1~2 种,开水泡代茶或煎服。

（2）将病人移向阴凉处,冷敷。再用生姜汁、韭菜汁、大蒜3~5 瓣捣烂取汁,灌服,

plicable to the treatment of premonitory signs of sun-stroke.

3) 50g of mung bean is decocted for oral taking, applicable to the treatment of interior accumulation of summer-heat.

4) 50g of Shigao (*Gypsum Fibrosum*) and 0.6g of Bingpian (*Borneolum*) are ground into fine powder. 1.5g each time and three times a day, applicable to the treatment of interior retention of summer-heat.

(3) External therapy

1) 50g of salt is used to rub the hands, feet, hypochondria, chest and back till the skin turns reddish and the patient feels comfortable, applicable to the treatment of interior retention of summer-heat.

2) 1g of Xixin (*Herba Asari*) and 3g of Yazaojiao (*Fructus Gleditsiae Abnormalis*) are ground into powder and blown into the nose of the patient to induce sneezing, applicable to the treatment of sudden syncope due to sunstroke.

2.7.5　Postpartum hypogalactia

　　Postpartum hypogalactia means that the parturient secretes a little or no milk in breast-feeding.

　　Postpartum hypogalactia is usually caused by constitutional asthenia of qi and blood in the parturient complicated by loss of blood and qi in labor; or by hypofunction of the spleen and stomach and insufficiency of the production of qi and blood; or by frequent mental depression; or by postpartum impairment due to emotional factors, disharmony between qi and blood as well as inhibited circulation of qi and blood in meridians and vessels. The clinical symptoms are scanty milk or no milk secretion.

　　适用于中暑先兆。

　　（3）绿豆50 g，水煎服，适用于暑热内蕴证。

　　（4）石膏50 g，加冰片0.6 g共研细末，每服1.5 g，每日3次，适用于暑热内闭证。

　　3. 外治法

　　（1）食盐50 g，擦揉患者手、足、胁、胸、背处，擦出红点为度，觉轻松即愈，适用于暑热内闭证。

　　（2）细辛1 g，牙皂角3 g，研粉，吹鼻得嚏，适用于中暑突然昏倒者。

第五节　产后缺乳

　　产后缺乳是指产妇在哺乳期内乳汁甚少或全无，亦称"乳汁不足"，或"乳汁不行"。

　　本病多因产妇素体气血虚弱，复因产时失血耗气，或脾胃虚弱，气血生化之源不足；或素性抑郁，或产后七情所伤，气血失调，经脉涩滞，乳汁运行受阻所致。临证以乳汁甚少，或全无为主要症状。

[Key points for diagnosis]

(1) Scanty or no secretion of milk after labor.

(2) The breast is soft without distension and pain. Under pressure, it secretes several drops of milk of thin texture. Or the breast is full-grown, but the mammary gland appears in mass. Under pressure, it is very painful and cannot secret milk.

(3) Hypogalactia should be differentiated from obstruction of milk due to crater nipple and rupture of nipple.

[Syndrome differentiation and treatment]

Hypogalactia is either asthenia or sthenia. Hypogalactia without distension and pain pertains to asthenia; while hypogalactia with hardness, distension and pain in the breast pertains to sthenia. The therapeutic principles are reinforcing asthenia and resolving sthenia. Usually nourishing qi to invigorate blood and soothing the liver to relieve stagnation are used in treating hypogalactia in combination with other drugs for promoting lactation according to the pathological conditions. Cares should be taken to prevent breast abscess.

(1) Syndrome of asthenia of qi and blood

Main symptoms: Lack of milk or even no milk after labor, thin milk, soft breasts without distension, spiritual lassitude, poor appetite, lusterless complexion, light-colored tongue with scanty fur, thin and weak pulse.

Therapeutic methods: Nourishing qi and blood in combination with drugs for promoting lactation.

Prescription and drugs: Modified Tongru Dan composed of 12g of Dangshen (*Radix Codonopsis Pilosulae*), 12g of Huangqi (*Radix Astragali*), 10g of Danggui (*Radix Angelicae Sinensis*), 9g of Maimendong (*Radix*

【诊断要点】

（1）产后排出的乳汁量少，甚或全无，不够喂养婴儿。

（2）乳房检查松软，不胀不痛，挤压乳汁点滴而出，质稀。或乳房丰满乳腺成块，挤压乳汁疼痛难出。

（3）排除因乳头凹陷和乳头皲裂造成的乳汁壅积不通，哺乳困难。

【辨证论治】

乳汁缺少，证有虚实，乳房柔软，不胀不痛者为虚；乳房坚硬，胀痛者为实。治疗以虚者补而通之，实者化而通之为原则，根据不同病证分别采用补气益血、疏肝解郁法，并适当配伍通乳之品。且须注意乳痈的防治。

一、气血虚弱证

主要证候　产后乳少，甚或全无，乳汁清稀，乳房柔软，无胀满感，神倦食少，面色少华，舌淡，苔少，脉细弱。

治　法　补气养血，佐以通乳。

方　药　通乳丹加减：党参12 g，黄芪12 g，当归10 g，麦门冬9 g，木通6 g，桔梗6 g，甘草5 g，猪蹄1对。

Ophiopogonis）, 6g of Mutong（*Caulis Akebiae*）, 6g of Jiegeng（*Radix Platycodi*）, 5g of Gancao（*Radix Glycyrrhizae*）and 2 pig trotters.

Modification: For dizziness and palpitation, 10g of Gouqizi（*Fructus Lycii*）, 10g of Danshen（*Radix Salviae Miltiorrhizae*）and 6g of roasted Zaoren（*Semen Ziziphi Spinosae*）are added; for anorexia and abdominal distension, 6g of Chenpi（*Pericarpium Citri Reticulatae*）and 5g of Muxiang（*Radix Aucklaneliae*）are added.

（2）Syndrome of liver qi stagnation

Main symptoms: Inhibited secretion of milk with thick texture or no secretion of milk, distension, hardness and pain in the breasts, mental depression, distension and distress in the chest and hypochondria, poor appetite, or mild fever, normal conditions of the tongue, thin and yellow tongue fur, taut and thin or taut and rapid pulse.

Therapeutic methods: Soothing the liver and relieving stagnation, activating collaterals and promoting secretion of milk.

Prescription and drugs: Modified Xiaru Yongquan San composed of 10g of Danggui（*Radix Angelicae Sinensis*）, 10g of Chishaoyao（*Radix Paeoniae Rubra*）, 10g of Baishaoyao（*Radix Paeoniae Alba*）, 6g of Chuanxiong（*Rhizoma Chuanxiong*）, 9g of Shengdihuang（*Radix Rehmanniae*）, 6g of Chaihu（*Radix Bupleuri*）, 6g of Qingpi（*Pericarpium Citri Reticulatae Viride*）, 6g of Chenpi（*Pericarpium Citri Reticulatae*）, 9g of Tianhuafen（*Radix Trichosanthis*）, 9g of Loulu（*Radix Rhapontici*）, 5g of Jiegeng（*Radix Platycodi*）, 5g of Baizhi（*Radix Angelicae*）, 5g of Mutong（*Caulis Akebiae*）, 9g of roasted sliced Shanjia（*Squama Manitis*）, 9g of Wangbuliuxing（*Semen Vaccariae*）and 5g of Gancao（*Radix Glycyrrhizae*）.

加　减　头晕心悸者,加枸杞子10 g,丹参10 g,炒枣仁6 g;纳呆腹胀者,加陈皮6 g,木香5 g。

二、肝气郁滞证

主要证候　产后乳汁涩少,浓稠,或乳汁不下,乳房胀硬疼痛,情志抑郁,胸胁胀闷,食欲不振,或身有微热,舌正常,苔薄黄,脉弦细或弦数。

治　法　疏肝解郁,活络通乳。

方　药　下乳涌泉散加减:当归10 g,赤芍药10 g,白芍药10 g,川芎6 g,生地黄9 g,柴胡6 g,青皮6 g,陈皮6 g,天花粉9 g,漏芦9 g,桔梗5 g,白芷5 g,木通5 g,炙山甲片9 g,王不留行9 g,甘草5 g。

Modification: For loose stool, Shengdihuang (*Radix Rehmanniae*) and Tianhuafen (*Radix Trichosanthis*) are deleted, while 10g of roasted Baizhu (*Rhizoma Atractylodis Macrocephalae*) and 6g of roasted Muxiang (*Radix Aucklaneliae*) are added; for restless sleep in the night, Baizhi (*Radix Angelicae*) and Chuanxiong (*Rhizoma Chuanxiong*) are deleted, while 6g of roasted Yuanzhi (*Radix Polygalae*) and 9g of roasted Zaoren (*Semen Ziziphi Spinosae*) are added; for severe distension and pain in the breasts, 5g of Juluo (*Vascular Aurantii Citri Tangerinae*), 40g of Sigualuo (*Retinervus Luffae Fructus*) and 10g of Xiangfu (*Rhizoma Cyperi*) are added for regulating qi and dredging collaterals as well as eliminating stagnation and stopping pain; for distension and hardness in the breast, local pyretic sensation and tenderness, 10g of Baijiangcao (*Herba Patriniae*), 15g of Pugongying (*Herba Taraxaci*) and 10g of Chishaoyao (*Radix Paeoniae Rubra*) are added for clearing away heat and cooling blood as well as dispersing stagnation and abating swelling.

[Other therapeutic methods]

(1) Chinese patent drugs

1) Shiquan Dabu Pill: 6g each time and twice a day, applicable to the treatment of hypogalactia due to asthenia of qi and blood.

2) Xiaoyao Pill: 6g each time and three times a day, applicable to the treatment of hypogalactia due to liver depression and qi stagnation.

3) Lujiao Powder: 4g each time and twice a day, applicable to the treatment of agalactia due to asthenia of kidney yang.

4) Yongquan Powder: 3g each time and 3 times a day, applicable to the treatment of hypogalactia due to stagnation of qi and blood.

加　减　大便偏溏者,去生地、天花粉,加炒白术10 g,煨木香6 g;夜寐甚差者,去白芷、川芎,加炙远志6 g,炒枣仁9 g;若乳房胀痛甚者,酌加橘络5 g,丝瓜络40 g,香附10 g以增理气通络、行滞止痛之力;乳房胀硬结块,局部生热,触痛者,酌加败酱草10 g,蒲公英15 g,赤芍药10 g以清热凉血,散结消肿。

【其他疗法】

1. 中成药

(1) 十全大补丸　每次服6 g,1 日 2 次,适用于气血虚弱证缺乳。

(2) 逍遥丸　每次服6 g,1 日 3 次,适用于肝郁气滞证缺乳。

(3) 鹿角粉　每次服4 g,1 日 2 次,适用于肾阳虚乳汁不下。

(4) 涌泉散　每次服3 g,1 日 3 次,适用于气血壅滞证缺乳。

(2) Empirical and folk recipes

1) Zengru Decoction: 10g of roasted sliced Shanjia (*Squama Manitis*), 1 carp and 10g of Wangbuliuxing (*Semen Vaccariae*) are decocted for oral taking, applicable to the treatment of agalactia due to blood asthenia and liver depression.

2) Qiu Xiaomei's Empirical Decoction: 12g of Danggui (*Radix Angelicae Sinensis*), 9g of Lujiaoshuang (*Cornu Cervi Deglatinatum*), 10g of sliced Chuanshanjia (*Squama Manitis*) (to be decocted first), 9g of Wangbuliuxing (*Semen Vaccariae*), 9g of Tianhuafen (*Radix Trichosanthis*) and 1.5g of Tongcao (*Medulla Tetrapanacis*) are decocted for oral taking, applicable to the treatment of agalactia due to kidney asthenia.

3) 90g of Mutong (*Caulis Akebiae*) and 1 pig trotter is decocted for oral taking, applicable to the treatment of agalactia in various syndromes.

4) 250g of Chixiaodou (*Semen Phaseoli*) is decocted for oral taking, applicable to the treatment of agalactia due to asthenia of qi and blood.

5) 6g of roasted Gualouren (*Semen Trichosanthis*) is ground into powder and taken orally with wine, applicable to the treatment of agalactia due to blood stasis and cold coagulation.

2. 单验方

（1）增乳方　炙山甲片10 g,鲫鱼(去鳞肠)1 尾,王不留行10 g,水煎服,适用于血虚肝郁之缺乳。

（2）裘笑梅验方　当归12 g,鹿角霜9 g,穿山甲片(先煎)10 g,王不留行9 g,天花粉9 g,通草1.5 g,水煎服,适用于肾虚瘀阻之缺乳。

（3）木通 90 g,猪前蹄1只,炖汤服,适用于各证缺乳。

（4）赤小豆250 g煮服,适用于气血虚弱证缺乳。

（5）炒瓜蒌仁6 g研末,酒送服,适用于血瘀寒凝乳汁不下。

2.8 Female genital organ tumor and other diseases

第八章 女性生殖器官肿瘤及其他

2.8.1 Hysteromyoma

第一节 子宫肌瘤

Hysteromyoma, a most commonly seen benign tumor of female reproductive system, is formed with hyperplasic uterine smooth tissue, also known as leiomyoma of uterus, occupying over 90% of gynecological tumor and often seen among women from the age of 30 to the period before menopause, especially among women at the age of 40-50.

Hysteromyoma is usually caused by emotional upsets, stagnation of liver qi, unsmooth flow of qi and inhibited circulation of blood; or by invasion of wind-cold-dampness into the uterus and struggle with blood; or by sexual activity during menstruation; or by insufficiency of the spleen and kidney, asthenia of yang-qi, dysfunction of the spleen in transformation, retention of dampness and fluid into phlegm in the uterus. Stagnation of the uterine vessels and dysfunction of the thoroughfare and conception vessels as well as failure of newly produced blood to flow in the vessels may change menstruation or lead to sudden profuse uterine bleeding. Consequently anemia may be caused. So in TCM it pertains to the conceptions of abdominal mass, profuse menstruation and sudden profuse uterine bleeding.

[Key points for diagnosis]

(1) Progressive increase of menstruation, prolonged

子宫肌瘤是女性生殖系统最常见的良性肿瘤,主要由子宫平滑肌组织增生所致,又称为子宫平滑肌瘤,占妇科良性肿瘤的 90% 以上,多发生于30 岁以上至绝经前的妇女,一般 40～50 岁发病率最高。

本病多由情志不遂,肝气郁积,气机不畅,血行滞涩;或经期产后血室正开,风寒湿邪,侵袭胞宫,与血相搏结;或经期产后余血未净,伤于房劳,余血败精,交结内阻而成;亦有脾肾不足,阳气虚弱,脾运失健,水湿不化,凝聚成痰,痰瘀阻于胞中,而成癥瘕。瘀阻于胞脉,冲任失调,新血不得归经,而致月经改变,或崩中漏下。又可继发贫血。故中医归属"癥瘕"、"月经过多"、"崩漏"之范畴。

【诊断要点】

(1) 进行性月经增多,经

menstruation, or irregular uterine bleeding and even secondary anemia as well as symptoms of bladder and rectum pressure when tumor is enlarged.

(2) Gynecological examination: Irregular enlargement, hardening, normal movement and no tenderness of the uterus.

(3) Type B ultrasonic examination, hysteroscopy and abdominoscopy are helpful for accurate diagnosis.

(4) It should be differentiated from gravid uterus, ovary tumor, metrauxe, adenomyosis, pelvic inflammatory mass and deformity of uterus.

[Syndrome differentiation and treatment]

Hysteromyoma is mainly classified into syndrome of qi stagnation and blood stasis, syndrome of qi asthenia and blood stasis, syndrome of mixture of phlegm and stasis, syndrome of cold coagulation and blood stasis as well as syndrome of yin asthenia and liver hyperactivity. The basic therapeutic principle is resolving stasis and dissipating stagnation. The therapeutic methods used are regulating qi, resolving phlegm, warming yang, nourishing yin and replenishing qi to be selected according to differentiation of syndrome and treatment in or not in menstruation. Drugs are selected according to syndrome differentiation of conditions in and not in menstruation. Treatment of integrated traditional Chinese and western medicine can be used if necessary.

(1) Syndrome of qi stagnation and blood stasis

Main symptoms: Mass in uterus, irregular profuse or scanty menstruation with dark color and clot, distending pain or stabbing pain in the lower abdomen, alleviation of pain after removal of the clot, discomfort in hypochondria, mental

期延长,或有不规则的子宫出血,甚者可继发贫血。肌瘤增大时可见膀胱和直肠压迫症状。

(2) 妇科检查:子宫不规则的增大,质地硬,活动度尚好,无触痛。

(3) B超、宫腔镜、腹腔镜可协助明确诊断。

(4) 与妊娠子宫、卵巢肿瘤、子宫肥大症、子宫腺肌病、盆腔炎性包块、子宫畸形鉴别。

【辨证论治】

本病临床表现主要分为气滞血瘀证、气虚血瘀证、痰瘀互结证、寒凝血瘀证及阴虚肝旺证。治疗以化瘀散结为基本治则,根据辨证及经期或非经期分别采用理气、化痰、温阳、滋阴、补气等法。必要时采用西医手术治疗。

一、气滞血瘀证

主要证候　胞中结块,月经先后无定期,量或多或少,色暗红,有块,少腹胀痛或刺痛,块下痛减,胸胁不舒,情志

depression, blackish tongue, thin and moist tongue fur, deep and taut pulse.

Therapeutic methods: Soothing the liver and eliminating stagnation, resolving stasis and dissipating retention.

Prescription and drugs: Modified Xuefu Zhuyu Tang composed of 10g of Chaihu (*Radix Bupleuri*), 10g of Xiangfu (*Rhizoma Cyperi*), 10g of Zhike (*Fructus Aurantii*), 10g of Chenpi (*Pericarpium Citri Reticulatae*), 10g of Chuanxiong (*Rhizoma Chuanxiong*), 10g of Baishaoyao (*Radix Paeoniae Alba*), 15g of Sanleng (*Rhizoma Sparganii*), 15g of Ezhu (*Rhizoma Curcumae*), 6g of Chuanlianzi (*Fructus Toosendan*), 10g of Shanzha (*Fructus Crataegi*) and 10g of Yujin (*Radix Curcumae*).

Modification: For hard mass, 20g of roasted Biejia (*Carapax Trionycis*) (to be decocted first) and 15g of Kunbu (*Thallus Laminariae seu Eckloniae*) are added; for severe pain, 10g of Yanhusuo (*Rhizoma Corydalis*), 10g of Ezhu (*Rhizoma Curcumae*) and 8g of Jianghuang (*Rhizoma Curcumae Longae*) are added; for cold pain in lower abdomen, 5g of Xiaohuixiang (*Fructus Foeniculi*) and 5g of Paojiang (*Rhizoma Zingiberis*) are added; for profuse menstruation and incessant profuse uterine bleeding, 5g of Sanqi powder (*Radix Notoginseng*), 10g of roasted Puhuang (*Pollen Typhae*) and 10g of Xueyutan (*Crinis Carbonisatus*) are added; for severe blood stasis, squamous skin and blackish complexion, Dahuang Zhechong Wan is added; for severe lower abdominal pain, 10g of Yanhusuo (*Rhizoma Corydalis*) and 6g of prepared Moyao (*Myrrha*) are added.

(2) Syndrome of qi asthenia and blood stasis

Main symptoms: Mass in uterus, early profuse

抑郁,舌黯,苔薄润,脉沉弦。

治　法　疏肝行滞,化瘀散结。

方　药　血府逐瘀汤加减:柴胡10g,香附10g,枳壳10g,陈皮10g,川芎6g,白芍药10g,三棱15g,莪术15g,川楝子6g,山楂10g,郁金10g。

加　减　若积块坚牢者,加炙鳖甲(先煎)20g,昆布15g;疼痛剧烈者,加延胡索10g,莪术10g,姜黄8g;小腹冷痛者,酌加小茴香5g,炮姜5g;月经过多,崩漏不止者,加三七粉5g,炒蒲黄10g,血余炭10g;若血瘀甚者,兼肌肤甲错,面目黯黑,加用大黄䗪虫丸;若少腹痛甚者加延胡索10g,制没药6g。

二、气虚血瘀证

主要证候　胞中结块,月

menstruation with light color, thin texture and large blood clot, prolapsing pain in the lower abdomen, profuse leukorrhea with white color and thin texture, weakness of limbs, lack of strength, no desire to speak, light-colored tongue with thin and white fur, weak, thin and unsmooth pulse.

Therapeutic methods: Nourishing qi and strengthening spleen, resolving stasis and dissipating mass.

Prescription and drugs: Modified Buzhong Yiqi Tang combined with Xuefu Zhuyu Tang composed of 15g of Dangshen (*Radix Codonopsis Pilosulae*), 10g of Huangqi (*Radix Astragali*), 12g of Baizhu (*Rhizoma Atractylodis Macrocephalae*), 5g of Shengma (*Rhizoma Cimicifugae*), 15g of Chenpi (*Pericarpium Citri Reticulatae*), 10 g of Chishaoyao (*Radix Paeoniae Rubra*), 15g of Sanleng (*Rhizoma Sparganii*), 15g of Ezhu (*Rhizoma Curcumae*), 15g of Shanyao (*Rhizoma Dioscoreae*), 15g of Zhike (*Fructus Aurantii*), 15g of Kunbu (*Thallus Laminariae seu Eckloniae*) and 10g of Taoren (*Semen Persicae*).

Modification: For profuse menstruation, 30g of Yimucao (*Herba Leonuri*) and 15g of Qiancao (*Radix Rubiae*) are added; for cold sensation in the body and cold limbs as well as morning diarrhea, 10g of Roudoukou (*Semen Myristicae*) and 15g of Yinyanghuo (*Herba Epimedii*) are added.

(3) Syndrome of mixture of phlegm and stasis

Main symptoms: Uterine mass, occasional pain, or profuse menorrhea with dull color, thick texture and clot, profuse leukorrhea with white color and sticky texture, stiffness and oppression in chest and hypochondria, obesity, purplish tongue with white and greasy fur, thin and soft or deep and slippery pulse.

经先期,量多,色淡,质稀,有大血块,小腹坠痛,带下量多,色白,质稀,四肢乏力,少气懒言,舌淡,苔薄白,脉虚细而涩。

治　法　补气健脾,化瘀散结。

方　药　补中益气汤合血府逐瘀汤加减:党参15 g,黄芪10 g,白术12 g,升麻5 g,陈皮15 g,赤芍药10 g,三棱15 g,莪术15 g,山药15 g,枳壳15 g,昆布15 g,桃仁10 g。

加　减　若月经过多者,经期加益母草30 g,茜草15 g;若兼形寒肢冷,五更泄泻者,加肉豆蔻10 g,淫羊藿15 g。

三、痰瘀互结

主要证候　胞中结块,时或作痛,经量或多,色暗红,质稠有块,带下量多,色白,质粘腻,胸脘痞闷,形体肥胖,舌暗紫,苔白腻,脉细濡或沉滑。

Therapeutic methods: Regulating qi and resolving phlegm, breaking stasis and eliminating mass.

Prescription and drugs: Modified Kaiyu Erchen Tang composed of 10g of prepared Banxia (*Rhizoma Pinelliae*), 10g of Chenpi (*Pericarpium Citri Reticulatae*), 15g of Fuling (*Poria*), 10g of Qingpi (*Pericarpium Citri Reticulatae Viride*), 10 of Xiangfu (*Rhizoma Cyperi*), 6g of Chuanxiong (*Rhizoma Chuanxiong*), 10g of Ezhu (*Rhizoma Curcumae*), 6g of Muxiang (*Radix Aucklaneliae*), 10g of Binglang (*Semen Arecae*), 10g of Cangzhu (*Rhizoma Atractylodis*) and 6g of Gancao (*Radix Glycyrrhizae*).

Modification: For yellowish leukorrhea due to transformation of heat from accumulation of dampness, 15g of Baijiangcao (*Herba Patriniae*), 10g of Mudanpi (*Cortex Moutan Radicis*) and 15g of Hongteng (*Caulis Sargentodoxae*) are added; for evident asthenia of spleen, Binglang (*Semen Arecae*) is deleted while 12g of Baizhu (*Rhizoma Atractylodis Macrocephalae*) and 12g of Dangshen (*Radix Codonopsis Pilosulae*) are added.

(4) Syndrome of cold coagulation and blood stasis

Main symptoms: Uterine mass, delayed menstruation, profuse menorrhea with blackish color and blood clot, cold pain in the lower abdomen, spasm, alleviation after removal of the clot, profuse leukorrhea with white color and thin texture, cold limbs, light-purplish tongue with thin and white fur, deep and tense pulse.

Therapeutic methods: Warming the uterus and dispersing cold, resolving stasis and dissipating mass.

Prescription and drugs: Modified Shaofu Zhuyu Tang composed of 10g of Xiaohuixiang (*Fructus Foeniculi*), 6g of Ganjiang (*Rhizoma Zingiberis*), 12g of Yanhusuo (*Rhizoma Corydalis*), 10g of Moyao (*Myrrha*),

治　法　理气化痰,破瘀消癥。

方　药　开郁二陈汤加减:制半夏10 g,陈皮10 g,茯苓15 g,青皮10 g,香附10 g,川芎6 g,莪术10 g,木香6 g,槟榔10 g,苍术10 g,甘草6 g。

加　减　若湿蕴化热,带下色黄者,加败酱草15 g,牡丹皮10 g,红藤15 g;若脾虚明显者,上方去槟榔,加白术12 g,党参12 g。

四、寒凝血瘀证

主要证候　胞中结块,月经后期,量少,色黑红,有血块,小腹冷痛,拘急,块下痛减,带下量多,色白,质稀,四肢不温,舌淡紫,苔薄白,脉沉紧。

治　法　暖宫散寒,化瘀散结。

方　药　少腹逐瘀汤加减:小茴香10 g,干姜6 g,延胡索12 g,没药10 g,当归15 g,川芎6 g,肉桂6 g,赤芍药10 g,蒲

15g of Danggui (*Radix Angelicae Sinensis*), 6g of Chuanxiong (*Rhizoma Chuanxiong*), 6g of Rougui (*Cortex Cinnamomi*), 10g of Chishaoyao (*Radix Paeoniae Rubra*), 10g of Puhuang (*Pollen Typhae*) (to be wrapped) and 10g of Wulingzhi (*Faeces Trogopterorum*).

Modification: For complication of phlegm and dampness, 10g of Baijiezi (*Semen Sinapis*) and 15g of Shancigu (*Bulbus Iphigeniae*) are added; for complication of yang asthenia, 10g of sliced Lujiao (*Cornus Cervi*), 15g of Shudihuang (*Rhizoma Rehmanniae Praeparata*) and 15g of Niuxi (*Radix Achyranthis Bidentatae*) are added.

(5) Syndrome of yin asthenia and liver hyperactivity

Main symptoms: Uterine mass, delayed and scanty menstruation, or early profuse menstruation with red color, scanty leukorrhea, or dry sensation in the vagina, dry mouth and irritating sensation in the eyes, feverish sensation in the palms, soles and chest, flushed cheeks, vertigo, purplish red tongue with thin and yellow fur, thin and taut pulse.

Therapeutic methods: Nourishing yin and blood, resolving stasis and dissipating mass.

Prescription and drugs: Modified Zhibai Dihuang Tang composed of 10g of Danggui (*Radix Angelicae Sinensis*), 12g of Shengdihuang (*Radix Rehmanniae*), 15g of Shashen (*Radix Adenophorae*), 12g of Gouqizi (*Fructus Lycii*), 10g of Maimendong (*Radix Ophiopogonis*), 6g of Chuanlianzi (*Fructus Toosendan*), 15g of Kunbu (*Thallus Laminariae seu Eckloniae*), 12g of Baishaoyao (*Radix Paeoniae Alba*) and 10g of Xiakucao (*Spica Prunellae*).

Modification: For profuse early menstruation, 10g

黄(包)10 g,五灵脂10 g。

　加　减　若兼痰湿者,加白芥子10 g,山慈姑15 g;若兼阳虚者,加鹿角片10 g,熟地黄15 g,牛膝15 g。

五、阴虚肝旺证

　主要证候　胞中结块,月经后期,量少,或先期量多,色红,带下甚少,或阴中干涩,口干目涩,五心烦热,两颊潮红,头晕目眩,舌紫红,苔薄黄,脉细弦。

　治　法　滋阴养血,化瘀散结。

　方　药　知柏地黄汤加减:当归10 g,生地黄12 g,沙参15 g,枸杞子12 g,麦门冬10 g,川楝子6 g,昆布15 g,白芍药12 g,夏枯草10 g。

　加　减　若月经先期量

of Daji (*Herba seu Radix Cirsii Japonici*), 10g of Xiaoji (*Herba Cephalanoploris*) and 10g of roasted Huaihua (*Flos Sophorae*) are added; for severe dry mouth and throat, 10g of Shihu (*Herba Dendrobii*), 10g of Wuweizi (*Fructus Schisandrae*) and 10g of Yuzhu (*Rhizoma Polygonati Odorati*) are added.

[Other therapeutic methods]

(1) Chinese patent drugs

1) Guizhi Fuling Pill: 9g each time and twice a day, applicable to the treatment of blood stasis syndrome.

2) Wuxiang Pill: 6g each time and three times a day, applicable to the treatment of qi stagnation and blood stasis.

3) Jiuqi Xintong Pill: 9g of big honey-coated pill each time, 3g of small honey-coated pill each time, twice or three times a day, applicable to the treatment of cold coagulation and qi stagnation syndrome.

4) Dahuang Zhechong Pill: 10g each time and twice a day, applicable to the treatment of blood stasis syndrome.

(2) Empirical and folk recipes

1) Liu Yunpeng's prescription for hysteromyoma during menstruation: 9g of Danggui (*Radix Angelicae Sinensis*), 9g of Gandihuang (*dry Rhizoma Rehmanniae*), 9g of Baishaoyao (*Radix Paeoniae Alba*), 9g of Qiancao (*Radix Rubiae*), 9g of Liujinu (*Herba Artemisiae Anomalae*), 9g of charred Puhuang (*Pollen Typhae*), 9g of Chuanxiong (*Rhizoma Chuanxiong*), 15g of Danshen (*Radix Salviae Miltiorrhizae*), 12g of Ejiao (*Colla Corii Asini*) (to be melted for decocting), 12g of Yimucao (*Herba Leonuri*) and 15g of Zicaogen (*Radix Lithospermi*) are decocted for oral taking.

多者加大蓟10 g,小蓟10 g,炒槐花10 g;若口燥咽干甚者,加石斛10 g,五味子10 g,玉竹10 g。

【其他疗法】

1. 中成药

（1）桂枝茯苓丸　每次服9 g,1 日 2 次,适用于血瘀证。

（2）五香丸　每次服6 g,1 日 3 次,适用于气滞血瘀证。

（3）九气心痛丸　大蜜丸每服9 g,小蜜丸每服3 g,1 日 2～3 次,适用于寒凝气滞证。

（4）大黄䗪虫丸　每次服10 g,1 日 2 次,适用于血瘀证。

2. 单验方

（1）刘云鹏子宫肌瘤行经期方　当归9 g,干地黄9 g,白芍药9 g,茜草9 g,刘寄奴9 g,蒲黄炭9 g,川芎9 g,丹参15 g,阿胶(烊化)12 g,益母草12 g,紫草根15 g,水煎服。

2) Liu Yunpeng's prescription for hysteriomyoma not in menstruation: 9g of Danggui (*Radix Angelicae Sinensis*), 9g of Chuanxiong (*Rhizoma Chuanxiong*), 9g of dry Dihuang (*Radix Rehmanniae*), 9g of Chishaoyao (*Radix Paeoniae Rubra*), 9g of Baishaoyao (*Radix Paeoniae Alba*), 9g of Taoren (*Semen Persicae*), 9g of Honghua (*Flos Carthami*), 9g of Sanleng (*Rhizoma Sparganii*), 15g of Kunbu (*Thallus Laminariae seu Eckloniae*), 15g of Danshen (*Radix Salviae Miltiorrhizae*), 15g of Liujinu (*Herba Artemisiae Anomalae*) and 5g of Biejia (*Carapax Trionycis*) are decocted for oral taking, applicable to the treatment of hysteromyoma in blood stasis syndrome.

（2）刘云鹏子宫肌瘤非经期方：当归9g,川芎9g,干地黄9g,赤芍药9g,白芍药9g,桃仁9g,红花9g,三棱9g,昆布15g,丹参15g,刘寄奴15g,鳖甲5g,水煎服,适用于血瘀证子宫肌瘤。

2.8.2 Oophoritic cyst

Oophoritic cyst is a commonly encountered tumor in gynecology, either benign or malignant. The following discussion may focus on benign type. Oophoritic cyst is usually caused by dysfunction of the viscera, disharmony between qi and blood, invasion of wind and cold right after labor or during menstruation, retention of blood stasis during menstruation and labor that inactivate kidney yang; or by interior impairment due to emotional changes, stagnation of qi and interior retention of phlegm, fluid and stasis.

[Key points for diagnosis]

（1）Mass in the lower abdomen, or accompanied by abdominal distension, abdominal pain, lumbago, pressure symptoms, pain and disturbance of menstruation.

（2）Gynecological examination shows mass beside the uterus with evident margin or mobility.

（3）Cytological examination, puncture with thin needle for biopsy, type B ultrasonic examination, radiological

第二节 卵巢囊肿

卵巢囊肿是妇科常见肿瘤,有良性和恶性之分。本文主要对卵巢良性肿瘤加以叙述。中医属"肠覃"、"积聚"范畴。多由脏腑失调,气血不和,因新产、经行不慎,伤于风冷,寒湿内侵,经产余瘀阻滞,又致肾阳不振;或情志内伤,气机阻滞,痰饮夹瘀内留所致。

【诊断要点】

（1）临证以下腹部肿块,或伴有腹胀、腹痛、腰痛、压迫症状、疼痛、月经紊乱等为主要症状。

（2）妇科检查见子宫旁肿块,边界清楚,或可活动。

（3）细胞学检查、细针穿刺活检、B超、放射学诊断、腹

examination, abdominoscopy and tumor signifiers can be used as supplementary examinations of benign and malignant tumor.

(4) Benign ovarian tumor should be differentiated from oncological changes of ovary, oviduct and ovary cyst, hysteromyoma, gravid uterus and ascites; malignant ovarian tumor should be differentiated from endometriosis, inflammation of pelvic connective tissue, tuberculous peritonitis, tumor outside birth canal and metastatic ovarian tumor.

[Syndrome differentiation and treatment]

Clinically oophoritic cyst is classified into syndrome of qi stagnation and blood stasis, syndrome of phlegm and dampness retention and syndrome of stagnation of virulent dampness and heat. The therapeutic principle is softening hardness and eliminating mass. The therapeutic methods used are promoting qi flow, resolving phlegm and clearing away heat and draining dampness.

(1) Syndrome of qi stagnation and blood stasis

Main symptoms: Cystic mass in the lower abdomen, abdominal distension and pain, dull complexion, spiritual lassitude, dry mouth without desire to drink water, dry lips, unsmooth urination and defecation, purplish tongue, taut and thin pulse.

Therapeutic methods: Promoting qi flow and activating blood, softening hardness and eliminating mass.

Prescription and drugs: Modified Qizhi Xiangfu Wan combined with Xuefu Zhuyu Tang composed of 12g of Cangzhu (*Rhizoma Atractylodis*), 12g of Baizhu (*Rhizoma Atractylodis Macrocephalae*), 9g of Danggui (*Radix Angelicae Sinensis*), 10g of Chishaoyao (*Radix Paeoniae Rubra*), 10g of Taoren (*Semen Persicae*), 0.5g of Hupo powder (*Succinum*) (to be taken orally), 10g of

腔镜检查、肿瘤标志物可辅助检查良、恶性肿瘤。

(4) 良性卵巢肿瘤应与卵巢瘤样病变、输卵管卵巢囊肿、子宫肌瘤、妊娠子宫、腹水等相鉴别;恶性卵巢肿瘤须与子宫内膜异位症、盆腔结缔组织炎、结核性腹膜炎、生殖道以外的肿瘤、转移性卵巢等肿瘤相鉴别。

【辨证论治】

本病临床主要分为气滞血瘀证、痰湿凝结证及湿热郁毒证。治疗以软坚消癥为原则,根据病情分别采用行气、化痰、清热利湿法。

一、气滞血瘀证

主要证候 下腹有囊性肿块,巨大囊肿可见腹胀腹痛,面色晦暗,神疲乏力,口干不欲饮,唇燥,二便不畅,舌紫暗,脉弦细。

治 法 行气活血,软坚消癥。

方 药 七制香附丸合血府逐瘀汤加减:苍术12 g,白术12 g,当归9 g,赤芍药10 g,桃仁10 g,琥珀粉(吞)0.5 g,木香10 g,山楂10 g,生鸡内金6 g,炒枳壳5 g。

Muxiang (*Radix Aucklaneliae*), 10g of Shanzha (*Fructus Crataegi*), 6g of crude Jineijin (*Endothelium Corneum Gigeriae Galli*) and 5g of roasted Zhike (*Fructus Aurantii*).

Modification: For constipation, 6g of Dahuang (*Radix et Rhizoma Rhei*) (to be decocted later) is added; for red tongue with scanty fur, 9g of dry Dihuang (*Radix Rehmanniae*) and 15g of roasted Guiban (*Plastrum Testudinis*) are added.

(2) Syndrome of phlegm and dampness coagulation

Main symptoms: Obesity, chest and epigastric oppression and pain, occasional nausea, leukorrhagia, white and greasy tongue fur, taut and slippery pulse.

Therapeutic methods: Resolving phlegm and promoting qi flow, softening hardness and eliminating symptoms.

Prescription and drugs: Modified Haizao Yuhu Tang composed of 12g of Haizao (*Sargassum*), 12g of Kunbu (*Thallus Laminariae seu Eckloniae*), 12g of Xiakucao (*Spica Prunellae*), 9g of Shichangpu (*Rhizoma Acori Graminei*), 9g of Danxing (*Arisaema cum Bile*), 30g of crude Muli (*Caro Ostreae*) (to be decocted first), 9g of Cangzhu (*Rhizoma Atractylodis*), 9g of Ezhu (*Rhizoma Curcumae*), 9g of Sanleng (*Rhizoma Sparganii*), 10g of Taoren (*Semen Persicae*), Chishaoyao (*Radix Paeoniae Rubra*), 10g of crispy Shanzha (*Fructus Crataegi*), 10g of roasted Liuqu (*Massa Medicata Fermentata*) and 3g of Rougui (*Cortex Cinnamomi*) (to be decocted later).

Modification: For relative predominance of cold, 9g of prepared sliced Fuzi (*Radix Aconiti Praeparata*) and 9g of Baijiezi (*Semen Sinapis*) are added and the quantity of Rougui (*Cortex Cinnamomi*) is added to 5g.

加 减 大便秘结者,加大黄(后下)6 g;舌红苔少者,加干地黄9 g,炙龟版(先煎)15 g。

二、痰湿凝结证

主要证候 形体较胖,胸脘闷痛,恶心时作,带下较多,舌苔白腻,脉弦滑。

治 法 化痰行气,软坚消癥。

方 药 海藻玉壶汤:海藻12 g,昆布12 g,夏枯草12 g,石菖蒲9 g,胆星9 g,生牡蛎(先煎)30 g,苍术9 g,陈皮6 g,莪术9 g,三棱9 g,桃仁10 g,赤芍药10 g,焦山楂10 g,焦六曲10 g,肉桂(后下)3 g。

加 减 偏寒者,加制附片9 g,白芥子9 g,肉桂改为5 g。

(3) Syndrome of stagnation of virulent dampness and heat

Main symptoms: Lower abdominal mass, abdominal distension or pain or fullness, or irregular vaginal bleeding, even accompanied by ascites, dry stool, yellow urine, burning sensation in urination, dry mouth, bitter taste in the mouth and no desire to drink water, deep-red tongue with thick and greasy fur, taut and slippery or rapid and slippery pulse.

Therapeutic methods: Clearing away heat and draining dampness, eliminating toxin and dissipating mass.

Prescription and drugs: Modified Qingre Lishi Jiedu Tang composed of 30g of Banzhilian (*Herba Scutellariae Barbatae*), 30g of Longkui (*Herba Solani*), 30g of Baihuasheshecao (*Herba Hedyotis Diffusae*), 10g of Chuanlianzi (*Fructus Toosendan*), 30g of Cheqiancao (*Herba Plantaginis*), 30g of Tufuling (*Rhizoma Smilacis Glabrae*), 15 Qumai (*Herba Dianthi*), 30g of Baijiangcao (*Herba Patriniae*), 30g of Biejia (*Carapax Trionycis*) and 10g of Dafupi (*Pericarpium Arecae*).

Modification: For predominant virulent heat, 15g of Longdancao (*Radix Gentianae*), 15g of Kushen (*Radix Sophorae Flavescentis*) and 15g of Pugongying (*Herba Taraxaci*) are added; for severe ascites, 10g of Shuihonghuazi (*Fructus Polygoni Orientalis*) and 10g of Youhulou (*Gryllus testaceus Walker*) are added.

[Other therapeutic methods]

(1) Chinese patent drugs

1) Guizhi Fuling Pill: 6g each time and twice a day, applicable to the treatment of ovarian cyst of phlegm and dampness retention syndrome.

2) Dahuang Zhechong Pill: 1 pill each time and

三、湿热郁毒证

主要证候 小腹部肿块,腹胀或痛或满,或不规则阴道出血,甚至伴有腹水,大便干燥,尿黄灼热,口干口苦不欲饮,舌暗红,苔厚腻,脉弦滑或滑数。

治 法 清热利湿,解毒散结。

方 药 清热利湿解毒汤:半枝莲30 g,龙葵30 g,白花蛇舌草30 g,川楝子10 g,车前草30 g,土茯苓30 g,瞿麦15 g,败酱草30 g,鳖甲30 g,大腹皮10 g。

加 减 若热毒盛者加龙胆草15 g,苦参15 g,蒲公英15 g;若腹水多者加水红花子10 g,油葫芦10 g。

【其他疗法】

1. 中成药

(1)桂枝茯苓丸 每次服6 g,1 日 2 次,适用于痰湿凝结证卵巢囊肿。

(2)大黄䗪虫丸 每次

twice a day, applicable to the treatment of ovarian cyst of blood stasis syndrome.

3) Huazheng Huisheng Pill: 1 pill each time and twice a day, applicable to the treatment of ovarian cyst of blood stasis syndrome.

(2) Empirical and folk recipes

1) Chuanshanjia Powder: Chuanshanjia (*Squama Manitis*), Ezhu (*Rhizoma Curcumae*), Sanleng (*Rhizoma Sparganii*), Heichou (*Semen Pharbitidis*), Wulingzhi (*Faeces Trogopterorum*), Yanhusuo (*Rhizoma Corydalis*), Niuxi (*Radix Achyranthis Bidentatae*), Danggui (*Radix Angelicae Sinensis*), Chuanxiong (*Rhizoma Chuanxiong*), Dahuang (*Radix et Rhizoma Rhei*), Danshen (*Radix Salviae Miltiorrhizae*), and Rougui (*Cortex Cinnamomi*) etc. are ground into powder that is taken orally 3g each time and twice a day, applicable to the treatment of ovarian tumor.

2) 9g of Danggui (*Radix Angelicae Sinensis*), 9g of Baishaoyao (*Radix Paeoniae Alba*), 9g of Chuanlianzi (*Fructus Toosendan*), 9g of Yanhusuo (*Rhizoma Corydalis*), 9g of Xuduan (*Radix Dipsaci*), 12g of Hongteng (*Caulis Sargentodoxae*), 6g of Chaihu (*Radix Bupleuri*) and 6g of Yujin (*Radix Curcumae*) are decocted for oral taking, applicable to the treatment of ovarian cyst of qi stagnation and blood stasis syndrome.

3) 9g of Danggui (*Radix Angelicae Sinensis*), 6g of Chuanxiong (*Rhizoma Chuanxiong*), 6g of Zelan (*Herba Lycopi*), 6g of Sanleng (*Rhizoma Sparganii*), 6g of Ezhu (*Rhizoma Curcumae*), 6g of Yanhusuo (*Rhizoma Corydalis*), 12g of Zishiying (*Fluoritum*), 9g of Taoren (*Semen Persicae*), 9g of roasted Wulingzhi (*Faeces Trogopterorum*), 9g of roasted Puhuang (*Pollen Typhae*), 9g of prepared Xiangfu (*Rhizoma Cyperi*), 9g of Lizhihe (*Semen Litchi*), 4.5g of Liangtoujian (*Rhi-

（3）化癥回生丹　每次服 1 粒，1 日 2 次，适用于血瘀证卵巢囊肿。

2. 单验方

（1）穿山甲散　穿山甲、莪术、三棱、黑丑、五灵脂、延胡索、牛膝、当归、川芎、大黄、丹参、肉桂等，研末，每服 3 g，每日 2 次，适用于卵巢肿瘤。

（2）当归 9 g，白芍药 9 g，川楝子 9 g，延胡索 9 g，续断 9 g，红藤 12 g，柴胡 6 g，郁金 6 g，水煎服，适用于气滞血瘀证卵巢囊肿。

（3）当归 9 g，川芎 6 g，泽兰 6 g，三棱 6 g，莪术 6 g，延胡索 6 g，紫石英 12 g，桃仁 9 g，炒五灵脂 9 g，炒蒲黄 9 g，制香附 9 g，荔枝核 9 g，两头尖 4.5 g，熟大黄 4.5 g，干姜 4.5 g，水煎服，适用于妇女小腹癥瘕。

zoma Anemones Raddeanae), 4.5g of prepared Dahuang (*Radix et Rhizoma Rhei*) and 4.5g of Ganjiang (*Rhizoma Zingiberis*) are decocted for oral taking, applicable to the treatment of lower abdominal mass in women.

4) Soft-Shelled Turtle Paste: The paste is warmed soft to apply to the abdomen, applicable to the treatment of ovarian cyst of qi stagnation and blood stasis syndrome.

2.8.3 Prolapse of uterus and vaginal wall

Hysteroptosis means that the uterus descends along the vagina or even completely comes out of the vaginal orifice, often complicated by protrusion of the posterior and anterior walls of the vagina. Hysteroptosis is usually caused by early labor, dystocia, prolonged labor, overstrain in labor and increase of abdominal pressure due to various kinds of work; or by excessive sexual life, multiparity and impairment of the uterine collaterals; or by weak constitution and asthenia of qi and blood to maintain the organs in the original position; or by asthenia-cold in uterus; or by downward migration of liver fire and damp-heat. The main clinical symptoms are aching pain and prolapsing sensation in the lumbosacral region and protrusion of something out of the vaginal orifice.

[Key points for diagnosis]

（1）Accurate diagnosis can be made according to medical history and examination.

（2）Gynecological examination: Detect the degree of hysteroptosis, the degree of protrusion of posterior and anterior walls of viginia and laceration of perineum as well as stress incontinence.

（3）It should be differentiated from protrusion of

（4）甲鱼膏 加温软化，贴敷脐腹,适用于气滞血瘀证卵巢囊肿。

第三节 子宫及阴道壁脱垂

子宫脱垂是指子宫从正常位置沿阴道下降,宫颈外口达坐骨棘水平以下,甚至子宫全部脱出于阴道口以外,常合并有阴道前壁和后壁膨出。本病多因临盆过早,难产,产程过长,产中用力太过,及各种增加腹压的劳动;或房劳多产,损伤胞络;或体质较差,气血虚弱,不能收摄;或子脏虚冷;或肝火湿热下注等所致。临证以腰骶部酸痛和下坠感,阴道口有物脱出等为主要症状。中医属"阴挺"范畴。

【诊断要点】

（1）根据病史和妇科检查可以诊断。

（2）妇科检查可判断子宫脱垂的程度而予以分度。同时了解阴道前、后壁膨出及会阴撕裂的程度,有无张力性尿失禁。

（3）须与膀胱膨出、阴道

bladder, cyst of vaginal wall, inversion of uterus, submucosal myoma of uterus or myoma of cervix uteri.

[Syndrome differentiation and treatment]

Clinically it is either of qi asthenia syndrome or of kidney asthenia syndrome. The therapeutic principle is to nourish asthenia and to elevate sinking. The therapeutic methods usually used are nourishing qi and elevating ptosis, nourishing the kidney and stopping prolapse. Severe hysteroptosis should be treated with the treatment of integrated traditional Chinese and western medicine.

（1）Qi asthenia syndrome

Main symptoms: Downward migration of uterus, or protrusion of uterus from the vaginal orifice, aggravation after overstrain, prolapsing sensation in the lower abdomen, spiritual lassitude, lack of strength and no desire to speak, frequent urination, or profuse leukorrhea with white color and thin texture, pale complexion, light-colored tongue with thin fur, slow and weak pulse.

Therapeutic methods: Nourishing qi and elevating prolapse.

Prescription and drugs: Buzhong Yiqi Tang composed of 30g of Huangqi (*Radix Astragali*), 30g of Dangshen (*Radix Codonopsis Pilosulae*), 15g of Baizhu (*Rhizoma Atractylodis Macrocephalae*), 10g of Danggui (*Radix Angelicae Sinensis*), 5g of roasted Gancao (*Radix Glycyrrhizae*), 5g of Chenpi (*Pericarpium Citri Reticulatae*), 5g of roasted Shengma (*Rhizoma Cimicifugae*), 5g of Chaihu (*Radix Bupleuri*), 3 slices of Shengjiang (*Rhizoma Zingiberis Recens*) and 5 Dazao (*Fructus Jujubae*).

Modification: For profuse leukorrhea with whitish color and thin texture, 10g of Shanyao (*Rhizoma Dioscoreae*), 10 g of Qianshi (*Semen Euryales*) and 10g of

壁囊肿、子宫内翻、子宫粘膜下肌瘤或宫颈肌瘤相鉴别。

【辨证论治】

本病临床主要分为气虚证及肾虚证。治疗以"虚者补之，陷者举之"为原则，根据病情分别采用益气升提，补肾固脱法。重度脱垂宜中西结合治疗。

一、气虚证

主要证候　子宫下移，或脱出阴道口外，劳则加剧，小腹下坠，神倦乏力，少气懒言，小便频数，或带下量多，色白质稀，面色少华，舌淡，苔薄，脉缓弱。

治　法　补气升提。

方　药　补中益气汤：黄芪30 g，党参30 g，白术15 g，当归10 g，炙甘草5 g，陈皮5 g，炙升麻5 g，柴胡5 g，生姜3片，大枣5枚。

加　减　若带下量多，色白质稀者，酌加山药10 g，芡实10 g，桑螵蛸10 g。

Sangpiaoxiao (*Oötheca Mantidis*) are added.

(2) Kidney asthenia syndrome

Main symptoms: Downward migration of uterus, or protrusion of uterus from the vaginal orifice, prolapsing sensation in the lower abdomen, frequent urination, aching sensation in the loins and flaccidity of legs, vertigo and tinnitus, light-colored tongue with thin fur, deep and thin pulse.

Therapeutic methods: Nourishing the kidney and stopping prolapse.

Prescription and drugs: Modified Dabuyuan Jian composed of 3 - 10g of Hongshen (*Radix Ginseng Destillata*), 10g of Shanyao (*Rhizoma Dioscoreae*), 10g of Shudihuang (*Rhizoma Rehmanniae Praeparata*), 10g of Duzhong (*Cortex Eucommiae*), 10g of roasted Danggui (*Radix Angelicae Sinensis*), 10g of Shanzhuyu (*Fructus Corni*), 9g of Gouqizi (*Fructus Lycii*), 6g of roasted Gancao (*Radix Glycyrrhizae*), 12g of Jinyingzi (*Fructus Rosae Laevigatae*), 12g of Tusizi (*Semen Cuscutae*) and 12g of Ziheche (*Placenta Hominis*).

Modification: For protrusion of uterus from the vaginal orifice, contusion, secondary damp-heat symptoms, local swelling and ulceration, profuse leukorrhea wth yellow color like pus and foul odor, 10g of Huangbai (*Cortex Phellodendri*), 10g of Cangzhu (*Rhizoma Atractylodis*), 10g of Tufuling (*Rhizoma Smilacis Glabrae*) and 10g of Cheqianzi (*Semen Plantaginis*); for severe case, Longdan Xiegan Tang can be used.

(3) Damp-heat syndrome

Main symptoms: Protrusion of uterus out of the vaginal orifice with ulceration on the surface, profuse leukorrhea with yellow color like pus and foul odor, swelling

二、肾虚证

主要证候　子宫下移,或脱出阴道口外,小腹下坠,小便频数,腰酸腿软,头晕耳鸣,舌淡,苔薄,脉沉细。

治　法　补肾固脱。

方　药　大补元煎:红参3～10 g,山药10 g,熟地黄10 g,杜仲10 g,炒当归10 g,山茱萸10 g,枸杞子9 g,炙甘草6 g,金樱子12 g,菟丝子12 g,紫河车12 g。

加　减　若子宫脱出阴道口外,摩擦损伤,继发湿热证候者,局部红肿溃烂,黄水淋漓,带下量多,色黄如脓,有臭秽气味,轻者加黄柏10 g,苍术10 g,土茯苓10 g,车前子10 g,重者用龙胆泻肝汤。

三、湿热证

主要证候　子宫脱出阴道口外,表面红肿溃烂,黄水淋漓,带下量多,色黄如脓,臭

pain in anus or loose stool, burning sensation in anus, yellow urine, burning sensation and pain in urination, dry mouth and bitter taste in the mouth, red tongue with yellow and greasy fur, soft and rapid pulse.

Therapeutic methods: Clearing away heat and dampness, nourishing qi and invigorating the kidney.

Prescription and drugs: Modified Longdan Xiegan Tang composed of 6g of Longdancao (*Radix Gentianae*), 10g of Zhizi (*Fructus Gardeniae*), 10g of Huangqin (*Radix Scutellariae*), 10g of Cheqianzi (*Semen Plantaginis*) (to be wrapped for decocting), 6g of Mutong (*Caulis Akebiae*), 10g of Zexie (*Rhizoma Alismatis*), 10g of Shengdihuang (*Radix Rehmanniae*), 10g of Danggui (*Radix Angelicae Sinensis*), 3g of Gancao (*Radix Glycyrrhizae*) and 5g of Chaihu (*Radix Bupleuri*).

Modification: For profuse leukorrhea with purplish and blackish color or with multiple color, 10g of Cebaiye (*Cacumen Platydadi*), 10g of Chishaoyao (*Radix Paeoniae Rubra*) and 3g of Sanqi powder (*Radix Notoginseng*) (infused in boiled water for oral taking) are added for cooling blood and stopping blood.

(4) Birth injury syndrome

Main symptoms: History of dystocia or birth injury, hysteroptosis, prolapsing sensation in the lower abdomen, lack of strength and no desire to speak, aching and weak sensation in the loins and knees, frequent urination, vertigo, palpitation, light-colored tongue and thin pulse.

Therapeutic methods: Invigorating qi, nourishing blood and elevating prolapse.

Prescription and drugs: Enriched Bazhen Tang composed of 10g of Shudihuang (*Rhizoma Rehmanniae Praeparata*), 10g of Baishaoyao (*Radix Paeoniae Alba*), 10g of Danggui (*Radix Angelicae Sinensis*), 10g

秽,肛门肿痛或大便溏泄,肛门有灼热感,小便黄赤,灼热而痛,口干口苦,舌红,苔黄腻,脉濡数。

治　法　清利湿热,益气补肾。

方　药　龙胆泻肝汤:龙胆草6g,栀子10g,黄芩10g,车前子(包煎)10g,木通6g,泽泻10g,生地黄10g,当归10g,甘草3g,柴胡5g。

加　减　若带下量多,色紫晦黯,或如败酱,或赤白相间,加侧柏叶10g,赤芍药10g,三七粉(冲服)3g以凉血止血。

四、产伤证

主要证候　有难产或产伤史,子宫脱垂,小腹下坠,气短懒言,腰膝酸软,尿频,头晕,心悸,舌淡,脉细。

治　法　补气养血升提。

方　药　八珍汤加味:熟地黄10g,白芍药10g,当归10g,川芎10g,党参20g,白术10g,茯苓10g,甘草10g,三七

of Chuanxiong (*Rhizoma Chuanxiong*), 20g of Dangshen
(*Radix Codonopsis Pilosulae*), 10g of Baizhu (*Rhizoma
Atractylodis Macrocephalae*), 10g of Fuling (*Poria*),
10g of Gancao (*Radix Glycyrrhizae*), 3g of Sanqi powder (*Radix Notoginseng*) (infused in boiled water for
oral taking), 25g of Zhike (*Fructus Aurantii*) and 10g
of Shengma (*Rhizoma Cimicifugae*).

Modification: Right after labor, 15g of Yimucao (*Herba Leonuri*) is added for contracting uterus to stop bleeding.

[Other therapeutic methods]

(1) Chinese patent drugs

1) Buzhong Yiqi Pill: 6 - 9g each time and three
times a day, applicable to the treatment of hysteroptosis
of spleen asthenia and qi sinking syndrome.

2) Wuzi Bushen Pill: 6g each time and three times a
day, applicable to the treatment of hysteroptosis of kidney
asthenia and lack of consolidation syndrome.

3) Longdan Xiegan Pill: 5g each time and three
times a day, applicable to the treatment of hysteroptosis
of liver meridian damp-heat syndrome.

(2) Empirical and folk recipes

1) 60g of Mianhuagen (*Cotton root*) and 30g of
Zhike (*Fructus Aurantii*) are decocted for oral taking,
applicable to the treatment of hysteroptosis of qi asthenia
and sinking syndrome.

2) 15g of Zhike (*Fructus Aurantii*) and 15g of
Chongweizi (Fructus Leonuri) are decocted for oral taking, applicable to the treatment of hysteroptosis of various syndromes.

(3) External therapy

1) 50g of Zhike (*Fructus Aurantii*), 25g of Huangqi (*Radix Astragali*), 25g of Yimucao (*Herba Leonuri*)
and 10g of Shengma (*Rhizoma Cimicifugae*) are decocted for fumigation and washing or rinsing and washing,

粉(冲服)3 g,枳壳25 g,升麻
10 g。

加　减　新产后可酌加
益母草15 g以缩宫止血。

【其他疗法】

1. 中成药

（1）补中益气丸　每次
服6～9 g,1 日3次,适用于脾
虚气陷证子宫脱垂。

（2）五子补肾丸　每次
服6 g,1 日 3 次,适用于肾虚
失固证子宫脱垂。

（3）龙胆泻肝丸　每次
服5 g,1 日 2～3 次,适用于肝
经湿热证子宫脱垂。

2. 单验方

（1）棉花根60 g,枳壳
30 g,水煎服,适用于气虚下陷
证子宫脱垂。

（2）枳壳15 g,茺蔚子
15 g,水煎服,适用于各证子宫
脱垂。

3. 外治疗法

（1）枳壳50 g,黄芪25 g,
益母草25 g,升麻10 g,水煎,1
日 1 剂,分早晚熏洗或浸洗,
用于气虚证。

one dose a day and applicable to the treatment of qi asthenia syndrome.

2) 50g of Zhike (*Fructus Aurantii*), 25g of Yimucao (*Herba Leonuri*), 10g of Shengma (*Rhizoma Cimicifugae*) and 50g of Jinyingzi (*Fructus Rosae Laevigatae*) are decocted for fumigation and washing or rinsing and washing, one dose a day and applicable to the treatment of kidney asthenia syndrome.

3) 60g of crude Zhike (*Fructus Aurantii*) and 10g of Lianpengke (*Receptaculum Nelumbinis*) are decocted for fumigation and washing, applicable to the treatment of hysteroptosis in various syndromes.

4) 15g of Danshen (*Radix Salviae Miltiorrhizae*), 9g of Wubeizi (*Galla Chinensis*) and 9g of Kezirou (*Fructus Chebulae*) are decocted for fumigation and washing, applicable to the treatment of hysteroptosis of various syndromes.

5) 30g of Jinyinhua (*Flos Lonicerae*), 30g of Zihuadiding (*Herba Violae*), 30g of Pugongying (*Herba Taraxaci*), 30g of Shechuanzi (*Fructus Cnidii*), 6g of Huanglian (*Rhizoma Coptidis*), 15g of Kushen (*Radix Sophorae Flavescentis*), 10g of Huangbai (*Cortex Phellodendri*) and 10g of Kufan (*Alumen*) are decocted for fumigation and washing, applicable to the treatment of hysteroptosis of damp-heat syndrome.

6) Songhua Liuyi Powder is sprinkled over the uterus body or ulcerated area over the cervix, applicable to the treatment of hysteroptosis with ulceration.

7) 20 - 50 Bimazi (*Semen Ricini*) are ground into paste which is spread over a piece of white cloth and applied to Baihui (GV 20). If the uterus begins to ascend, the paste over the cloth is taken off and applied to the region 1 - 3 cun below the navel, applicable to the treatment of hysteroptosis of various syndromes.

（2）枳壳50 g，益母草25 g，升麻10 g，金樱子50 g，水煎，1日1剂，分早晚薰洗或浸洗，用于肾虚证。

（3）生枳壳60 g，莲蓬壳10 g，煎水薰洗，适用于各证子宫脱垂。

（4）丹参15 g，五倍子9 g，诃子肉9 g，煎水趁热薰洗，适用于各证子宫脱垂。

（5）金银花30 g，紫花地丁30 g，蒲公英30 g，蛇床子30 g，黄连6 g，苦参15 g，黄柏10 g，枯矾10 g，煎水薰洗坐浴，适用于湿热证子宫脱垂。

（6）宫体或宫颈破溃处用松花六一散外搽，适用于子宫脱垂破溃者。

（7）蓖麻子20～50粒，捣如泥，摊于白布上，贴百会穴。如子宫上收时，将药膏揭下贴脐下1～3寸处，适用于各证子宫脱垂。

Postscript

The Compilation of *A Newly Compiled English-Chinese Library of TCM* was started in 2000 and published in 2002. In order to demonstrate the academic theory and clinical practice of TCM and to meet the requirements of compilation, the compilers and translators have made great efforts to revise and polish the Chinese manuscript and English translation so as to make it systematic, accurate, scientific, standard and easy to understand. Shanghai University of TCM is in charge of the translation. Many scholars and universities have participated in the compilation and translation of the Library, i. e. Professor Shao Xundao from Xi'an Medical University (former Dean of English Department and Training Center of the Health Ministry), Professor Ou Ming from Guangzhou University of TCM (celebrated translator and chief professor), Henan College of TCM, Guangzhou University of TCM, Nanjing University of TCM, Shaanxi College of TCM, Liaoning College of TCM and Shandong University of TCM.

The compilation of this Library is also supported by the State Administrative Bureau and experts from other universities and colleges of TCM. The experts on the Compilation Committee and Approval Committee have directed the compilation and translation. Professor She

后　记

《(英汉对照)新编实用中医文库》(以下简称《文库》)从2000年中文稿的动笔,到2002年全书的付梓,完成了世纪的跨越。为了使本套《文库》尽可能展示传统中医学术理论和临床实践的精华,达到全面、系统、准确、科学、规范、通俗的编写要求,全体编译人员耗费了大量的心血,付出了艰辛的劳动。特别是上海中医药大学承担了英语翻译的主持工作,得到了著名医学英语翻译家、原西安医科大学英语系主任和卫生部外语培训中心主任邵循道教授,著名中医英语翻译家、广州中医药大学欧明首席教授的热心指导,河南中医学院、广州中医药大学、南京中医药大学、陕西中医学院、辽宁中医学院、山东中医药大学等中医院校英语专家的全力参与,确保了本套《文库》具有较高的英译水平。

在《文库》的编撰过程中,我们始终得到国家主管部门领导和各中医院校专家们的关心和帮助。编纂委员会的国内外学者及审定委员会的

Jing, Head of the State Administrative Bureau and Vice Minister of the Health Ministry, has showed much concern for the Library. Professor Zhu Bangxian, head of the Publishing House of Shanghai University of TCM, Zhou Dunhua, former head of the Publishing House of Shanghai University of TCM, and Pan Zhaoxi, former editor-in-chief of the Publishing House of Shanghai University of TCM, have given full support to the compilation and translation of the Library.

With the coming of the new century, we have presented this Library to the readers all over the world, sincerely hoping to receive suggestions and criticism from the readers so as to make it perfect in the following revision.

Zuo Yanfu

Pingju Village, Nanjing

Spring 2002

专家对编写工作提出了指导性的意见和建议。尤其是卫生部副部长、国家中医药管理局局长佘靖教授对本书的编写给予了极大的关注，多次垂询编撰过程，并及时进行指导。上海中医药大学出版社社长兼总编辑朱邦贤教授，以及原社长周敦华先生、原总编辑潘朝曦先生及全体编辑对本书的编辑出版工作给予了全面的支持，使《文库》得以顺利面世。在此，一并致以诚挚的谢意。

在新世纪之初，我们将这套《文库》奉献给国内外中医界及广大中医爱好者，恳切希望有识之士对《文库》存在的不足之处给予批评、指教，以便在修订时更臻完善。

左言富

于金陵萍聚村

2002 年初春

A Newly Compiled Practical English-Chinese Library of Traditional Chinese Medicine

（英汉对照）新编实用中医文库

Basic Theory of Traditional Chinese Medicine	中医基础理论
Diagnostics of Traditional Chinese Medicine	中医诊断学
Science of Chinese Materia Medica	中药学
Science of Prescriptions	方剂学
Internal Medicine of Traditional Chinese Medicine	中医内科学
Surgery of Traditional Chinese Medicine	中医外科学
Gynecology of Traditional Chinese Medicine	中医妇科学
Pediatrics of Traditional Chinese Medicine	中医儿科学
Traumatology and Orthopedics of Traditional Chinese Medicine	中医骨伤科学
Ophthalmology of Traditional Chinese Medicine	中医眼科学
Otorhinolaryngology of Traditional Chinese Medicine	中医耳鼻喉科学
Chinese Acupuncture and Moxibustion	中国针灸
Chinese Tuina (Massage)	中国推拿
Life Cultivation and Rehabilitation of Traditional Chinese Medicine	中医养生康复学

Publishing House of Shanghai University of Traditional Chinese Medicine
530 Lingling Road, Shanghai, 200032, China

Diagnostics of Traditional Chinese Medicine
Compiler-in-Chief Wang Lufen   Translator-in-Chief Li Zhaoguo   Bao Bai
(A Newly Compiled Practical English-Chinese Library of TCM General Compiler-in-Chief
Zuo Yanfu)

ISBN 7 - 81010 - 657 - 0/R • 623   paperback
ISBN 7 - 81010 - 682 - 1/R • 647   hardback

Printed in Shanghai Xinhua Printing Works

图书在版编目(CIP)数据

中医妇科学 / 谈勇主编；李照国，成培莉主译. —上
海：上海中医药大学出版社，2002
（英汉对照新编实用中医文库/左言富总主编）
ISBN 7 - 81010 - 657 - 0

Ⅰ.中... Ⅱ.①谈...②李...③成... Ⅲ.中医
妇科学-英、汉 Ⅳ.R271.1

中国版本图书馆 CIP 数据核字(2002)第 047655 号

中医妇科学   主编 谈 勇 主译 李照国 成培莉

上海中医药大学出版社出版发行　　　　（零陵路 530 号 邮政编码 200032）
新华书店上海发行所经销　　　　　　　　　　　上海新华印刷厂印刷
开本　787mm×1092mm　1/18　印张 15.333　字数 366 千字　印数 1—3 600
版次 2002 年 10 月第 1 版　　　　　　　印次 2002 年 10 月第 1 次印刷

ISBN 7 - 81010 - 657 - 0/R • 623　　　　　　　定价 36.70 元